FLOATING & FISHING
Oregon's
Wilderness River Canyons

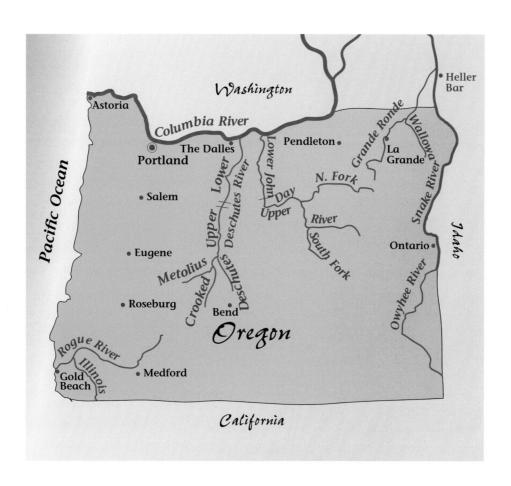

Melinda Allan

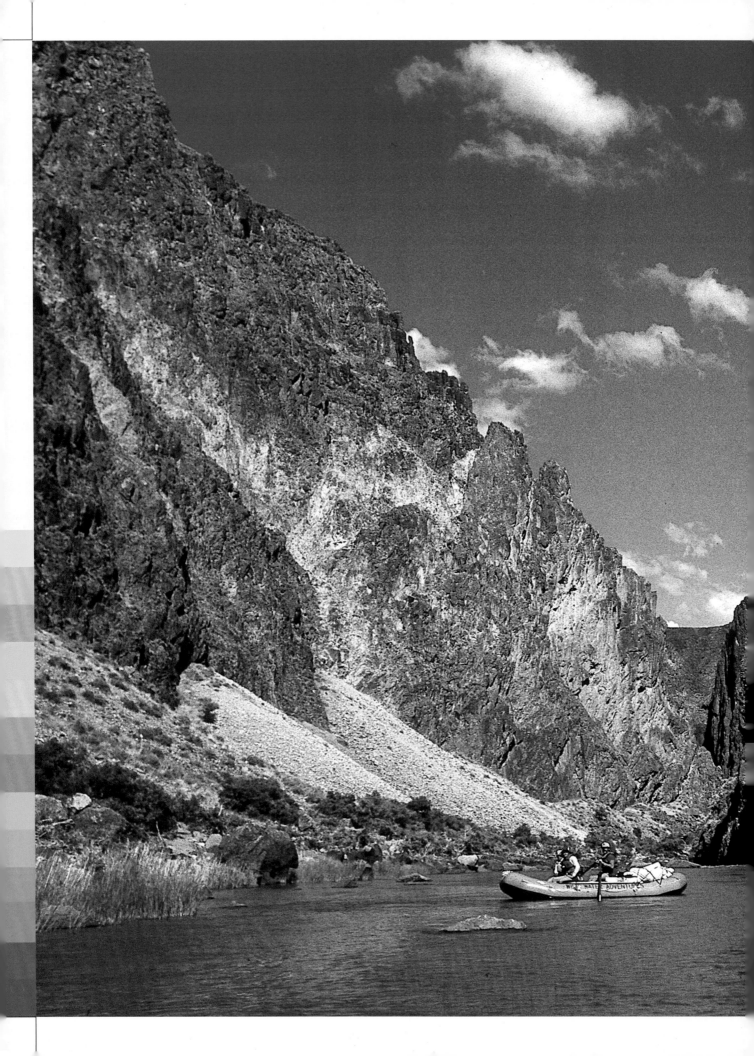

FLOATING & FISHING
Oregon's
Wilderness River Canyons

MELINDA ALLAN

A *Frank* **mato**
PORTLAND

Dedication

To "Ma and Pa Shuttle," (aka Marjorie and William Law, my husband's parents), who helped with long Owyhee River shuttles and reservoir tows, fed us dinner when we were too busy to remember to eat, and even helped set up gear. Mom and Dad believed in us and our fledgling business when everyone else thought we would fall on our faces, and assisted us all they could. I am forever grateful for their support, and their love as a substitute family when I lost my mother in 1991.

And for my husband, Al, who thought a five-day river trip down one of Idaho's biggest flooded-out streams would be the perfect honeymoon, even for a bride who had been on only a few day trips (sorta like taking your first backpack trip up Mt. Everest). I will remember the mice in the Forest Service cabin (better than the monsoons happening outside!), the warp in the "unbreakable" frame, skinny-dipping while 16 professional boatmen on a training trip cruised by, waving, and of course The Big Flip at Wolf Creek Rapid, after our support raft passed us by. I think this was the first time Al realized women can cry a lot, especially when they are petrified, cold, and determined not to get back in the boat that just tossed them out.

WARNING

BOATING: This book is not meant for navigational purposes. Before proceeding down any river or stretch of river, boaters should visually check the water first. It should be remembered that all the rivers in this book are subject to floods and high water and their currents and courses change frequently. Extreme caution is advised at all times, as is the use of Coast Guard-approved personal floatation devices (pfds).

FISHING REGULATIONS: Fishing regulations often change, especially due to the complexities of managing steelhead and salmon populations. Check the Oregon Sport-Fishing Regulations booklet before each season, and before fishing a new piece of water.

Frank Amato Publications, Inc.

P.O. Box 82112, Portland, Oregon 97282

503•653•8108 • www.amatobooks.com

All photos by Melinda Allan unless otherwise noted. (Oregonriverbum@aol.com)

Book and Cover Design: Kathy Johnson

Printed in Hong Kong

ISBN: 1-57188-321-5 • UPC: 0-81127-00155-2

2 4 6 8 10 9 7 5 3 1

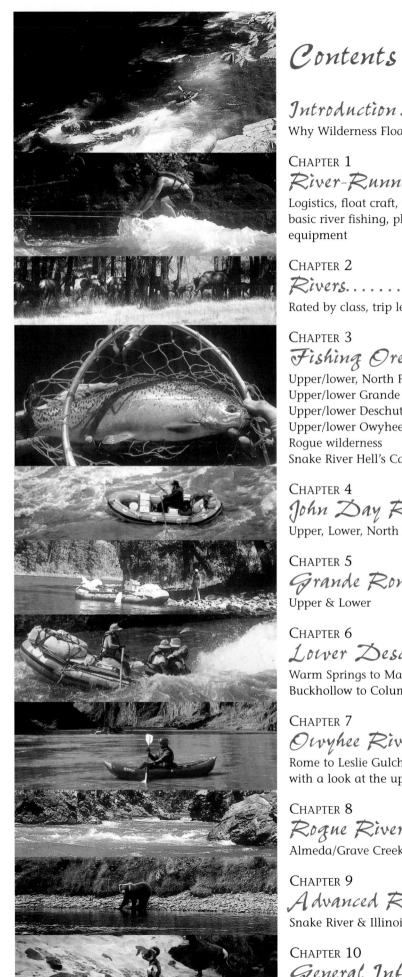

Contents

INTRODUCTION

Why Wilderness Floats?

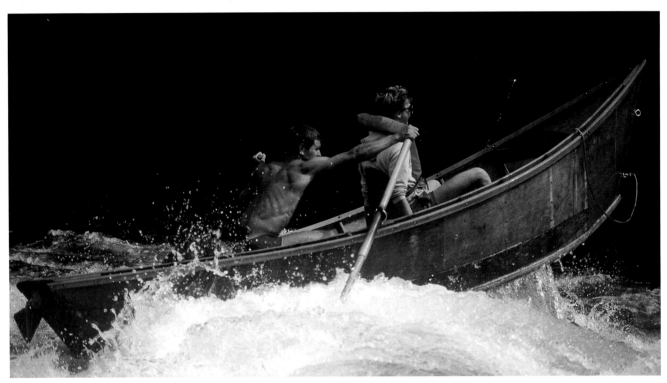

This macho rower is plowing through a hydraulic that can easily flip a driftboat. Driftboat "drivers" should avoid heavy hydraulics whenever possible, as their boats can flip and sink (since they usually have little flotation). Experienced driftboaters can tackle bigger waters with the addition of flotation such as inner tubes or Styrofoam blocks tied into the boat. Mr. Macho compounds the risk by not wearing a life jacket, and having his passenger in a cheap "horse collar" life jacket.

POISED ON THE BRINK OF A ROCKY CLASS II+ RAPID, I backpaddled to hold my little boat against the strong current's grasp. With fishing rod held firmly between my knees, I maneuvered the inflatable kayak to keep my lure off the rocky bottom and spinning. Suddenly, the river underneath me exploded with dual forces: I'd hooked a muscular trout, while my boat had been sucked into the rapid. I was able to crank the reel a few times before surrendering to the river's power. My double-bladed paddle windmilled frantically, dodging rocks and blasting through waves, with the trout being towed right along with me.

The inside curve of the river shallowed quickly, threatening shoals, so I headed for river left, where the outer banks were higher, the water deeper, the current stronger. This route delivered me to the tail-out, where I spun around in the calm eddy to view the maze of spray and stone I'd just run. Then I remembered my fish. I reeled in the trout, a sturdy 12-incher, none the worst for its whitewater ride. I flipped the trout carefully off my Rooster Tail and watched it swim away. Wild fish, wild ride.

The slopes of the Grande Ronde River canyon rose sharply on both sides; I was in one of the deepest and most rugged gorges in North America, fishing and exploring by sitting back and letting the current carry me and my gear. The river was low, with lots of rock dodging, but with water so clear that bumps and shoals were easily "read" from the boat.

Once, I was a backpacker. I struggled to carry 40 pounds of basic necessities up and down hills. Then I learned to row a raft. Before long, I was rowing cargo boats with a half-ton or more of gear. Even that small inflatable kayak can float a hundred pounds of gear in addition to a paddler. Some of our Oregon rivers are at the bottom of very rugged terrain, but the river provides easy access to those with a good boat and knowledge of how to maneuver it.

I have had numerous knee surgeries ending with total knee replacement. So backpacking is no longer practical for me, but running up to Class IV whitewater has become almost instinctual for me. I've even rafted wilderness rivers such as the Rogue while I was on crutches.

Rowing and paddling are great alternatives to hiking even if you don't have knee or hip problems. (Shoulders don't actually support the weight of floating craft, and so do not develop the overuse common to runners and other athletes whose body weight pounds the pavement. Occasional muscle strain in shoulders or back is possible; however, careful use of oars and paddles can prevent injuries.)

By letting the power of moving water work for you, what seems a grueling upper body sport—rowing or paddling whitewater—soon evolves into a practical method, using fewer muscles and coordination, somewhat like a combination of playing tennis and learning to drive a stick shift, for efficient transport for both you and your gear, as well as all of your dreams: wild adventure, big fish, great scenery, interesting pioneer and Native American history, wildlife almost tame enough to touch...everything you want in an escape from civilization.

With more capacity for weight and bulk, river craft can carry an amazing assortment of luxury items: four-inch-thick queen-size air mattresses (with a foot pump for quick inflation), propane-powered hot shower makers, cast-iron Dutch ovens for pioneer-style baking, a library of hardcover books, furniture such as folding chairs, cots

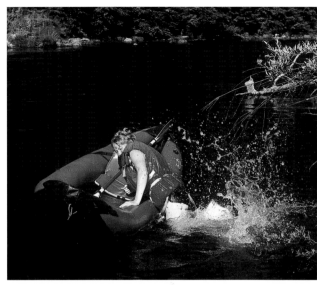

Knowing self-rescue is important for all boaters, but especially for canoeists and kayakers. This woman knows how to use the self-bailing floor as a lifeline to hold onto, to use for reflipping her inflatable kayak, and for leverage to climb back inside a slippery craft. The art of self-rescue can be practiced in calm waters during warm weather, or in a swimming pool (especially for kayakers).

Many women master the art of rowing, especially in lighter and more maneuverable driftboats or catarafts. It's not unusual to see women rowing half-ton cargo rafts on rivers such as the Rogue and Deschutes. By knowing how to use the river's current to move a load, a skilled rower uses minimal muscle. In addition, rowers can employ their entire body to move their craft, including strong legs and back as well as biceps.

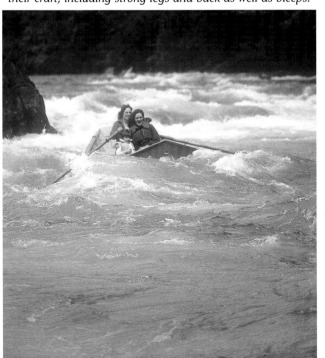

and tables, stovetop espresso makers, even hand-cranked blenders for mixing that necessary under-the-stars margarita.

Floating wilderness whitewater rivers offers unparalled opportunities for personal challenge and solitude, or, if you prefer, building teamwork and savoring friendships. A clean run of a rapid generates a solid feeling of accomplishment. You can escape civilization, while leaving little trace of your presence (float boats don't even leave tracks). Utilizing low-impact camping techniques, no one will ever know where you stayed.

Why Oregon rivers? Oregon, with our State Scenic Waterways act, counts more protected rivers and streams than any other state (over 40 of them). Most of Oregon's multi-day runs are suitable for the intermediate boater, so with a modest amount of training and practice, just about anyone can be floating these rivers safely. Most intermediate-level Oregon rivers are very forgiving, especially for the rafter or catarafter. And, while many popular Western rivers have access restricted by permit lotteries to prevent overcrowding, in Oregon, only two rivers require such permits, and none are required in the off-season. Additionally, there are many shorter trips close to civilization where boaters can rehearse for more remote trips.

What's more, our varied terrain has produced a useful variety of practice waters. We have fast-flowing, rocky rivers that hone "technical" river-running skills, as well as slower rivers for beginners to learn how to eddy-hop, identify hazards further in advance, navigate a rock garden with ease and flair, and gain confidence. We have

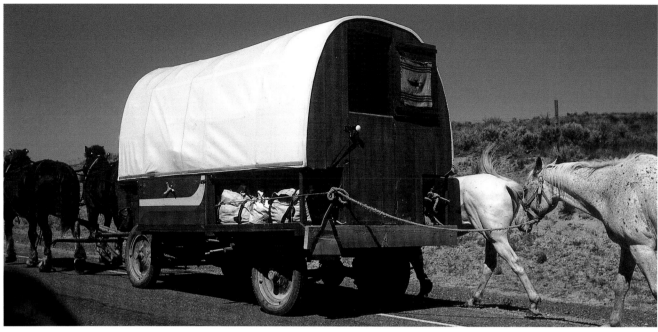

Getting there is half the fun. In the John Day backcountry, a sheepherder's wagon travels at Amish pace along the shuttle road. Oregon "scenic byways" may contain other surprises for the city slicker, including herds of cattle or sheep covering the roadway, so drive with caution.

Unwelcome in any camp is poison oak, a common pest along many Oregon rivers. On the west side of the Cascades, this irritating weed sports oak leaf shapes, and grows in bushes or vine-like formations wrapped around trees, sometimes reaching eight to ten feet high. On the east side, the leaves appear more "ivy-like" but possess the same invisible oil that causes skin to break out in nasty blisters, turn red, and itch like crazy. Prevention is easier than treatment; remember the saying "leaflets three, let it be" and wash any skin that contacts the plant with strong soap or special poison oak removers. In particular, avoid rubbing eyes after contact or throwing the plant into fires; this can cause temporary blindness. Antihistamines can soothe the itch and swelling.

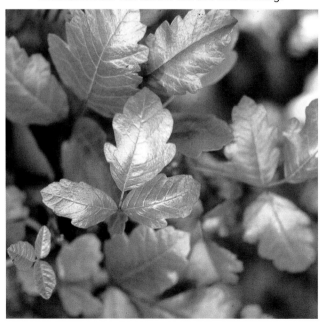

rivers that roar to flood stage at predictable times, allowing boaters to master "big water" skills, even a few rivers that run as "big water" all summer long. With a few years' experience on mostly user-friendly Oregon rivers, boaters can look beyond the state to the challenge of exotic, expert-rated expeditions such as the Colorado through Grand Canyon, the famous whitewater of Idaho, perhaps even remote rivers in far-away corners of South America or Asia. We have plenty of day trips to develop float/fishing and whitewater skills within easy reach of a road before venturing into the wilds.

Of course, river fishing in Oregon is fantastic. Hooking a fish at the head of a busy rapid is just one fishing challenge awaiting the float boater. Another is the chance to hook a fish as big as your boat, quite capable of towing you both upstream. On most Oregon rivers, you can fish right from your boat, covering as much as ten to twenty miles of great fishing waters in a day or two—much more coverage than you could ever attempt on foot. Even as we lose more public access to roads leading into canyons, floating and fishing while drifting through private property remains legal. Also, Oregon's wild rivers will remain forever wild and free flowing. All of the wilderness floats described here are State of Oregon—designated Scenic Waterways. The Rogue was one of the first eight rivers designated as a federally-protected Wild & Scenic River.

Fishing from a floating craft, particularly on larger rivers, is a technique so effective that it has been banned on Oregon's Deschutes River to save a fantastic native redside rainbow trout and wild steelhead fishery. Our other wilderness rivers still allow fishing from boats, so the conscientious angler will practice catch and release of all wild fish, as well as trophy fish, when possible. On the other hand, saving a few medium smallmouths or hatchery trout for dinner is acceptable. The aroma of fresh bass or catfish fillets fried in butter or alongside bacon is the best reason to get out of bed in the morning.

Oregon's rivers are unsurpassed in beauty. The very essence of canyons and gorges is spectacular, sculpted rock walls. All Oregon rivers are different, and each has its own personality: some are in forested canyons, others at the base of open hillsides; several are desert gorges, with water colors ranging from turquoise to turbid, clear to heavily silted. The gradient, or rate of elevation loss, of each river differs —some are continuous rapids, most "pool and drop" where a rapid is followed by a quiet pool for recovery.

For sighting wildlife, the quiet approach of a float craft is unsurpassed. Sneaking up to bighorn rams butting heads in the fall isn't unusual if you know where to go. Bird watchers can go crazy with all the water-loving birds that don't have to be talked: the great blue heron, green heron, osprey or "fish hawk", bald and golden eagles, marsh and red-tailed hawks, waterfowl from Canada geese to harlequin ducks and cinnamon teals, the kingfisher, ouzel, nighthawk, cormorant, canyon wren, swallows with their mud nests on cliff walls. Then there are the songbirds: western meadow lark, red-winged blackbird, western tanager, warbling vireo. Many birds just visit canyons: the peregrine and prairie falcons, American kestrel, magpie, great horned owls, sage grouse, chukar, turkey vulture.

Big game, besides bighorn sheep, includes blacktail, whitetail and mule deer, Rocky Mountain and Roosevelt elk, antelope, cougar, bobcat, and black bear. Coyotes prowl and howl Oregon's canyons. Small river bank wildlife is common: mink, muskrat, beaver (bank beaver, which don't build dams across major rivers, but dig burrows into the river banks, are most frequently encountered), playful river otters, racoons, and, yes, skunks.

Wilderness river campsites cover a wide range of experiences. From Greeley Bar on the Owyhee, the desert night sky—far from city lights—is stunning, with the Milky Way flowing like a river in space. Seeing Hale-Bopp comet blazing above was a special treat for me one spring, as was viewing a rare showing of Northern Lights from a natural hot springs tub. On the Rogue's Tate Creek, campers can scramble through a pretty streambed and climb up a rope to experience a natural water slide, then swim in a river eddy with endangered Western pond turtles the size of dinner plates. That clanging at three a.m. is probably a black bear raiding your kitchen!

Oars have the advantage of leverage over paddles,
due to their length and elevation in oarstands (and allowing the entire body to work them).
However, in some rapids, paddlers can help the rower by digging in and pulling the bow (front) of the boat through,
increasing momentum. "Paddle assist" technique is recommended on Class V rivers such as the Illinois, but can also be employed
on easier waters. A strong paddler with a "guide stick" or long heavy paddle can help a rower with turns as well as momentum.

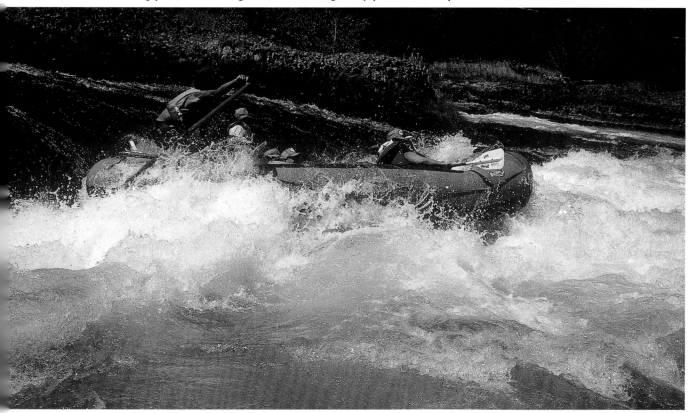

CHAPTER 1

River-Running Basics

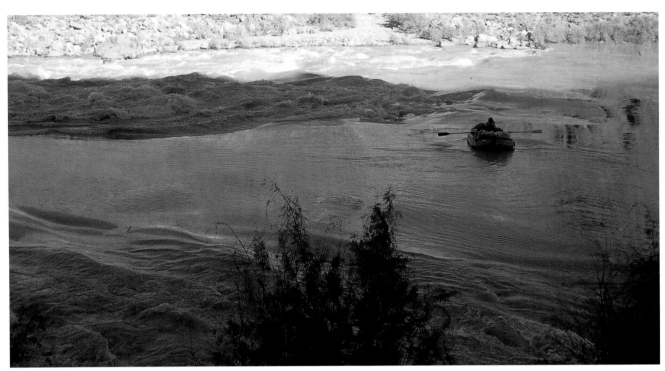

A classic "tongue" or slick at the top of a simple rapid. Such a formation usually offers the best and safest route through a rapid, generally leading into big standing waves for an adrenalin rush. Learn to look for the downstream-pointing V shape that marks a tongue. (A V-shape that points upstream indicates a rock; avoid it.) Fishing in the slick can be productive.

Logistics

LONG BEFORE A RIVER TRIP LAUNCHES, THE BOATER must plan and prepare for the trip—hence, logistics. Not only what type of boat is best for the boater's skill level, the conditions of the river to be floated, or the most productive ways to fish a river, but also how many miles to float, where to camp, how a shuttle is accomplished, what hazards are present, when is the optimal season for floating, and what will the river be like at the particular water level you happen to encounter, which regulations apply to all rivers or just certain rivers, and so forth.

Logistics present a great argument for taking a commercial guided trip, especially a fishing trip. Someone else handles the planning and preparation, the readying of gear and shuttles, knows all the best fishing holes and what lures or flies to use (and usually provides them for you), you just show up with clothes and a fishing license. You can row if you wish on the flat water, for building skill, or not row at all. Planning can also be an exciting part of the adventure, more fun than work if you're not a river guide.

Choosing a river to float means comparing your skill level with the river's classification of difficulty. If you have done only day trips, adding camping is more complicated than it appears. All of Oregon's wilderness rivers have a minimum rating of Class II+, not just because of the rapids, but because the rivers in this book flow through remote country, where help is far away and cell phone signals won't reach out of deep canyons. Of modern gadgetry, even satellite phones can fail deep in a gorge, and GPS systems are not precise—depending on quality—plus there are batteries to consider. Remember radio signals travel in straight lines, so they may not be able to penetrate a deep canyon unless the satellite is straight overhead. Climbing to a high location may help bring in a signal, but plan on being self-reliant.

Going with a more experienced group is a good way to start; you can develop rowing or paddling skills under their direction. Following a more experienced boater's "lines" (routes) through rapids is a standard learning technique, since you don't have to read the water as well—just watch the other boat, and copy his or her moves. The boater to be followed should be aware of this, so that he/she will choose an obvious line and safer routes. If the other boater is not a member of your group, but you are unsure of the route, ask if you can follow.

Oregon's many day trips are good training grounds. The McKenzie, besides having the most hatchery fish planted, also boasts wild redside trout, summer steelhead and spring chinook, all within an hour or less from Eugene and Springfield. The upper run is good for practicing on technical water, while the middle run can build beginner confidence with Class IIs and fishing from the boat. Practice for tougher rapids by running Brown's Hole and Martin's Rapid, two top hydraulics. The North Umpqua, Clackamas and North Santiam also offer good runs for training.

The North Umpqua is an excellent training ground for running all kinds of whitewater. It offers big water conditions during the rainy and snowmelt season November to June; its record for high water level is tremendous for what is in mid-summer a smaller stream, compared to the Rogue or Deschutes: 265,000 cubic feet per second in December of Oregon's big flood year, 1964.

In summer, there is much pinballing action on the North Umpqua, perfect for technical water training. Many experienced whitewater boaters train on the North Umpqua, with some holding the opinion that if you can run the NU at any water level that is sane—below 12,000 cfs or when the logs aren't floating down it—then you have the skills to run any river in the country.

Rating The Rapids, Rating The Trips

In Oregon, rapids are rated on the International Scale of Whitewater Difficulty, with Class I (one) as moving flat water with no or minor obstacles and Class VI (six) as unrunnable (usually a big waterfall or other extreme water hazard). Class II is a rapid that requires maneuvering but is suitable for a beginning boater, while Class II+ rapids demand more experience. Canoes, driftboats, and other open craft may "swamp" (fill up with water, sink, or be out of control due to the tremendous weight of the extra water) even in Class II. Class III and IV rapids may require the boater to "scout" (look over the route before running it, from shore or by standing up in the boat to increase visibility). Maneuvering becomes increasingly complex. Risks increase, the chances of having an overboard (accidental swimmer), a boat wrapped (stuck for hours or until "mechanical advantage" is applied) or even overturning (flipping) increases. (See pages 26-27 for rating charts.)

The ratings of Oregon rapids vary as to the condition of the river when you float, and who is rating them (an expert boater tends to dismiss Class II+ rapids as "nothing" but a less-experienced boater might hit rocks or flip sideways in a wave). In general, most rapids are more difficult for open canoes and driftboats, both of which may swamp, even in fairly straightforward waves or small hydraulics. Rafts and catarafts are much more forgiving of beginners' mistakes, while covered canoes and kayaks (both the traditional hardshell kayak and the hybrid inflatable kayak) can take on almost any type of water, limited only by the skill and daring of the individual boater.

I have taken the conservative view and rate rivers according to the degree of difficulty from the perspective of someone new to the river and/or a whitewater greenhorn. Even the most nervous novice can ride up to Class IV with a guide at the oars, and many boaters are able to run rapids a bit above their skill level by following an experienced boater closely.

Rating the individual boater's skill and then matching him or her to an appropriate river is a better way to decide what class of rivers to run. For example, a Class I boater is a total novice, starting out on flat but moving water on slower rivers. A Class II boater is an informed beginner who knows basic methods of moving his or her craft, has been instructed in whitewater safety, and can read obvious river features such as exposed rocks or big waves, and can land in a large eddy.

A Class II+ is an experienced beginner who can choose correct routes on easier water, or follow another's route on harder water.

The intermediate boater, in addition to having the ability to navigate Class III rapids, recognizes and avoids less-obvious but dangerous hazards such as "strainers" (downed trees that let current pass through, but trap unwary boaters), logjams, bridge pillars, turbulent eddies and reversals. The intermediate boater is beginning to learn to make decisions "on the fly" (route-finding from the boat, rather than scouting every minor drop from shore) and how to handle fast-moving water. This boater also understands verbal or written directions on how to run a rapid, such as negotiating an S-curve or what to expect along a U-shaped bend. Using the current by placing the boat at an angle is almost instinctive for the Class III+ boater.

Logistics is the planning and execution of expedition details: getting to the river, having a fun and safe trip, knowing where you are and how many miles you must make each day, major rapids and other hazards, fish and how to catch them, seasonal variations in water levels, permit requirements, and so forth. Then there are equipment requirements (fire pans, porta-potties, and garbage removal are required on all wilderness rivers; kitchen water must be strained, drinking water must be filtered or otherwise purified).

All the trips are described by the following criteria:

River

The river that can be floated and is in a wilderness setting, such as the lower 100 miles of the Deschutes. Includes history, how the river was named, wildlife, etc.

River-Running Basics

Section

Most rivers are divided into runnable and unrunnable sections, or sections where the road parallels the river, as opposed to wild stretches without road access. Some rivers have two or more segments which can be run separate or as one long trip (example: upper John Day, lower John Day, North Fork John Day). Note that the Grande Ronde, John Day, and Deschutes rivers are all run along their "lower" sections—however, these are then divided into "lower upper" and "lower lower." To avoid confusion I refer simply to upper and lower sections.

Sectioning may also be used to refer to state and/or federal designations of protected portions: the "scenic" run has a road alongside it, while the "wild and scenic" stretch has no vehicular access.

Fishing, public access, weather, hatches, water temperatures, etc. can vary wildly. For example, ask the average fly angler about fishing on the Owyhee River and she will answer that the river is an excellent tailwater fishery, where she caught a large brown trout, using a size 22 midge pattern. However, the tailwater is below the dam, from cold reservoir water (remember your basic river physics: water drawn from the bottom of a lake or reservoir is always colder than surface water).

Our angler would be surprised to learn that about 70 miles upstream, I am catching dozens of bass in very warm water while floating beneath thousand-foot-high cliffs. Instead of driving on an access road and walking down to the Owyhee River, I have it right under my boat.

The Deschutes has many sections, from flat canoeing water to raging torrents. The best float-in fishing is the lower 100 miles of the river. This time, the wilderness float begins just below a dam, so the entire river is a tailwater fishery, with a year-round standard water temperature.

Central Oregon's Crooked River has a wonderful tailwater fishery, located—you guessed it—right below the dam (located above Prineville). But the trout tend to be small (anglers boast of hooking six-inchers on a gnat imitation). Stop for a gaze over the gorge where the Crooked flows, at Ogden State Park, and you'll see long quiet pools that get a bit stagnant in summer. The water's murkier, due to irrigation use and natural mica particles suspended (like glacial silt). Yet, if you climb 300 feet down and place your lure where the current dumps into the head of the pools, line will go ripping off your reel as you battle a redside trout with shoulders like a linebacker.

Moral: Research your river carefully. If no one is floating the Deschutes River at Lower Bridge, it's because irrigation water has been diverted, creating a river of rocks with a bit of water tossed in. More importantly, though, is that parts of the upper Deschutes have Class VI waterfalls that are potential death traps. So, while the walk-in

Aptly named, a "boulder garden" is a scattering of rocks amid strong current, an easy place to flip, wrap, crash, fall overboard or become crushed should you get "between a rock and a hard place (the boat)." This Class V rock slalom features powerful currents with few eddies. Less difficult stone mazes can be negotiated with careful planning and maneuvering, often utilizing eddy water behind rocks to pivot or slow the boat by catching their upstream-moving currents with an oar. Scouting from shore is usually necessary to find a safe route. In gentler waters, fishing behind the rocks is excellent.

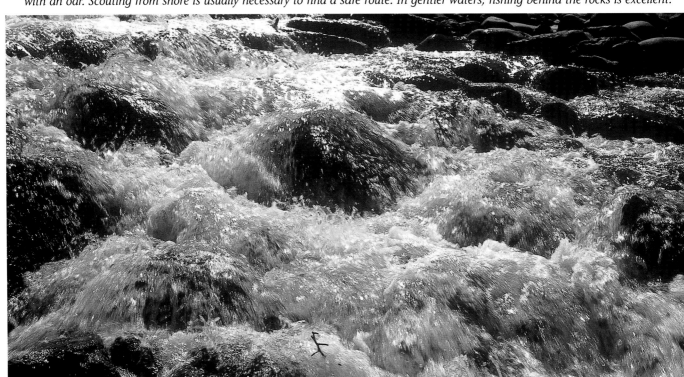

fishing is choice, you will not want to take a boat, at least not until your low-water skills are finely honed and you have a very good map showing the locations of the waterfalls.

Location

Oregon is a big state with many different terrains and climate zones, so this category helps define not just where the river is located, but its runoff level and weather. Central Oregon refers to the High Desert with its juniper trees and sagebrush, between the Cascades and the eastern boundary of the Great Basin (Burns and east), north to the Columbia River, east to Bend and Wasco County.

Southwest Oregon is warmer than Portland or Eugene, which is why the Rogue attracts many boaters from the large population centers. Southeastern Oregon, east of Burns, is remote even for highway driving, the location of the spectacular Owyhee Canyonlands.

Northeast Oregon is the land of "Oregon's Little Switzerland", the Wallowa Mountains, often compared to the European Alps, another lesser-visited area which features the Snake in Hells Canyon and its wilderness tributary, the Grande Ronde (the Owyhee is also a tributary of the Snake).

Personality

Each river has its own personality, or character, including types of terrain encountered on the float, and how elevation loss affects the river. A river canyon such as the Rogue is defined as forested as few open meadow lands exist. On the other hand, the Owyhee is arid desert canyon, with almost no trees other than a few hackberries and small junipers.

The nature of the river current is part of its character: usually pool and drop (rapids are followed by long quiet stretches), or technical/busy (rapids follow one another with few breaks in the action). History, both natural and human, and unique features contribute to each river's description.

Difficulty

How the river section is rated in terms of whitewater difficulty. This considers the isolation of the area (more difficult, as getting help may take days instead of minutes), temperature of water (hypothermia greatly increases risk should someone go overboard or be repeatedly splashed), and the possibility of portaging rapids and/or walking around/out of the canyon.

Other factors to keep in mind are the distances between camps, wind slowing the drift time, wildfires erupting, the number of other boaters available to render assistance, the length of a swim through a particular rapid, high water or flood stage (which increases coldness of water and swiftness of current), low water (slows float time, forces dragging over gravel bars, makes strong winds worse), storms, dangerous animals, etc.

Our wild river canyons have stayed undeveloped by roads and trails mostly due to their sheer ruggedness—something to keep in mind when determining which river matches your boat and your skills.

Gradient

Gradient is the term for how many feet per mile a river drops. Rivers with slower gradient, such as the upper John Day at eight to nine feet per mile, are easier than those with a faster gradients, such as the upper Grande Ronde's 21-22 feet per mile. On a slow gradient, the boat drifts at a more modest pace, allowing the boater more time to see obstacles, scout from the boat, find a landing spot, and choose the proper entry to a rapid. How fast is the river going? If a person on shore can keep up by walking, it's about 2-3 mph. If our hypothetical follower must run, the current is 4-6 mph. If faster than human legs, the current could be up to 12-15 mph.

However, slow gradient is not a guarantee of easy water. Some rivers lose elevation in several big drops, rather than continuously—the Snake is just 10 feet per mile gradient, but has large volume Class IV and V rapids. In general, none of Oregon's multi-day river trips have a high gradient rating (above 30 feet per mile) except during spring floods. Lesser gradients also mean more time to cover mileages, especially when a headwind is blowing hard.(Fishing these moderate currents, on the other hand, is easier.)

Mileage/Days

The total number of miles between the suggested launch point and the recommended take-out site, plus the minimum time it takes to float the stretch comfortably. Most float craft can travel five to 20 miles in one day (kayaks and canoes being faster than inflatables, while stops/slowdowns for fishing skew average float times). For serious fishing, add at least one day to the minimum listed, preferably two or more. Rushing down a 65-mile river in 3 days, traveling from "can't see to can't see", and the constant worry of missing a shuttle rendevous, work, or other obligation—all these ruin what would be a pleasant 5- or 6-day trip.

This section also includes popular alternate put-ins and take-outs, to make the trip shorter or longer, or to compensate for non-optimum water levels. In low water, particularly, boaters will want to launch at sites below rapids that have become unrunnable at lower levels, and sites with fewer miles between because lower levels take longer to float.

Average Float Levels/Seasons

The optimum water levels most boaters will find easiest and most comfortable, plus what time of year these levels are likely to occur. Most Oregon rivers rise in the spring, occasionally very rapidly and without notice. Tie boats double and set a watch if the river seems to be rising quickly, so no one is caught off-guard asleep in a floating tent.

Beginners should stick to the optimum levels until their experience with high/low water increases. Driftboats and open canoes, as well as rafts 12 feet or smaller, usually require optimum levels for safe floating.

To determine the existing flow of any river in this book, contact the River Forecast Center in Portland (503/261-9246) and follow the push-button-phone directions to reach the river levels you wish. The government website is www.usgs.gov for all rivers, http://Oregon.usgs.gov for the state. Many other websites offer access to the water level sites, even some commercial outfitter sites.

High-Water Season

Flood stages usually occur November through April, sometimes later in spring, when a combination of heavy snowpack and warm spring rains or very hot weather convert a quiescent stream into a raging torrent. With high-elevation snowpacks such as the Grande Ronde, big water occurs as late as June. In some areas, when the river rises overnight, boaters should stay in a safe place until water levels drop (think of being in a 3,000-foot-high gorge with no beaches or landing spots!). The Illinois, listed here as an advanced trip, has killed boaters who tackle water levels beyond the listed safe upper level of 3,000 cfs. However, high water on easier rivers (such as the John Day) is much easier to run, offering good experience that builds confidence in handling higher water.

In extreme water, logs and debris will wash down rivers, posing a hazard to navigation. The water will be colder than expected. Rocks will be covered over, but may also form new and unexpected hydraulics. Eddies transform into fierce whirlpools. Camps are often flooded out. Slowing the boat's speed or finding a place to stop will be more difficult. Sometimes low bridges or cable crossings will be close calls, or you might even have to duck. Faster thinking and route planning is required; high water will hone your boating skills and build your confidence, providing you don't have a bad experience, such as a flipped boat or runaway raft. Balance thrills with a solid dose of caution.

Learn the basics of channel choosing for all river conditions, but especially high water. Directions are river right and river left as you face downstream. Right of center does not mean run the center. Look for the "tongue", a V-shape pointing downstream, also known as a "slick" or "V-slick" for its smooth, even appearance. (An "upstream-pointing V" indicates a rock at the tip of the V.) Stay on the inside of river bends, as the stronger currents on the outside bend take you into trouble: deadly strainers, cliff walls, boulders. Don't get too far inside as shallows or washboards (hodgepodge of rocks) occur there. Memorize the oar routine: Face the danger, angle the boat, and pull with both oars.

Stay in the middle of the river when possible, where there is less friction and more current, plus fewer obstacles. Learn to land your boat quickly and safety (backferrying is necessary in strong current—face away from the shoreline, set your angle, and pull on both oars to make the eddy). Look far downstream. Learn to work with strong current, not against it. Pick open channels that you can see the bottom of, not blind side channels that may be blocked. Choose quickly at the top of islands or you may wind up grounded. Look for the channel that drops first, has more whitewater, is obviously wider, or is recommended/taken by other boaters.

The classic signs of approaching big drops are a "horizon line" (the river appears to disappear at the top of the rapid), a long, slow section as water "pools up" as would water behind a dam, a loud noise, spray or mist, boulders appearing to block the channel, other boaters pulled over to "scout" from shore (decide on a route before committing to the rapid), even a warning sign that says "Falls Ahead!" Boaters have actually ignored such signs.

Despite these risks, navigating high river levels is exhilarating, turning a conventional float into a grand adventure. Every boater who aspires to run wilderness whitewater should become familiar with the effects that high water levels have on their local rivers, so that should an unexpected flood occur, the boater will know how to handle the challenge.

And, if high water drops suddenly, you might even pick up abandoned fishing lures and other treasures while walking the river banks. A beat-up Rapala minnow I found on the Deschutes after a long season of big water finally dropped to normal levels snared a 20-inch smallmouth bass on a low-water John Day trip.

Low-Water Season

Here is the exact opposite of the flood—river levels so low, managing agencies might even post a warning sign to keep uninformed boaters off the river. Chief among concerns is the extra time and physical effort required to pull, tow, push, and grunt your boat off the rocks or gravel bars it will surely become stuck on. A three-day trip can easily take four or five days (even if you're not worried, the folks back home might be).

The constant getting out, pushing, and getting back into the boat is both tiring, and frustrating. Plus, you can count on the wind blowing upstream, against your efforts to make time, with less current to assist.

On the other hand, because most boaters avoid rivers when they are too low to easily float, the fishing can be outstanding. A cold spring float transforms into a warm bass haven with the arrival of summer weather. Another benefit is solitude. Favorite camps are most likely open.

Running low water will sharpen your river-reading skills. Keep in mind that deep water favors the high bank and the outside bend. Low banks or gravel bars, or riffles, and the inside bends, indicate shallow water. When

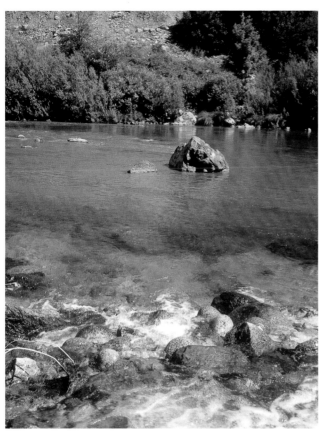

Especially in spring, Oregon rivers can flood, turning a beautiful clear stream into ugly, unfishable muck, sometimes in just a few hours. Summer thunderstorms can also raise the river and muddy the water. In such conditions, look for clear side streams entering the river. Fish will move towards the cleaner water to feed, and will be better able to view your offering. Unexpected dam releases are rare, but can also raise river levels and spoil fishing. Rapids may also increase in size, power and difficulty. Always tie your boat up when you pull ashore!

choosing a channel around an island, the best channel is the one that has the most favorable characteristics of a passable channel: the channel drops first, the channel has visible waves (not riffles), the channel has more water and faster current heading towards it, the channel is on the outside of the bend. Use the eddies behind rocks, even the tiny pocket water, to draw your craft into the deeper water of the eddy. A skilled boater will seldom have to get out and push, saving strength for making miles, catching fish, and enjoying the scenery.

When you must run a riffle or float over a gravel bar, use an aggressive approach. Line up on what seems to be the deepest spot, then start a hard push (or straight backwards pull, if you're confident and don't freak out when running blind). Begin this in the deep water and continue, non-stop, until the boat clears the shallows. The momentum caused by stronger rowing and paddling propels the craft through segments where it's too shallow to

dip a blade to move the boat. Most inflatables can handle a "draft" or minimum water level of four to six inches; lightly loaded inflatable kayaks can almost drift a heavy dew! (Well, almost!)

Sometimes low water includes ice if you float in winter. Call for information from the managing agency, but also call locals who drive shuttles to find out if the river is frozen solid, full of icebergs, or mostly open. I learned many new tricks while floating the Grande Ronde during an exceptionally cold November. For instance, when rowing in slush, wiggle the blades to create room to stroke, and be sure to pull the blades through the oarlocks often to knock ice loose, ice adds a lot of weight to the oars. Carry a hatchet to chop your boat loose from its parking lot in a frozen eddy. And if you carry pop, choose high-sugar types which take longer to freeze than those with low sugar.

If stuck on a rock (and not about to wrap), have everyone jump up and shift their weight toward the side of the boat that is the "least stuck" on the rock. Don't jump out, even shallow currents are strong enough to knock you down and you could "pin" (trap) a foot on an undercut rock. Getting out of the boat to push it free should be the last choice. Additionally, be careful when wading; push from the upstream side, to avoid being sandwiched between a "rock and a hard place", with the hard place being the boat, swamped with much water weight.

You can also try a "sea anchor" to work one end loose by tying an object to a rope less than 20 feet long from bow or stern, whichever side appears to have stronger and faster current to work with. A bail bucket with a sturdy handle will work; but if it doesn't, add more weight: drybags, rocket boxes (very large Army surplus ammo cans). Keep lines floating by having one person in charge of this task, to help prevent snagging on the river bottom. If the boat seems to want to stay overnight on the rock, it's time to break out the "Z-drag kit" (a collection of special floating ropes, ropes for fashioning Prusik knots, pulleys that fit the ropes, and carabineers that clip on and also screw tight, must have a minimum breaking point of one ton).

Try to never be sideways approaching a rock, lest you broach. Hit rocks bow or stern first if you can't avoid them. If you do broadside a rock in current, avoid a wrap by having everyone shift weight to the downstream (high side) or rock side of the boat.

Also, the safest channel in any water level is the channel you can see the most of, preferably one where you can see the confluence with the main stem. This is because logs or boulders can block minor channels that are blind from the upstream approach, and if a strong current is going directly into such obstacles, often there isn't room to dodge them. Drownings have occurred in such situations. Remember: when in doubt, scout it out!

River-reading skills also come in handy for ducking the wind. Stay close to the high banks when the wind is fierce. Stay in the current, any current, to help move your boat forward. A heavy boat with a dragging floor may actually move faster against the wind, because the floor has more contact with the current. Hard boats such as driftboats and canoes produce less friction, so they move much faster than inflatables, especially in windy or low water/slow gradient conditions. The sea anchor mentioned above helps keep a boat in current during windy conditions.

If the wind is really bad, you might want to wait it out. Tie up and have lunch, fish, tie a fly, hike, swim, read a book, or take a nap. Most winds come up in afternoon, especially on our desert rivers, so getting a very early start and camping just after lunch may be necessary. Go to bed early and get up before first light, so you can launch as soon as there is enough light to see. Reservoirs or long flat stretches with no rocks might be navigated at night, especially during a full moon, when the wind has died down.

If the going is very slow, which happens in low water conditions, you may have to put aside the rod and start making miles in order to keep to your schedule. That is why a particular float section can take two to five days or more. For fishing, try to do fewer miles in more days. A layover day in camp is nice, especially if the fishing is hot, people are tired or the weather is bad (often a storm,

especially in the desert, will blow over in a few hours or overnight).

Doing the Whitewater Limbo, or "How low can you go?", is a difficult dance to learn, but once you've conquered "sleepers" (small rocks just under the surface that give no warning, but snag your boat), powering over gravel bars, channel selection, following the outside bend and the high bank, and outwitting the Wind Tunnel from Hell, the feeling of mastery is exhilarating. I recall paddling after dark on a low-water John Day trip, navigating only by starlight, listening for the sounds of water pouring over rocks and wing dams that had to be avoided, and the great splashes of the unknown (beaver? steelhead? bullfrog?)—my head was spinning with a natural high. "Damn, I'm good!" I shouted to the empty canyon. "I can hear rocks coming!"

Craft For Oregon Wilderness Rivers
Driftboats

The traditional fishing craft in the Pacific Northwest—and Oregon in particular—has been the driftboat. These are so closely associated with fishing and guiding anglers on certain rivers that two styles have emerged, named for their habitat: the McKenzie driftboat, and the Rogue

The Deschutes River between Bend and the Billy Chinook reservoir is seldom run, due to numerous waterfalls, private property issues, and reduced flow by irrigation needs. This attempt to run at 300 cfs required much lining of boats along slippery-rocked shores, scrambling through a virtual "briar" patch of riparian brush. Levels here do freshen in fall after the growing season, but rapids are difficult (most waterfalls in this area are rated Class V+, expert level).

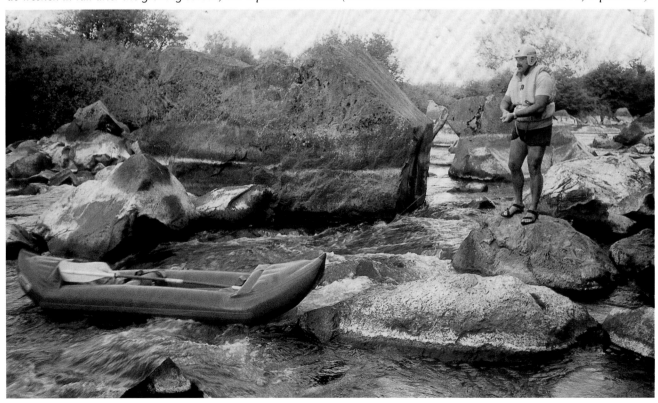

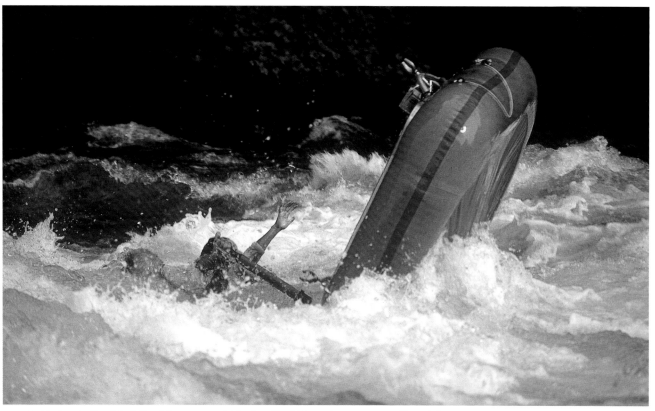

A 12-foot inflatable "flips" in a powerful hydraulic. This raft was too small and flimsy to tackle Class III waters safely. The boaters might have prevented overturning by performing a quick "highside" maneuver.

River driftboat. These days, the McKenzie driftboat is seen from Alaska to Montana, and even in Maine as well as in Oregon, floating its namesake river.

Driftboats are super-easy to control, requiring little strength provided they are loaded light. They are aesthetically pleasing, the curves of bow and stern matching the artistry of madrone trees, driftwood, and other natural shapes. Driftboats are the easiest craft to guide-fish—that is, to hold the boat in place by rowing backwards while the client fishes from the bow of the boat.

Working a lure while the boat is held against the current is sometimes called "plugging" and is a very effective technique for trout and steelhead. The plug is often a Hot Shot, but even a Roostertail will sometimes produce.

Additionally, driftboats are easy to anchor, plus you can stand up to cast your fly or lure. With a small electric motor, you can fish a hot spot repeatedly, or make time downstream to the takeout after messing around fishing, rather than arriving ignominiously in total darkness (on sections of river where motors are allowed).

These elegant craft do have their drawbacks, of course. They "clunk" when a rock is struck, especially the aluminum ones, so everyone within a mile knows you mis-read the river. A more serious mis-judgment of a rock resulting in collision can flip the boat, gouge a serious hole (causing the boat to fill with water or even sink out from under), or make the boat wrap. In extreme cases, the "hardshell" (translation: non-rubberized-fabric-and-

air construction) aspect of the driftboat can cause the boat to tip enough to dump a passenger or strike their head/body.

Aluminum is the strongest material, with almost no care required except for knocking out dents or patching the rare puncture. Wood and fiberglass models are quieter, but require maintenance. Plus, all driftboats must be ferried to the river on a special trailer with a winch to load the boat, and this trailer must also be shuttled to the end of the trip before the boat can be loaded.

They can carry only light loads, a 14-footer typically has one rower or guide with two clients in the bow. A 16-footer might have a third client in the stern (back) or some lightweight cargo. The boat sitting on its trailer takes up a fair amount of space in a backyard or garage. (This drawback turns into an advantage when the driftboat is kept loaded with fishing equipment, oars, anchor, life jackets, and so forth, ready to head for the river at a moment's notice.) Multiple driftboats may be stacked, like teacups, so if a friend owns one, yours will probably sit nestled inside it.

Because driftboats can disappear in heavy water—especially in big waves, backcurling waves, reversals and other hydraulics—their rowers must not only be exact in running complex rapids, they must be willing to forego the gung-ho attitude of many whitewater boaters and miss all the fun stuff. (A driftboat can be rigged with floation—such as inflated inner tubes—as one would an open canoe with blocks of Styrofoam, in order to float heavier waters more safely.)

The Dory Boat

Is a close second to the driftboat in terms of beauty and usefulness as a fishing craft. But being much heavier, rowing is harder, and holding in place for fishing doesn't work well. Dories are usually found only on very large rivers: the Snake, the Idaho Salmon, the Colorado in Grand Canyon, where their trained oarsmen "cheat" (slip by a bad spot on the edge) boat-flipping hydraulics. Dories deliver a lot of bounce for the buck, making for a great ride on wave trains, and are now available in self-bailing versions, permitting the rower to tackle even bigger waters head-on. Dories are not suitable for the smaller, tighter rivers found in much of Oregon (they can run the John Day, Grande Ronde and Owyhee at high water levels of 4,000+ cfs).

Rafts

The most versatile of all whitewater craft, 12- to 14-foot rafts can handle nearly all the major whitewater found in Oregon (with skill and a little luck), while carrying hundreds of pounds of gear, passengers/anglers in front, ice chests as seats for the rower, dry boxes that fit into a special frame, cargo slings and nets to keep dry bags off the floor and inside the boat, ammo cans and small ditty bags to keep personal gear handy, even special fishing frames with bucket seats for anglers and rod holders built in. Self-bailing floors keep feet and gear less wet as they drain the boat before it can swamp in heavy hydraulics.

For bigger groups or heavy gear (such as for a flotilla of small craft), a 16-foot raft can support over half a ton. The mechanical advantage provided by 9 to 10' oar lengths allows even a small oarsman/woman to maneuver such a cargo boat. "Lisa" was a young woman I met on a guided Grand Canyon-Colorado River 21-day trip, who rowed a super-heavy 18-foot cargo raft through many large and dangerous rapids, even though she was only 5'2".

Rafts must first be aired up, which can be a drawback, or they can be kept inflated and carried to the river site on a flatbed trailer. A good foot or arm-powered air pump must be carried at all times, just in case a tube loses air. Novices often fear an inflatable will rip open and sink, but this is extremely rare in quality modern rafts. Not only do the quality rafts have at least 4 separate air chambers (not counting the "thwarts" or side-to-side tubes, or the self-bailing floor, which is also inflated), their construction is of a very strong fabric (such as nylon, somewhat like the rip-stop nylon in your backpack or rain gear) coated with a leak-resistant seal (Hypalon, neoprene, or PVC derivations). Of course, carrying a good patch kit is in order, but on moderate rivers, most boo-boos may be fixed quickly and easily with duct tape.

Catarafts

Like their companion boat, the raft, catarafts require inflation to full pressure, plus a frame to keep the craft rigid and permit it to be rowed. The cataraft is simply two long inflated tubes that are joined in place on the long sides of a rectangular frame, using cambuckle straps. The frame may include a suspended floor (made of marine plywood, plastic mesh, or webbing) that serves to keep splashes out of your lap, besides keeping the rower from falling through the middle of the boat. The floor also allows for easy stand-up casting and scouting of rapids. Or, the floor can be removed in low-water conditions, allowing the technique of "Flintstoning" (walking while holding a side of the cataraft in each arm, as Fred Flintstone carries his car in the cartoon set in the Stone Age).

Catarafts are remarkably stable craft, permitting the advanced and daring rower to power through huge hydraulics and big waves. A cat' in the standard 12- to 14-foot range, in the hands of an expert, can tackle such whitewater as Oregon's upper Klamath (50 rapids rated Class II to V in 17 miles of river, with the five miles of Hell's Corner Gorge dropping nearly 100 feet per mile, or fpm).

They are often an affordable alternative to rafts, since the lack of a floor reduces the amount of material and hand-labor required. If you're handy with tools or torch, a frame can be made on the cheap using lumber or steel tubing, adding a plywood floor as a fishing and scouting platform. The set-up of tubes and frame, plus a multitude of straps, can be a pain. Many people leave their cats rigged on a trailer.

Small craft with twin pontoons—designed as personal fishing boats, more like a float tube propelled by little oars rather than fins—can be tiny, fragile things suitable only for floating through gentle waters. Others are larger and tough enough to carry gear and can tackle medium whitewater, especially low water conditions.

Again, check the construction before you head out for back of beyond. Thin vinyl "rubber ducky" oval-shaped inflatables from the discount store are the worst offenders (I have seen one such "boat" puncture after being set down on a gravel boat ramp!).

Inflatable Kayaks

These are a tried-and-true low-water fishing craft for whitewater, rock dodging, and dragging over gravel bars. Most quality IKs can carry several hundred pounds of gear and boater weight (large people may use a two-man, sometimes run backward). I have run these at very low levels on the John Day, Grande Ronde and Owyhee, and they work well. I would stagger under a 40-pound backpack, but a hundred pounds of gear in the back of a nine-foot IK lets me use the river current to power the gear and myself into remote areas. These little boats can scoot into tiny eddies or pocket water behind small rocks,

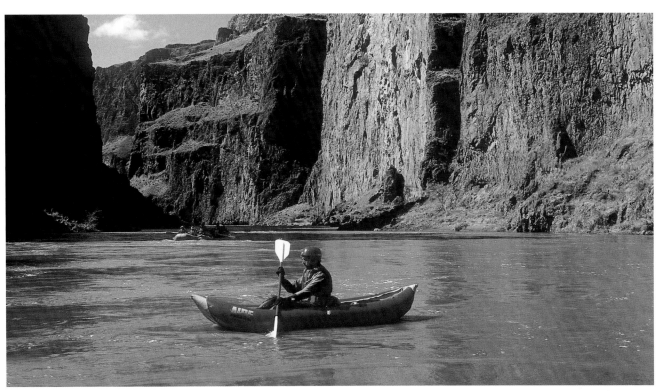

Red inflatable kayak in red gorge; adding a colorful boat or bright sweater to your pictures brings out more of the cliff colors.

for some fantastic solo experience fishing; much like float tubing, but with the added excitement of running whitewater.

Catyak

A hybrid between a cataraft and an inflatable kayak, two inflated tubes supported by a frame that is paddled, not rowed. Since paddles are shorter and easier to feather in at tight spots, lower water levels can be conquered in these craft. Also, without a floor, the Catyak doesn't get stuck on rocks as much. It is paddled with basic kayak paddling techniques.

Canoes and Hardshell Kayaks

The traditional craft for whitewater; however, their suitability for float fishing is limited. Open canoes swamp, are tippy, are not good at bouncing off rocks (except for the new hard plastic ones) and have limited gear capacity. Most of the trips in this book are for expert canoeists only, and a spray deck may be needed even at optimum water levels. (The American Canoe Association reports it's "convinced that occupant movement and weight shift plays a major role in half of all canoeing accidents" and "75% of all paddling-related fatalities involved canoeing" (according to *Paddle Dealer,* the trade magazine for paddle sports).

Kayaks are powerful craft in the hands of a pro, but carry the least gear of all whitewater craft, and are very unstable for beginners. If you aspire to learn the hardshell kayak, starting with a stable inflatable is best.

Basic Rowing

This book is intended to guide you through wilderness float fishing rivers, not instruct on boat-handling techniques. However, it's oriented to the oarboat rower, because this is the most common craft for float fishing, and the technique is not as instinctive as paddling.

But there are some easy tips that will help you learn faster. Bear in mind that some outfitters offer schools that teach rowing, or offer row-your-own boat trips with guides in lead boats to follow, plus there's the occasional driftboat salesman who will offer to teach you how to handle it.

Most oar boaters (rafts with frames, catarafts, driftboats and dories; Oregon river runners often refer to inflatables as "boats") run rivers facing downstream and pushing on both oars to move the boat (as paddlers face downstream, paddling forward). As you face downstream, your left is river left, and of course, the right bank is river right. Midstream is the middle of the river; if a description suggests taking the far right or left of center channel, divide the river into five sections (left, left of center, center, right of center, right). So "far right" means the channel next to the right-hand river bank.

This forward, or push, stroke is actually a rower's weakest stroke, using only the arms to move the boat. For more power, oarboats turn sideways to the current, and pull away from the obstacle they must miss. This is known as Face the Danger. The angle of the boat to the current determines how quickly the boat moves; a sharper angle is necessary in fast current. If this sounds confusing, just think: Face the danger, get the angle (diagonal to the current), pull with both oars until you have cleared the obstacle, then turn to face forward again.

Turning the oarboat is accomplished by pulling back on one oar on the side you need to turn to. Pushing forward on the opposite oar will achieve the same goal. Aspire to develop the double-oar turn, pulling on one oar while pushing on the other, which will swiftly and surely turn the oarboat. An example: To turn right, pull back on the right oar, or push forward on the left oar, or pull right while pushing left.

Try to always use both oars, and don't let them dangle (dangerous and may break an oar or jawbone). If holding the oars up constantly fatigues you, ship them into the boat or under your knees to take the weight off; this way, the oars are close by in case you need them.

If you can face the danger, turn the oarboat to a good angle and maintain it while pulling on both oars, then recover by turning forward—by instinct—you can run almost any rapid in the country. A river like the John Day in spring at optimum levels offers several good places to practice the turn and recover (such as the Class II+ Russo Rapid).

Oarboat Fishing

Again, the purpose here is not to teach you how to fly-fish or be a fishing guide, but to share methods that work for many float fishers. If you are new to fly-fishing, a wilderness river presents a different challenge than float tubing in a lake or standing on shore. For one, the boat may drift quickly through good water, and landing to fish may be the only option. Or on a slow section, you may have to beat the fish off with an oar! If you aspire to Class 4 (difficult fishing waters) angling, I recommend taking a trip with a fishing guide. You'll learn the flies and lures to use, where to fish on a particular river, and where to put the boat, in addition to seeing how a Dutch oven can produce excellent pineapple upside down cake.

To hold in the current for fishing, keep the boat straight and pull back on both oars repeatedly with careful, measured strokes. To set up anglers fishing from the bow (front), the best position to fish from, set up the oarboat at an angle facing an eddy line (the place where the slow upstream current meets the fast downstream current) so that the bow anglers can cast into the eddy, but the boat stays on the edge, so as not to frighten fish. Pluggers simply cast out a lure, then hold it in place, working it from side to side in the current, just below the surface and deeper down as well.

Fish will be found in eddies along shore, behind rocks, at the tailout or end of the upstream-moving current of an eddy, at the quiet water just below a rapid, and surprisingly enough, at the top of a rapid (where they often rest). Even a large steelhead, trout or bass can be hooked in pocket water (tiny eddies); while salmon and sturgeon prefer very deep water.

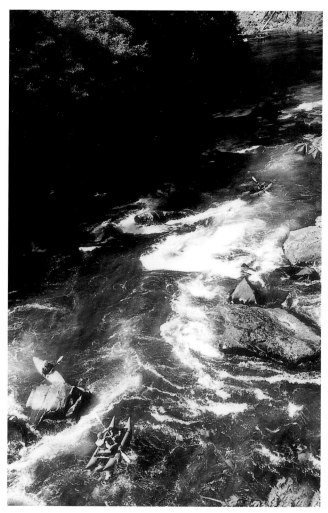

Twin tubes adjoined by a frame can be rowed, as a cataraft, or paddled, as this "paddle cat" or "Catyak". Both types are more maneuverable without a floor to cause drag, dodging boulders with ease. The paddle cat is lower to the river for an in-your-face experience; the cataraft has a higher frame, tubes and seat to accommodate the leverage and size of oars. Catarafts are more commonly employed in big rapids or for heavy loads and passenger carrying. Paddle cats are excellent in low-water conditions, rolling over gravel bars and sneaking past "sleeper" ledges. Note yellow "hardshell kayak" at bottom left waiting in eddy.

Watch the river as you float, noting gravel bars (the end is often good fishing) and the upstream V, which indicates a rock at the point of the V, so boats must dodge, but anglers should cast away at the entire V. A big downstream-pointing V (V-slick, tongue, slot) indicates deep water and is not often a good fishing site (although it's usually the best route for a drift craft).

Good anglers are needed to fish faster rivers with lots of pocket water. Without a way to stop or slow the oarboat, anglers cast into the eddy, work a line or fly slowly. Be ready to reel in quickly in shallows that will snag lures, and to get invisible fishing lines out of the way of the boat. It's pretty common for beginners to snag the lifeline (rope around the perimeter of the boat) with a hook or two.

The advantages of fishing from an oarboat are many, particularly when compared to shore fishing. You can cover many miles in a day, with many types of water: huge eddies, pocket water, currents below rapids that lead into pools, against cliff walls (great for rooting out a big bass), even throwing your line under logs, hanging brush, or bridge pillar eddies. Chances of snagging are reduced greatly because you are in front of the brush, not behind it, or to the side, as a bank angler. You don't have to wade or wear waders. You get to sit or stand, as you prefer. Novice fly fishermen can practice their cast without a tree in sight while floating slowly midstream. You can troll from the stern (back) or anchor in a good spot, land to shore to work more water or to spread out and get off by yourself for a while. You can plug for steelhead (with the boat held in moderate current, let lure and line out up to 20 feet from the boat, then work it back and forth across the current). Side-planing for salmon works on float craft as it does on motorized boats.

Most of the best fishing occurs early in the morning and late in the afternoon; but one of the reasons for this is that your shadow cast in mid-day frightens fish. From a boat, you can cast far beyond your shadow, catching fish off-guard. Bass hit all day long, and many other fish will strike anytime if they're hungry or if a hatch is present.

The hard part of oarboat fishing is getting someone to row while the others fish; this is why fishing guide services are so popular. If you are the only oarsman, don't get suckered into all the rowing. Start teaching others to row on Class I moving water, and talk them through small rapids. The oarsman can fish on calmer waters, but when facing upcoming maneuvering, the line should be reeled in, and the rod stowed in a safe place (in a pinch, between the knees will do, or install a rod holder where it won't interfere with rowing).

Paddling

Turning a Catyak or inflatable kayak is the same as with an oarboat: back stroke on the side of the boat in which direction you wish the boat to turn, or forward on the opposite side. However, here the similarity ends. Paddling's power stroke is forward, with backpaddling considered weaker. Angles to the current are just as important, even more so as too abrupt an angle may upset these small craft. Strong eddy fences—the visible line where competing currents meet—also pose problems.

A double-bladed paddle is employed, but there is no turning with both blades. The blades are usually feathered (set at opposite faces) with the paddler's strong hand (usually the right) gripping the paddle, and the weaker wrist rotating the left blade. This arrangement slices through wind better than paddles with both blades unfeathered (with both blades' flat surfaces set flat).

Paddles are available with a push-button in the middle that allows you to choose feathered or unfeathered blades; good for learning. Canoes, by the way, are almost always paddled with single-bladed paddles.

Paddle techniques are much the same for all long and narrow craft. The essentials: Keep the boat headed straight-on when running waves (sideways presents a large surface to the rapid, more to grab, flip or wrap against a rock); keep paddling in whitewater (momentum helps small boats get through waves and reversals), and lean forward in rapids (helps punch through waves).

Canoes are steered from the stern with a "J-stroke", where the blade is placed into the water forward of your position, pulled toward you, then angled out (usually in the shape of an L rather than a J when paddled on the right). The top hand must grasp the T-grip or pear shaped top of the paddle shaft for greater control, while the lower shaft is held by the other hand. Advanced strokes such as draw and pry, eddy turns, and so forth are best learned in a canoeing class.

On difficult waters, such as Oregon's Illinois River, oarboaters often utilize paddle assist—one or more passengers on an oarboat who help by paddling with canoe paddles, coordinating their strokes with the oarswoman/man. This is best accomplished from the bow. Rowers should call out commands that correspond with their strokes: "Backpaddle!" for pulling, "Forward!" for pushing. (I prefer not to say "Forward Paddle!" as in the cacophony of a rapid, this command is easily confused with "Backpaddle!").

Paddle Fishing

Similar to oarboat fishing, except the paddle craft is usually a solo boat and controlled by the paddler/angler during fishing. This is both exciting and frustrating, as depicted in my forced run through a long stretch of whitewater while holding the rod between my knees, towing a hooked trout along for the ride.

In a C-2 or two-person canoe, the stern paddler can steer the canoe to the edge of eddies, and even hold back in moving water, to assist an angler in the bow. A double-bladed kayak paddle comes in handy for this. Casting into eddies behind rocks and into tailwater amid rapids, obviously, is more difficult for the solo paddler, but also challenging and fun. Paddlers can land and fish from shore, or sit at the edge of a slow eddy. Trolling is good, too.

Permits

Advance permits drawn by lottery are required for floating the Rogue and Snake rivers most of the year. This requires choosing a date and submitting an application in the off-season, or drawing a launch permit that someone else has cancelled, and paying an application and/or user fee. Both rivers are open to all comers in the low-use season (October 16 to May 14 on the Rogue).

Boaters who operate commercially, that is, they charge a fee for their services beyond the regular expenses of private boaters (food, user fees, transportation and shuttle cost, rental of equipment, loss or damage to equipment), must have a commercial permit from the managing agency plus a commercial guide's license from the state (on top of liability insurance) to operate on all of the rivers listed here. (Of the rivers listed here, only the Owyhee is still open to new outfitters; the right to run commercially on the other rivers in this book must be purchased, with "substantial assets" such as equipment and mailing lists, from an existing business.)

To obtain a list of authorized outfitters, contact the managing agency for each river. Never float with an outfitter who doesn't have a permit from the federal agency in charge of a federally-protected river, as they do not have insurance on that river.

On some rivers where commercial outfitters operate, they are not allowed to receive a fee for escorting private boaters, with certain exceptions. A few outfitters do offer "whitewater school" and/or guide training, the chance to row most of the river (their boat or sometimes your own), and other learning opportunities for river novices.

For private anglers float fishing the rivers in this book, self-issuing permits are usually required (available at the put-in site, usually free and not needed in advance); on the Deschutes, a pay-in-advance boater pass is mandatory (the charge is per floater per day, more per day on weekends).

These conditions can change, however, so always contact the managing agency before planning your float to see if permits are necessary, where you can get them (sometimes by mail or Internet) and if there is a cost. Many state parks and recreation areas charge for camping, and some charge for overnight parking. Some privately-held parks charge access fees, too, and so do some land-owners.

Hazards

These include dangers not as obvious as whitewater. In truth, the drive to the river and back is more dangerous than the actual float. Careful boaters live long and healthy lives. Typical hazards beyond rapids include hypothermia from cold-water dunkings, river debris and natural or man-made dangers—logs or "strainers" in the current, bridge pillars, wrap-rocks, flip holes, loose lines on boats, and other risks (see safety check list). Dangerous animals: most hazardous of all is the honey bee and/or yellow jacket (more people die from an allergic reaction to them than die from snakebites), rattlesnakes (no other poisonous snakes are found in Oregon; our common timber rattler is shy and not highly poisonous, but the Great Basin rattlesnake is larger, meaner, and fortunately rare, only in desert areas), scorpions, black widow and brown recluse spiders, ticks—mostly for the diseases they carry—mosquitoes, too).

Bad drinking water is unexpected in Oregon's pure-looking mountain streams, but always filter and/or chemically treat all river, side stream, and creek water—regardless of how clear it looks. *Giardia*, a nasty intestinal pest, is found everywhere. Only spring water straight from the source is safe (other than tap/bottled water brought from home).

Some desert rivers may have farm chemicals in them from irrigation waters, and/or suspended silt: the John Day and Owyhee in particular. Let murky water settle in a bucket first before treating it. In addition, the Owyhee has mercury-poisoned fish, so practice a lot of catch and release on that river. Catfish have spines on their back that can cause a nasty puncture wound; handle them carefully.

The same hazards that increase the ratings of rapids should be kept in mind, especially isolation (even if there is a road, no cars or ranches may be along it, or it might be a 30-mile hike for help), over-reliance on technology—

Poisonous water hemlock is found along many wilderness rivers. Although this plant resembles a wild parsnip, eating a piece of root the size of your finger can kill a person, or even a large animal such as a cow. Identify the plant by its carrot-like foliage, purple streaks on the lower stalks, and strong odor. Children may be sickened just by putting the hollow stalks to their lips as a makeshift whistle. "Land" hemlock is similar, but grows in dry soil, often next to the edible wild carrot. Boaters should pack lots of food and not try to live off the land, inviting mistakes far from "911" assistance.

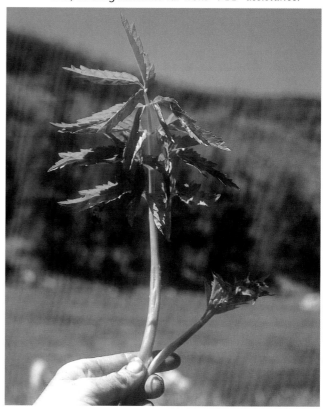

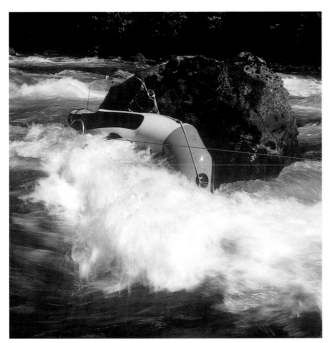

Any boat can "wrap" around a rock like a wet sheet if proper safety measures are not employed. Never "broach" or hit sideways—turn the boat to strike the rock bow or stern first if a collision is inevitable. Have all boaters move towards the rock—this means actually sitting on the rock side tube of a raft in someone's lap, if necessary! The shift of weight towards the rock lifts the upstream side, often causing the boat to pivot safely around the obstacle. Boaters must be cautious not to get between the rock and boat, or they can be pinned too. On some occasions, boats may be trapped for hours or days until the river rips them apart. Carry and know how to use a Z-drag rescue kit (a set of ropes and pulleys employed to increase the mechanical advantage of humans over the force of the river current).

cell phones do not work in many river canyons; in fact, even satellite phones don't work in some of the more remote areas. If you try to call for help, send your fittest member running up a hill for better reception (you must get a clear line to the satellite or tower that picks up your phone's signal).

Emergency equipment to carry is listed in the back of this book, but the minimum should be: spare oar/paddle, repair kit, first-aid kit, duct tape, work or sport gloves and waterproof adhesive tape (for blistered hands), throw-bag (a rope stuffed into a bag which, when tossed correctly, lands in front of a runaway passenger, and can also be used for rescue or lining), Z-drag kit (for salvaging a wrapped boat), whistle on each person's life jacket (to signal for help over the roar of rapids, required of each boat by state law), extra straps and rope (for jury-rigging), hand-powered pump for inflatables, bucket (for settling water and bailing).

Chlorox is useful for sanitizing dishes. Always carry extra clothing and rain gear and polyester fleece sleep-

ing-bag liner (in case someone's bag gets wet, or their clothing takes hours to dry), a tarp (keeps rain, sun off tent, kitchen), fire tools (folding shovel, container of water or bucket, axe; check fire regulations in the area you are floating). Some boaters keep injectable lidocaine and wire cutters in their first-aid kit (the first for numbing flesh to remove imbedded fish hooks, the second for cutting off the barb to extract a hook).

Don't even think of floating without a current map of the river and surrounding area (seal in plastic or have it laminated). In remote areas, bring emergency signaling devices for aircraft rescue (flare gun, flourescent orange cloth, plus matches/fire starter, steel mirror carried on your person). Select bright colors for safety. Equip vehicles for backcountry roads (spare, jack, full gas can, tools, spare fan belt, duct tape, etc.).

Make certain each passenger knows basic whitewater safety, even if they have to carry a cheat sheet as a reminder. Remind crew to bring along any necessary medications, and to let the group know about potential medical problems (diabetes, asthma, heart) and how to help them in a crisis. Keep all boats together. Elect the boater with the most experience as lead boat (nobody passes them) and the second-most experienced as sweep (no one gets behind them). Keep the boat in front of you and just behind you in sight at all times. If danger threatens (thunderstorm, for example), abandon fishing for safety.

Think before you buy gear—a dry bag with padded shoulder straps, for example, will be more suited to portage/walk-out situations than a cheap bag without even a handle. Pots with lids that fit boil water faster than open kettles, saving precious fuel. An aluminum Dutch oven cooks almost as well as a cast-iron version, but weighs a lot less. Gear should serve double duty whenever possible.

Know evacuation points on the river you plan to float, just in case. Two people alternating rowing can travel very fast when necessary (up to 50 miles per day). Remember that should an evacuation be necessary due to injury or illness, double or triple up the strongest boaters on one craft, and just row constantly, trading off, until civilization is reached. This is usually far faster and safer than climbing out of a sheer gorge or running along the river banks. Ranchers/farmers are sometimes available for assistance, but for emergencies only, they don't want their privacy and hard work interrupted for, say, a bad hangnail. Broken bones, yes.

The usual rule is to never boat alone, but I have done easy trips by myself in small craft, always wearing a life-jacket with signal device. A careful soloist may be better off than a bunch of novices who don't take the wilderness seriously.

Obviously, running whitewater and camping in remote places requires a clear head. Save alcohol for camp (it dehydrates you on hot days, anyway) and avoid illegal drug use. Drinking while controlling a boat is now considered illegal, as well as stupid. Under Oregon law, all children under 12 must wear a life jacket at all times while on the water. Under common sense, so should all adults.

Fishing

Check the current Oregon Department of Fish & Wildlife regulations before fishing, as the rules change every year. Contact the Portland Office at P.O. Box 59, Portland OR 97207-0059; 503/872-5268 or access their website at www.dfw.state.or.us. For non-hunters, wildlife watching tips are available. Out-of-state licenses are available by mail but not yet online.

Some basic fishing regulations are given for rivers where rules are unlikely to change, such as no angling from a floating device on the Deschutes, or using artificial flies or lures only, also on the Deschutes.

In this book fishing information on each river includes species available, how to fish in different seasons and varying water levels, what areas are most productive on each river, and brand names of lures/scents/flies/baits that work for me, other guides, and Joe Angler.

Pay attention to recommended water levels, float seasons and seasons for different species of fish (steelhead in June? Not likely on many rivers).

News reports on fishing and water conditions are available from ODFW, given in newspapers, available in Northwest-oriented fishing magazines, and on some websites. Locals or guides often call in current conditions to the newspapers. Most fly shops are glad to sell you flies recommended for the section of river you plan to float, while sporting goods stores can suggest the hottest lure the locals use, or the smelliest bait to tempt a river catfish.

Taking a guided fishing trip on a complex river such as the Rogue or Deschutes is highly recommended as a first step; not only will you learn the fishing holes and lures or flies, but you will get to see how an expert runs the rapids.

Managing Agency

This is the government agency in charge of maps, fire conditions, river regulations, water levels and hazards, permit applications for rivers where agencies restrict boater numbers, and so forth. This should be your first contact. Many have Internet sites. Some permit applications may be filed online, but most are still write-in/call-in lotteries.

River regulations on all of these rivers include mandatory use of a fire pan whenever building a fire, carrying an agency-approved porta-potty system, carrying a signaling device (whistle), carrying life jackets or PFDs (personal flotation devices) to fit all boaters (with boaters under 12 required to wear them at all times), taking out all trash, straining kitchen waste water, carrying out ashes, leaving archaeological sites alone (any site and

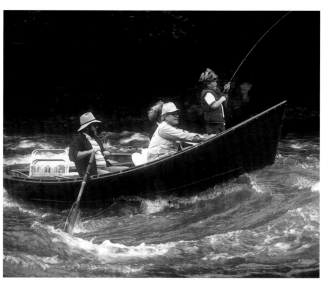

Surprisingly, many fish—trout and steelhead in particular— will strike in whitewater. Fishing at the top of a rapid is often so effective than even osprey use the technique. The Grande Ronde River is especially good for this technique. Rowers can slow the boat against the current to allow more casting time by pulling back on both oars.

artifacts over 50 years old), and occasionally may require more strict actions: carrying in your own wood (on rivers such as the Deschutes), fire season closures (no smoking except while on the boat or in a vehicle, no charcoal fires, and sometimes carrying fire tools). Check first before you are turned away at the launch site or are slapped with a $500 fine!

Shuttles

Rivers run in one direction. When you finish, you are dozens or even hundreds of miles by road from where you launched. Thus, the shuttle. Some boaters take two or more rigs and run their own shuttle, but with the price of gas and the even higher cost of your limited vacation time, consider hiring a commercial shuttle service. This is best with driftboats that must have a trailer to load (although many rafters now trailer their craft).

Current phone numbers are listed with each river, or you can get them from the managing agency. Nearly all shuttle drivers are safe and honest, but you should not leave any valuables in your rig, just in case. Do leave a spare set of keys for the shuttle (arrange for them to be locked inside the vehicle in an obscure location. If you're paranoid, have the shuttler mail them to your home— provide a stamped, addressed envelope.)

Be sure you and your driver know where and when the take-out is scheduled, so you will not arrive to find no car. Also, give your take-out time as earlier than you expect, so you have the option of quitting the trip sooner. Some shuttle services store your vehicle in a secure location as part of their service, or will even store your extra gear, bring you cold drinks, etc. Just ask around.

River Mileage And Highlights

Mileages from mile 0 (the put-in) to the take-out tend to be estimates, even under the best of circumstances, due to the constant changing of the rivers. Some rivers may move a quarter-mile or more each flood year. Some maps and guide books determine mileage from the mouth of the river, but I find it easier to figure miles floated. Times vary, but most boats can cover a river mile in three to fifteen minutes, depending on river discharge, gradient, type of boat (according to John Garren, a hardshell kayak that floats a distance in say, 1 minute, will take a raft 1.6 minutes to float, or a driftboat, 1.3). This estimate of time does not include off-river time or fishing time. Estimate the mileage you cover on day trips in your boat, then apply them to the overnight trips. Deduct off-river time from your estimates.

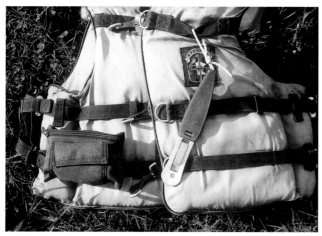

Many boaters wear a diver's knife on their PFD to cut or saw through lines (ropes) in an emergency. A line can become wrapped around a limb and underwater structure, holding the boater under water. A good river knife with serrated edges should be accessible by one hand for sawing through tough ropes.

I don't believe in carrying watches and timing your float down to the precise second, but sometimes this becomes a necessary evil when planning a longer trip. I prefer to rely on landmarks, such as unusual rock pinnacles, bridges, power lines, and other visual references to give me a general idea where I am on the river. Some GPS waypoints are available for major rapids, but precision is important, or you may accidentally enter a Class IV rapid without scouting.

To figure camps, split the river map into equal sections for the number of days you will be out, with shorter first days (to allow for unpacking and setup) and last days (unloading boats and carrying items to the trailer, time for driving, usually longer at the end of the trip). Plan your camp sites accordingly. For example, on the Rogue, when I am doing a 3-day trip, I plan on camping the first night somewhere in the Big Windy-Horseshoe

Bend area, about 1/3 of the distance. The second night needs to be within reach of the takeout for shuttling guests back to the beginning as well as unpacking and reloading, so that means camping below Blossom Bar Rapid, usually in the Brushy Bar-Tate Creek region. I pick a general region as the Rogue is a busy river and I want an area with many camps to choose from, rather than having to crowd in with others.

Beyond rapids and scouting sites, mileage lists also include highlights of the river stretch: scenic spots, history/pioneer cabins, wildlife unique to the area (bighorns on Owyhee, lower John Day, lower Deschutes, Grande Ronde), photo tips, hikes, wildflowers of the area, geology (from volcanic dikes to opals and gold), unique landmarks that let you know where you are (Johnny Cake Mountain on the North Fork John Day), and an occasional reference to River Mile (the mileage from the river's mouth).

Major rapids—those above Class II—are indicated, along with scouting sites, suggested routes at all three water levels, and special dangers, as well as some history (how the rapid was named), personal experiences, and anecdotes of bad runs. Rapids and rivers are rated for the beginner, so a very experienced boater may be insulted. Better bothered than buried, I say. Additionally, the routes suggested are used by many boaters, including myself, but you may prefer a different route. Evacuation points such as lodges and roads are also given, just in case.

Most rapids are named by the first to run the river. Official names are recognized by the BLM and Forest Service and recorded on maps. Other rapids have been named more recently, or have more than one name. Most minor rapids are not named (those rated Class II) and easier rapids are not listed or detailed on river mileages. If you can't run a Class I+ to II without instruction, you shouldn't be on a wilderness river without a guide or instructor. Some rapids and features are given personal names by myself or other boaters (such as Sentinel Canyon on the Owyhee, Hungry Rock on the John Day by guidebook writer Arthur Campbell, the Dungeon reversal on the upper Deschutes run).

The use of the term "rapids" to denote any stretch of whitewater has given way to the term "rapid" when describing a single drop or stretch. Thus, on the Deschutes you will have Whitehorse Rapid, which can also be called Whitehorse Rapids because there are numerous smaller drops following the main drop. But Boxcar Rapid, properly, is not Boxcar Rapids, because it's one drop.

When reading the mileage log, remember that "river right" is the right side of the river as you face downstream in your boat, while "river left" is the left side. If your boat is backwards, reverse the directions. River terms are indicated in quotation marks: "backferry" (with an explanation; to cross a river at an angle with the back of the boat pointed towards your destination).

Rivers

CHAPTER 2

Rivers
Rated by Class, Trip Length, Solitude, etc.

River Section	Miles	Length of Trip	Whitewater Classification	Fishing Difficulty	Solitude Rating
Deschutes River					
Warm Springs to Sherars Falls	50	2 to 5+ days	Class I to IV, Easy to expert	#4, No fishing from a floating device, no natural bait, single-point barbless hooks, anglers must wade strong currents. Watch for thick brush, deep water	#3. Very popular on weekends, mid-week is quiet, trains roll by, day and night
Warm Springs to Trout Creek	10	1	Class I+, Easy+,	#4, No fishing from a floating device, no natural bait, single-point barbless hooks, big wide river, strong currents to wade	#2. Very popular on weekends, trains, mid-week is quiet
Buckhollow to Macks Canyon	25	1 to 2+ days	Up to Class III+ for first 6 miles, then Class I Intermediates	No fishing from a floating device, no natural bait, single-point barbless hooks, big wide river, strong currents to wade	#3. (w/o jet boats) Road, float boat and jet boat access, can be crowded
Macks Canyon to Columbia River	25	1 to 2+ days	Five rapids in last 10 miles rated up to Class IV Expert	#4, No fishing from a floating device, no natural bait, single-point barbless hooks, big wide river, strong currents to wade	#4. (w/o jet boats) Access is by float boat, jet boat & trail can be crowded, jet boats alternate every other week
John Day River					
Service Creek to Twickenham	13	1 to 2+ days	II+ Slow current 1 major rapid	#2, Easy, obvious structure, bait OK.	#3+. Some ranches & roads, quiet, very deserted in off-season (July-Dec.)
Twickenham to Clarno	33	2 to 4+ days	II+ Slow current 2 major rapids	#2, Easy, obvious structure, bait OK	#3+. More remote, some ranches & very deserted in off-season (July-Dec.)
Service Creek to Clarno	47	3 to 4+ days	II+ Slow current 3 major rapids	#2, Easy, obvious structure, bait OK	#3+. Ranches, remote Big Bend is remote, quiet, very deserted in off-season (July-Dec.)
Clarno to Cottonwood	80	generally 5 days	1 rapid III-IV, faster current, 3 rapids II-II+	#2, Easy, obvious structure, bait OK	#4. Very remote,
North Fork, Dale to Monument	40	2 to 4+ days	lots, of rock dodging III+, very fast current	#4, Difficult, fast water, careful with native fish	#4. Very remote, a few ranches
Monument to Kimberly	15	1 to 3+ days	II+, slower current	#3, Difficult, fast water, careful with native fish	#2. Remote, some cabins, roads

Fishing Difficulty Ratings

1=very easy 6=near flooded out, fish all dead
Factors include:
A) Regulations (some prevent fishing from boats, which makes it difficult).
B) Difficulty of wading (deep water, fast current)
C) Availability of natural hatches & baits
D) Size of river & availability of pocket water, eddies, etc.

E) River clarity, esp. for fly-fishing
F) Species easy to catch (bass, catfish)
G) Purity of water (past chemical spills)
H) Dams (limit native fish, migratory fish)
I) Competition (how many people are fishing)
J) Quality of fish (wild preferable to hatchery)

olitude factors
– city water 6= unmapped wilds
actors include:
) Roads & how heavily traveled
) #'s of boaters, permit
   restrictions
) Dispersal of camps
) Location of intrusions such as
   bridges
) Train tracks with active trains
) Non-boating access
) Size of groups
   Location: proximity to large
   cities

International Scale of Whitewater Difficulty
Class I. Easy. 6 mph, small waves, wide routes around obstacles. Easy to hold boat in place
Class II. Medium. Larger waves, river bends, obstacles closer together, course usually obvious "tongue" in center. Easy recovery water.
Class II. Difficult. Maneuvering in rapids neccessary. Larger waves may swamp open boats. Faster currents make osbtacles harder to miss. Some hydraulics.
Class IV. Expert. Rapids are longer and rockier with bigger waves and usually requires scouting from shore. Hydraulics. Risk of wrapping/flipping boat, injury to overboards. Recovery water inadequate
Class V. Team of Experts. True waterfalls drop down 12-15 feet, waves up to 30 feet high, thorough scouting necessary. Risk of life and limb. Attempt only by experts in quality craft at optimum water levels. Powerful hydraulics.
Class VI. (Un-runnable). True waterfalls over 15 feet. Large hydraulics that may hold boater under water. Little or no recovery room. Often skill of boater makes no difference. Lining/portaging preferable.
(+) indicated rapid is usually more difficult than general rating, but less than next level (II+ is not III)

River section	Miles	Length of Trip	Whitewater Classification	Fishing Difficulty	Solitude Rating
Rogue River					
Hog Creek to Grave Creek	17	1 day	Class I to II+ pool & drop	#2, Fish from boat or bank	#2, Lots of amateur boaters & tour jet boats
Grave Creek to Foster Bar	38	2 to 5 days	Class II to IV Expert	#3, Fish from boat or bank, trail follows north bank along entire section, steelhead are wild	#4, Restricted to 120 people/day, no motors Grave Cr to Blossom B.
Owyhee River					
Three Forks to Rome		3 to 4 days	Up to Class V Portage Widow Maker, Expert	#3, Fish from boat or bank, very deep gorge, no real trail access, off-color water	#5, Limited access due to remote country and short runoff season
Rome to Leslie Gulch	65	4 to 6 days	Up to Class IV Expert, pool & drop, wrap rocks & holes	#3, Fish from boat or bank, deep gorges, no trails, extremely remote country, float in only, off-color water	#4+, Limited access due to remote country and short runoff season, almost empty after May 31
Grande Ronde & Wallowa Rivers					
Minam to Rondowa (only when road closures are open) Takeout at Rondowa	10	1 day	Class II to III Fast current, rocky rapids	#2+, (Grande Ronde) Fish from boat or bank, can be hiked along RR track, fly-fishing best here	#3, Train, seldom runs. Feeling of isolation, crowds disappear late July-Dec.
Minam to Troy	45.5	3 to 5 days+	Class II to III, mostly Class II Fast currents, rocky rapids	#2+, Fish from boat or bank, no trail access, lots of pocket water, eddies, fish strike in current	#3+, Popular during June & early July, weekends, crowds disappear late July-Dec.
Troy to Snake River	45	3 to 5 days+	Class II with one Class IV Current slows, fewer rocks	#2+, Fish from boat or bank, no trail access, need Washington license not far below Troy	#3, Popular during June & early July, weekends, crowds disappear late July-Dec.
Snake River					
Hell's Canyon Dam to Heller Bar	80	5 days+	Up to Class V, but also many miles of flat water Expert	#3+, Jet boat access, as well as float-in anglers, big wide river, hard to find pocket water. Many species	#3, Lottery drawing permit system controls access, jetboats
Illinois River					
Oak Flat to Rogue River	32	3 days	Up to Class V, many rapids, expert level river, logs in river, DANGEROUS AFTER HEAVY RAIN	#4, Varied nature of water flows makes fishing difficult. When river drops, clear turquoise pools for fly-fishing. Take care with endangered species	#4+, Can be popular during short access season, when river drops below 1,000 cfs, very isolated. Canyon access very difficult except by boat

CHAPTER **3**

Fishing on Oregon's Wilderness Rivers

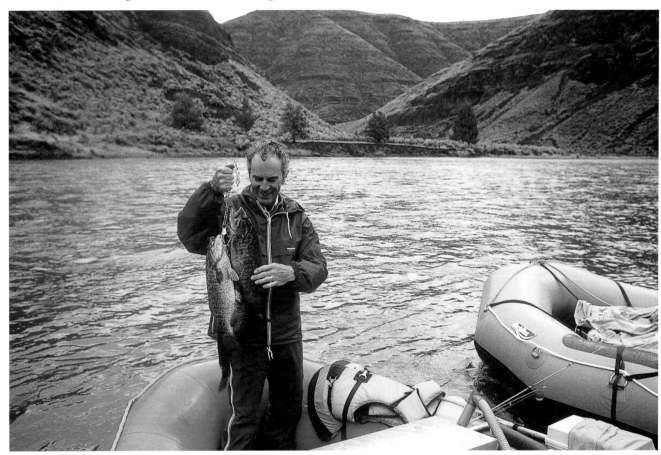

Another big bass in Hoot Owl Canyon. The river is still off-color.

Smallmouth Bass Fishing

Upper and Lower John Day, *Rated 2+

BRING NIGHTCRAWLERS TO GUARANTEE SUCCESS, especially early in the season when the river is high and muddy, but fishing from the boat over mostly slow pools and eddies makes catching bass easy for the beginner. Easily identified structures of bass habitat in this rock-laden canyon.

Lures and flies work better when water levels drop and clarity improves, usually late June. Lots of shore fishing, as well. Anglers report catching and releasing over 100 bass per day here. Trophies up to 8 pounds.

"For bass, I use a lot of dark colors," said Scott Cook. "They are better than light or flashy lures."

Snake, Rated 3

This is a very large river all summer long, with deep water, long pools interspersed with big rapids.

There is structure but it's a little harder to fish. Bass up to pounds, a few trophies. Head for the "little sister," John Day, f trophy bass. There are lots of bass on the Snake, though, entertain you while you wait for bigger fish of other species.

Upper and Lower Owyhee, Rated 3

The portion of this river above the reservoir is not common fished, so smallmouth bass readily take lures, but bring nigh crawlers and catfish baits as a backup.

Less accessible structure for bass fishing. Water condition often poor until late June, when the river becomes more difficu to run. Spectacular desert canyons, solitude, rock collecting, ar hot springs offset any disappointing angling.

Trout Fishing

Deschutes

Rated 4 for all fishing, since anglers can't fish from boats ar must wade strong currents, fight their way under overhangir

*See pages 26-27 for rating charts

brush, and watch for rattlesnakes. Fly fishing or artificial lures only.

Multiple factors, including dependence on landing to open shore, private property restrictions, and concentration of anglers on shore all contribute to difficulty. (Check current regulations.)

However, large and healthy populations of native redside trout are worth extra effort. Water clarity is excellent much of the year. Best trout fishing is above Sherars Falls, excellent day fishing around Maupin and Warm Springs to Trout Creek, to build confidence and skill for multi day float fishing. Hiring a fishing guide is recommended for novices, especially fly anglers.

Rogue, Rated 3

Fishing from the boat helps, but many trout are elusive. Half-pounders—immature steelhead—are counted as trout by ODFW (under 16 inches) and strike fiercely at lures, flies and baits beginning in early autumn (check regs for bait restrictions in fall). Bear in mind that the Rogue has rapids rated Class IV (expert) so a guided trip is recommended for the inexperienced.

Water is not as clear as colder rivers in summer except around side creeks.

North Fork John Day, Rated 4

Swift waters, hard to fish from boats on upper river. Fishing chances improve on lower reaches of the run as the river slows and pools more.

Native trout including redband are recovering from a chemical spill. Anglers must be cautious not to hook immature steelhead, and to catch and release carefully, as most trout are wild.

Grande Ronde, Rated as Class 2+ in season

Fishing from the boat is very successful after high spring levels drop, usually early July (below 3,000 cfs).

Trout are found above rapids, and in pools below, in pocket water, tailouts. Lots of pocket water amid swift riffles refine your technique. Lures are most effective on Grande Ronde, while flies work on Wallowa River.

Salmon/Steelhead Fishing

Rogue, Rated 4

Harder than trout or half-pounders, but worthwhile; watch for overly warm river water and fish the mouths of cold creeks. September and October usually better for steelhead; spring for chinook. Lower river has some competition from jetboats, a few anglers hike in, but the wilderness run is almost all for float fishers. Salmon runs have improved in last few years, with monsters caught near the mouth, but runs are still limited. Plunking from the bank, casting spinners, trolling and bait work; Hot Shots and plugs from boats too. Much action along with luxurious "camping" on guided angling trips that take

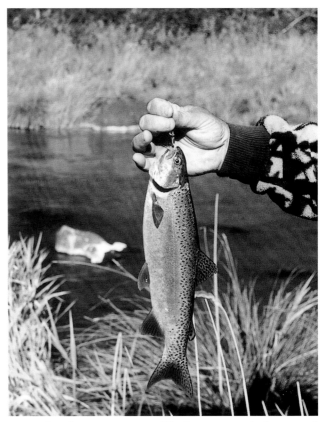

A nice hatchery trout, gone wild after years at the bottom of a desert canyon. A diet of fresh water shrimp and bugs will convert any junk-food fish into a lean, mean fighting machine. However, if you don't want to eat the fish, be sure to keep it in the water. (You can tell a live fish by the eyes; a dead fish's eyes stare straight, while the living fish looks downward, towards its river home.) Although fish in large reservoirs and lakes may grow to grotesque proportions, a river fish, even from the hatchery, fights through currents, developing a special feistiness flatwater fish will never experience.

advantage of wilderness lodges in strategic locations. Anglers on their own take advantage of making camp anywhere, not making miles to a certain spot.

Snake, Rated 4+

Big water fishing limits obvious steelhead habitat, dams impede historical runs of both species. Fishing for wide assortment of other species keeps anglers interested. Competition from jetboats.

Deschutes, Rated 4+

Summer steelhead anglers have a lot of competition from jetboats on opposite weeks on lower river, also walk-ins. Macks Canyon to Mouth contains some roadless areas, good especially midweek. Best bet is upper river later in summer and early fall, when fish have moved above Sherars Falls. The run features strong, sporty wild steelhead averaging 5 to 10 pounds. Guides help lessen the learning curve.

Remember that no angling from a floating device makes the fish harder to catch even in the best of conditions. But who can pass up the chance to fish one of the most productive wild steelhead runs in the nation? Plus side: River is almost always in good shape, clean and clear. Off-season fishing is good, even in winter. Many hatches even in fall.

Fall runs of wild chinook salmon are in good condition. Pelton Dam blocked upstream migration of spring chinook to upper spawning areas, so this season may be short or closed. The biggest draw for salmon is the opportunity to "egg plunk" below Sherars Falls, across from traditional Tribe salmon and steelhead netting territory. Check current regulations carefully.

John Day, Rated 2++

The steelhead runs in fall and winter are wild stock, with stray hatchery fish from other river systems available to take. The hottest month is usually November, not a good month for novices in the wilderness. Public access is limited, especially in the wilderness canyons, so float fishing when practical is very productive. Overlap of steelhead runs with smallmouth bass fishing in October, usually pleasant autumn weather, plus the sight of bighorn rams strutting, makes this stream a classic float, even when some riffles are only inches deep. (Closed for salmon to allow recovery of runs.)

Grande Ronde, Rated 3

Fall and winter steelhead runs, pick up as irrigators return water to the river after crop harvests. Many a nice steelhead has been caught during an elk hunting float. Best steelheading is closer to mouth, where Oregon and Washington meet (dual licenses needed). Expect cold conditions and possible ice in extreme weather; winter floating is more common in the drier lower canyon than through upper-elevation forests. Season is usually April-November, check regulations. (Closed for salmon.) Great wildlife in off-season includes wintering bald eagles, elk herds, cougar.

Sturgeon Fishing

Snake, Rated 4

Channel catfish are popular, but lose to the real heavyweights, sturgeon up to 10 feet long. The fishery is catch and release, but who cares when you can challenge a fish bigger than you are, in a mile-deep canyon? Big rapids increase difficulty of entry except for skilled boaters, both float and under power. If you want to catch one of these behemoths on the Snake, a guide is highly recommended.

Rogue, Rated 4

Only a few deep holes offer opportunities for sturgeon. Sturgeon rising out of the depths to surface in the creepy Mule Creek Canyon stretch often surprise boaters.

Common Lures, Flies, Baits, Techniques Used on Oregon Rivers

Salmon, steelhead, large trout: Spoons, spinners, topwater wood plugs, Hot Shots, diving plugs, cured salmon egg clusters (or single bright red eggs, such as Red Hots), nightcrawlers, divers (Pink Lady, Dipsy Diver), floats (not bobbers, but special floats to keep lures and bait off the bottom), Side Planers for angling from shore, Action lures such as Kwik-Fish lures, Rapalas and other minnow imitations (Hot Shots, etc.). Hot Shots are so frequently used in Oregon that they are now a brand name "verb", as in "I caught this fish Hotshotting."

Most Oregon waters contain diverse foods for fish, and they will strike lures or flies that resemble nymphs (larvae of flying insects such as the caddisfly), crawdads, periwinkles (small water snails), scuds (tiny freshwater shrimp), and so forth. Get down on your knees by the river, look closely, and turn over some rocks to see what the fish are feeding on. Check brush for pupae (cocoon-like) and hatch bugs. Midges hatch all year long on some Oregon rivers.

Fish react to color (they may snub a light-hued lure, but strike at a black one), lures that flash and/or spin, or

Looking for steelhead on a cold muddy winter float trip, river guide Al Law shows off a beautiful bass. In five minutes we had dinner for 9!

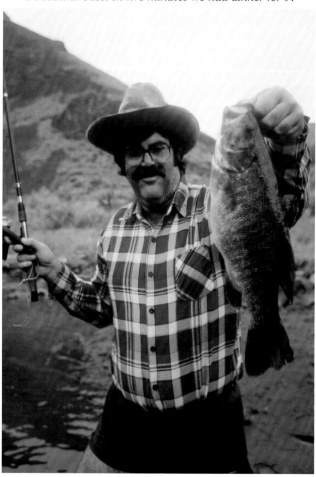

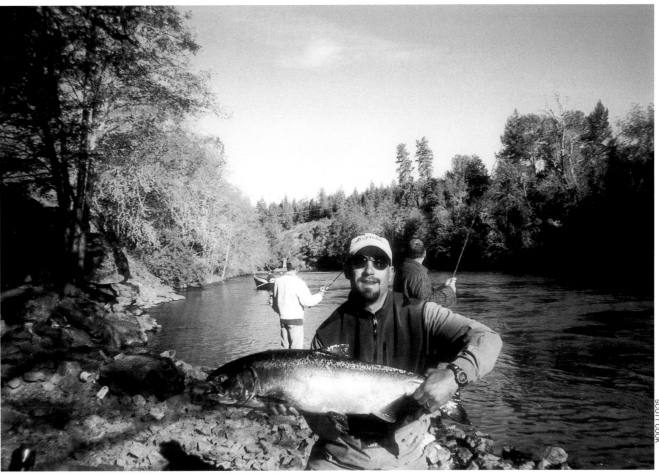

SCOTT COOK

Scott Cook happily displays a beautiful spring chinook salmon.

wobble. A large fish that isn't hungry or feeding, such as a salmon moving upstream or a trout in a small eddy, may strike a spoon aggressively, apparently defending their territory from the intruder. Lures are often made to resemble and move like a smaller fish that's injured, easy prey (the wobble and oversized eyes on a Wobble Wort tossed at a fish is much like tossing a fake mouse on a string to a cat). All of our major fish species are active predators as well as opportunistic.

"Roostertails are always a good one," says Nick Blomquist of G.I. Joes in Bend. "They work for trout and steelhead both." They also persuade smallmouth bass, and even catfish (on the Owyhee). Another recommended lure is the Wiggle Wort, used as a crank bait for steelhead. Black with silver specks is a productive color.

"Cast it upstream, sweep it back across the river (the same for Roostertails). Any type of spinner works: Blue Fox, Panther Martins." Spoons can be bounced or wobbled from a boat. For salmon, artificial egg clusters work. When scent is required in off-color water, he recommends Krill lure scent, and sometimes resorts to WD-40. For the bigger fish, use 6-to 8-pound line with an 8-foot rod.

"Fly fish the first two hours at the crack of dawn, before the sun hits the water," Craig Campbell of Fin 'n Feather advises. "Also fish the last two hours in the evening before the sun actually sets. During the day, the hardware guys continue to fish." Oregon rivers are at their clearest early and late in the day, plus that's when most hatches occur and the fish are actively feeding. Our smallmouth bass do hit all day long.

For bass waters (John Day, Owyhee, Snake), trout and steelhead lures work remarkably well. Using topwater wood plugs for bass is "a fascinating experience every angler should try... It's addictive," according to tackle sales company Luhr-Jenson (see appendix for more information on this and other angling techniques).

Guided fishing is almost always done in hardshell McKenzie or Rogue River driftboats, where the guide has total control of the boat and can anchor easily.

"Plugging" is paying out a line with a likely lure at the end, then moving it laterally. Novice fly-casters will find no more embarrassing moments with their fly snagged in a tree, since all vegetation is on the banks (with a few notable exceptions).

From the boat, trolling is very effective for bass. Tossing lures into pocket water, eddies, next to the river bank, at the edges of current, into shaded shallows, and so forth greatly increases your chances of success. Additionally, you can fish from shore in camp or pulling over (on public lands).

CHAPTER 4

John Day River Watersheds
UPPER, LOWER, AND NORTH FORK

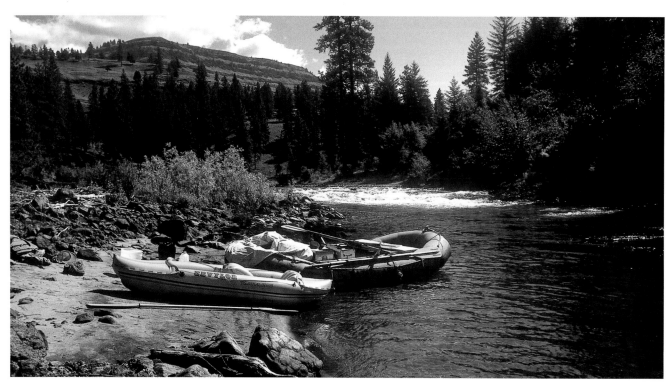

*Peaceful camp below fast rapids. Like the upper Grande Ronde, the North Fork John Day
has a gradient too fast to create many beaches.*

Overview

AT MORE THAN 280 MILES, THE JOHN DAY IS THE second-longest undammed river in the West (Idaho's Salmon is the longest at 425 miles). The John Day Dam is actually located on the Columbia River. An infamous stretch of whitewater on the as-yet-undammed Columbia, located west of Arlington at this dam site, was named Owyhee Rapids for a near-disaster of the steamer *Owyhee* (see Owyhee River section). Built in 1864, the large steamboat apparently grounded out on rocky shallows, a concept hard to comprehend when looking at the stagnant reservoir that is the modern Columbia. These rapids were inundated in 1968 with the completion of the John Day Dam.

The John Day delivers more than 750,000 tons of suspended silt a year (198 tons per mile), but only early in the season is the river murky. In very low water, waters are clear enough to see bottom. With its undammed reaches and huge silt load, wonderful camping beaches come and go at the whim of flood seasons. The only camps that are secure from season to season are the flat "terraces" in the junipers and sagebrush, but try to camp on sandy beaches when possible, to lessen your impact.

Few rivers are given a man's first and last name, but Mr. John Day earned a place in the history books by daring to head west. A backwoodsman from Virginia, Day (1771-1819) joined the John Jacob Astor overland party. Day and Ramsay Crooks fell behind the main party and were caught in bad winter conditions in the Blue Mountains in 1811-1812. Aided by Walla Walla Indians, they were directed to the Columbia River.

Near the mouth of the river that bears his name, Day and Crooks were met by hostile Indians who had just been cheated by a group of white men. Assuming Day was part of that group, they stole everything the men had, including all their clothes. Stark naked, Day and his men began the trek back to the Walla Walla Country and fortunately fell into Robert Stuart's party floating down the Columbia, who saved them from severe sunburn and humiliation. Fur-trapper Donald McKenzie (McKenzie River) reported Day's death in 1820 while in Snake River territory.

In 1805, Lewis and Clark had named this river Lepages after a member of their party. John Work used the name John Day River" in his 1825 journal. The Oregon Trail's covered wagon trains crossed the John Day at Scotts Ford by Rock Creek.

The John Day headwaters in northeast Oregon, draining from high-elevation snowpacks in the Wallowa-Whitman and Malheur National Forests. The main stem follows Highway 26 west from the town of John Day, then north along Highway 19 to Kimberly, becoming road-free at Service Creek and eventually flowing into the Columbia River near Rufus.

The North Fork of the John Day, a faster and rockier section, merges with the main stem at Kimberly. The John Day is considered floatable from Dale on the North Fork (near the mouth of Camas Creek) to the Cottonwood Bridge along Highway 206. Most boaters float from Service Creek to Clarno (upper) or Clarno to Cottonwood (lower). The stretch from Kimberly to Spray and/or Service Creek is paralleled by a road, less wild, but can also be floated, either as day or overnight trips, or as part of a two- to three-week adventure when there's enough water for your craft.

A few souls have drifted the mostly-private-lands stretch below the last public access at Scott Canyon off Highway 19 to the Columbia. Pooled waters stop the John Day's current for the last nine miles, from Tumwater Falls, which is not navigable, to the mouth. These last nine miles are a favorite fishing site for power boaters, offering bass, walleye and northern pike minnows—

trash fish with a state bounty on their heads when caught in the Columbia Basin—in addition to steelhead and salmon.

Personality

The John Day is a desert stream, winding through great volcanic-formed canyons with painted hills, ancient seashore and rainforest fossils, great basalt monoliths, some sandy beaches, lots of pioneer history, and friendly whitewater for the novice. Mule deer and coyotes are commonly seen, as are golden eagles, hawks and great blue heron.

Once known for its anadromous fish runs—migrating salmon and steelhead—the John Day is now famous throughout the nation as a fantastic smallmouth bass fishery, with catches in the state-record books: 6- to 8-pound fish are in the river. These fish are crafty, as to reach this size, they've evaded predators for many years. Action is often fierce, with occasional double fish (two bass on one treble hook, or two bass landed to the same boat at the same time), and claims of 50 to 100 fish hooked per day during hot streaks, particularly in summer, are not exaggerated.

However, the John Day is in no way a bass pond where beer-guzzling anglers cruise in motored barges using fish finders. Rather, this is still a wild river canyon with sufficient rapids and fluctuating water levels that almost eliminate motorized use (motors are presently still allowed, but only above the Clarno Bridge, and are impractical most of the year). The John Day is very much a whitewater stream, mostly Class II, but with enough surprises to wreck the occasional canoe, as well as deter the traditional john boat used to float-fish slow, calm bass rivers.

Cathedral Rock concludes your tour of the inner gorge. Now the countryside opens up and ranches will be seen.

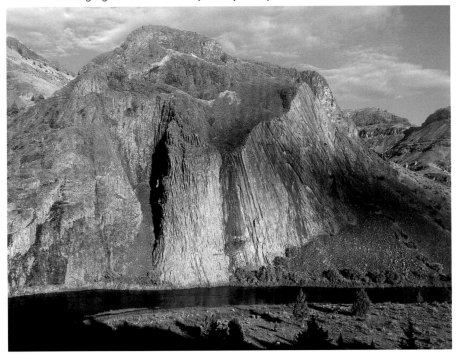

Fishing

The growth of this bass fishery is amazing given that there was virtually no warm weather fishery on the John Day until 80 bass were released at Service Creek and Kimberly in 1971. Now some estimate the bass population at 1,000 fish per mile. The bass do not interfere with salmonids or their fry, as these coldwater fish use the river only as a migration corridor, spawning in high-elevation headwaters. Most bass average 10 to 12 inches long. Releasing fish over 12 inches long will improve the trophy fishing in future years.

Numerous trash fish, mostly the northern pike minnow (formerly, squawfish) were present in the river in 1971; they have greatly declined since that time, with help from the bass (in one study, 24% of the John Day smallmouths' May diet was non-game fish, 0% was salmonids). Pike minnows are very destructive of salmonoid fry, so the bass are actually improving the coldwater fishery.

The ODFW divides the John Day into two management strategies, a Basic Yield stretch accessed by roads, where overlap between smallmouth bass and anadromous fish occurs, and a Quality Fishery, from Tumwater Falls upstream to Service Creek (the roadless, float-in area only). Basic is to provide "a variety of sizes of fish to anglers" while "Quality Fishery areas are managed to increase the abundance of mid to large-sized fish. The goal for the Quality Fishery area in the John Day River is to have at least 20% of the fish caught by anglers to be over 12 inches." (John Day River Smallmouth Study, by Tim Unterwegner, ODFW.)

For a snowmelt-fed desert river, the main stem John Day is big and broad in spring, but fish are found in their usual habitats, so concentrate on these rather than fishing aimlessly. Low water concentrates the fish more into deep pools and pocket water. Water conditions vary with the level, from dark and muddy in early spring to almost clear in the skinny trickle of late summer.

As an undammed river flowing free, the John Day's gravel bars, beaches and rocks change constantly, but smallmouth habitat is typical of most bass-producing rivers: dominated by cliff walls at the water's edge, rock ledges, boulders, deep pools, grassy shoals, bridge piers, and gravel bars. Bass fishing methods include using spin casting with fake baits, trout lures, real baits, and even steelhead lures; plus fly-fishing with the usual flies, both dry and wet.

Watching a smallmouth bass explode to the surface after your grasshopper imitation is truly an incredible experience, as is having one almost run off with your rod after you set it down for "just a moment". Before smallmouths came along, river anglers in Oregon were salmonid fishers, bass were strange green invaders from The East with no place among the mighty migratories. Many anglers have now converted and fish religiously for river bass. It certainly helps that the bass's main season on the John Day makes waders unnecessary and it's not doing what it usually does in Oregon—raining.

Plus, they are easy to catch and release, with tougher lips than the more delicate trout. To hold a bass, grasp one side of its jaw firmly with one hand. This seems to hypnotize the fish into temporary stillness, allowing easy removal of the hook. A captured bass will strike again and again, and larger bass will often chase a smaller hooked one right to your boat. Additionally, smallmouths taste great when filleted and fried in butter or bacon grease. Use one- to two-pounders for this; release smaller and larger fish (take photos and weigh to confirm trophies when possible).

Bass in this high-desert stream readily take the same baits, lures and flies that other bass do: pork rind crankbaits (especially in colder water); plastic lizards, grubs and worms (sometimes with added scents); traditional trout lures such as Roostertails; the Rapala, Kwikfish and other minnow imitations; topwater plugs,"power worms"; nightcrawlers and other live baits; flies that imitate insects (both terrestrial and water-dwelling), mice, and tiny freshwater shrimp (sometimes called krill or scuds); and especially, crawfish imitations, since crawfish constitute a significant portion of the John Day smallmouth's diet (as much as 44% in April). Surface poppers tossed around gravel bars and rocks work wonders in very low, warm waters.

For floaters in spring, they access "more water and bigger fish," says Scott Cook of Fly and Field Outfitters in Bend. "You can also do well in summer, but access is tougher." If the river is dark, use a dark-colored fly or lure. "Darker is better than light or flashy," Cook says. "Fish are constantly looking up; their eyes are on top of their head." He recommends black Woolly Buggers and Purple Poppers (a fly that sits on top of the water, then pops as you move it, the fish are attracted to both sight and noise). "The fish really school up. If you catch one, there

Petroglyphs are rock carvings; the pictographs on the upper John Day run are painted on, while these are etchings. It took many a moon to scrape an intricate design into these hard rocks—do not add your name or deface the drawings in any way.

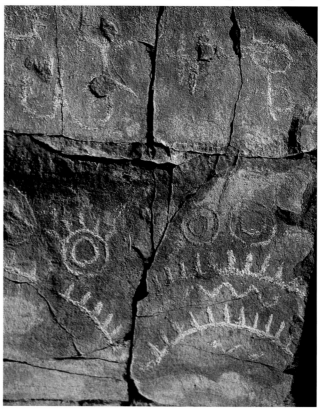

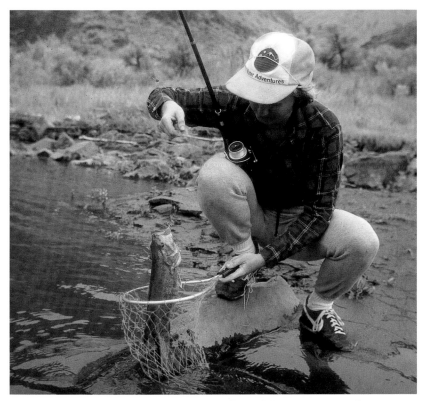

The author lands her first wild river smallmouth bass in Hoot Owl Canyon.

Lure selection depends heavily on four factors: water level, water temperature, clarity, and season. On average, for example, bass are eating 25% fish in the month of June, but no fish in April. The best month, statistically, for insect imitations is July, when 26% of their diet is bugs. This is also when the river is clear enough to begin serious fly-fishing.

Color is a matter of concern. At times, bass will take only black lures (a black, two-inch twin-tailed grub can work wonders when the mood is right). Guides have been known to carry Magic Markers to turn all lures black. Sometimes green is the magic color. Red and similar shades may appear crawfish-like to a bass. Once a hot lure is established, try to keep it out of the rocks!

Bass are the attention-getters these days, but the John Day also remains a stellar stream for salmonids. According to the ODFW, the John Day's wild run of spring chinook is the largest remaining in the Columbia Basin. Additionally, the steelhead population is one of the largest in the entire Columbia Basin.

The John Day boasts a great fall-winter steelhead run (September through April). Access by river floating after October may be difficult due to icebergs, below freezing temperatures, and other winter conditions in addition to low water (the John Day rises mainly from spring snowmelt, although fall rains and release of irrigation water causes some autumn rise).

John Day steelhead average four to six pounds. At the beginning of the fall run, fly-fish around Cottonwood Bridge with Purple Perils, Woollies and other traditional steelhead flies. (Remember this segment is difficult to access by boat, see end note.) In colder, murkier water, use drift techniques and don't be ashamed to use a night-crawler and Corky. They may move into the river as soon as mid-August.

Steelhead move into the main float-in section as January rolls around. They reach the Service Creek-Clarno section in February and March. Once warmer weather arrives, steelhead move up to the North Fork, where they can be fished for in optimum waters that occur around May, or in low-water conditions in summer. The John Day has no hatchery program—officially, most of the steelhead are wild, but a few hatchery specimens do sneak in from other river systems. Peak catches are in November. Salmon fishing is closed to protect remaining wild runs.

Trout are present in the river, as are channel catfish, which can be caught in deep pools near camps—great for youngsters and for the frying pan.

are 50 more. When they spawn in spring, they're really hungry."

Purple, black and blue colors, plus the Woolly Bugger, are also favored in off-colored water by other fly anglers. When the water clears, a rust or cinnamon brown offering will work.

Poppers on the surface will bring a bass blasting to the surface in hot pursuit. He uses grasshopper, cricket and other shoreline bug imitations.

"Those John Day bass aren't that picky," asserts Daniel Coleman of The Hook Fly Shop in Sunriver (a resort community south of Bend). He also recommends Woolly Buggers and poppers.

Always remember to fish all structure on the John Day below Kimberly: eddies behind rocks and boulders, cliff walls at water's edge, gravel bars, underwater ledges, backwaters around "islands" that have gone dry in one channel, bridge pillars, even ranching pipes. Work eddies that have grassy or brushy banks, as well, as bass wait here for bugs to come for dinner.

"John Day bass are pretty easy to take on the surface," asserts Craig Campbell of Bend's Fin 'n Feather shop. "Grasshoppers, Muddler Minnows—you don't need anything else." He suggested hitting a grassy bank with a bug imitation, then bouncing it into the river, mimicking the movement of a real bug. "All hell breaks loose. It's very easy to catch a hundred fish a day. Fish both banks. Put a crawdad (imitation) down deep, and they just smash it."

Upper John Day

Service Creek to Clarno

Location

North-central Oregon; From Interstate 84, go south from Arlington on Oregon Highway 19 through Fossil to Service Creek, or south from Biggs Junction on U. S. Highway 97 to Oregon Highway 206 to Condon and then south on Highway 19 to Service Creek. Or, from Prineville, east on Highway 26 and north on 207 to Service Creek. There are long stretches of highway, sometimes winding, slow roads, with few services.

Personality

Desert canyon, remote area with some ranches, limited public road access to inner canyon. The Big Bend canyon area is isolated and beautiful, with plentiful camps; great for photography and hiking. Painted-on Native American drawings known as pictographs are located at the end of the wild canyon section, which are very rare (paintings usually don't survive the test of time). Wildlife includes mule deer, coyote, birds of prey, great blue heron, antelope and chukar.

In early spring, waterfowl nest along the river; most often Canada geese, mallard and an occasional teal. Do not approach or disturb waterfowl in pairs, their nests, or their young (the parents may abandon their duties). Although nearby hillsides are famous for dinosaur fossil finds (and protected by National Monument status), few fossils are found along the river, although there is nice quartz near the pictographs, some agate and jasper.

Difficulty Class II+

Three rated rapids at optimum levels; all dump into cliff walls and require the ability to back ferry, some smaller rocky rapids rate as Class I+ or II depending on water levels. Major rapids may be lined or portaged. Many novices float this area. Landowners have challenged the navigability of the John Day, meaning that boaters must be careful to camp or stop only on public lands and avoid using private road access without permission.

Gradient

8-9 feet per mile

Mileage/Days

There are 3 trip options.

Service Creek to Clarno, 47 miles, 3-4+ days

This stretch is the most popular and includes three Class II+ rapids (Russo, Homestead, Burnt Ranch) plus some easier Class II rapids with rocks and shallows to dodge.

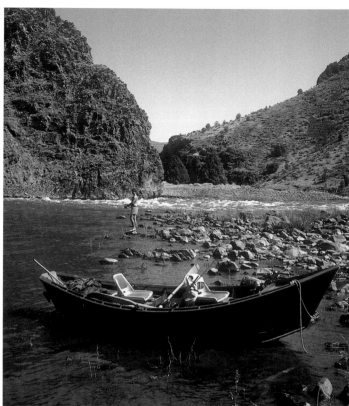

Driftboat at rest at the bottom of Homestead Rapid. This rapid is quite "sticky" beginning in mid to late June.

Twickenham to Clarno, 33 miles, 2+ days

A good option when water levels are lower, or to increase fishing/floating time further from civilization. Putting in below Service Creek avoids Russo, one of the Class II+ rapids.

In very low water, or for a quicker trip, put in 8 miles downstream of the Twickenham bridge at Priest Hole (a primitive BLM campsite/launch). Access downstream at Cherry Creek is limited due to private land. Access below Burnt Ranch Rapid is being developed by the BLM. A public access upstream of Clarno offers a takeout in low water to avoid drifting the very slow Clarno Pool.

Service Creek to Twickenham, 13 miles, 1+ days

Popular with anglers as a day trip, this run can be done as an overnight trip, good for greenhorns, with only one Class II+ rapid (and less isolation than the lower stretches).

Twickenham is a day-only access site surrounded by ranches; please respect their lands and do not camp, litter, build a fire or block roads. Have your vehicle shuttled promptly. For legal camping, a gravel road leads downstream eight miles to Priest Hole, on public lands, which also offers an alternate put-in. Camping is available at Service Creek and Shelton Wayside, but not at Clarno or the nearby John Day Fossil Beds National Monument. Motels are available in Fossil, Madras and the Columbia Gorge.

Craft

The upper John Day is Oregon's best wilderness canyon run for canoes, also good for driftboat novices. Even funky little craft such as discount-store rubber duckies thrive (although a flimsy vinyl inflatable should never travel solo, they just rip and tear too easily, leaving their occupant stranded in the middle of nowhere). Well-built rafts and catarafts can take any water levels. Paddle-cats, small catarafts and inflatable kayaks are popular craft for low water (driftboats and canoes will clang and bang at levels under 1,000 cfs).

Permits

Self-issuing at most put-ins. Note that fire season begins June 1 and lasts into October—no campfires or charcoal permitted.

Hazards

Two rapids rated Class II, one rapid rated Class II+; all three rapids have current pushing strongly into rock walls (use "face the danger" in an oar craft), rocks and gravel bars, shallow channels on sides of islands present at average levels, rattlesnakes in warm weather and ticks in early season, both found in brushy or grassy areas. Black widow spiders may be found in and around old buildings. Avoid camping near ranches or on private lands. Expect strong winds especially in afternoon; make your miles in the morning. Storms blow up fast; anchor tents and boats, carry rain gear and tarp/rain fly, warm clothes, stove wind shield. March through June, expect freezing temperatures at any time, in addition to storms. Always bring and use sunscreen, hat, coverups, socks: the sun is intense.

Old wagon wheels left behind after a movie was filmed in the John Day Canyon. Alas, the wood was so dry that a lightning strike nearby started a blaze that consumed all but the rims. The scenic background impressed Denver Dixon, a maker of Westerns, to film here in 1928.

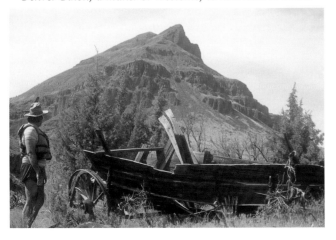

Average Float Levels/Seasons

Optimum flow for driftboats is 3-4,500 cfs. Average flow in spring is 2,000-6,000 cfs, occurring late April through early June. Gauge: Service Creek (River Forecast Center in Portland.)

High-Water Season

The John Day headwaters in mountains as high as 9,000 feet, so snow-fed runoff may happen anytime during warm or wet weather. A usual big water flow is 8,000-30,000+ cfs, usually March-April, although boaters could face a flow of 10,000+ cfs in May with heavy snowmelt and warm rain or very hot weather. In high water, the river is much faster and muddier, harder to read. In extreme conditions, boaters may have to duck or portage highway bridges. Beaches, islands and gravel bars are under water. Tie boats securely. The record high level occurred in January, 1964 (a notorious flood year) with a peak of 39,400 cfs.

Many rapids wash out, while others will grow bigger standing waves. The river is reasonably straight-forward at most higher levels once the rocks are covered. Rafts 14 feet and longer will have no problems, but those in canoes and driftboats should exercise caution, as empowered currents will exert more force than anticipated. In extreme conditions, watch for floating logs and other debris, as well as low bridges and power lines. The best advantage to high water is being able to make miles easily; doing the upper and lower river in three or four days becomes a sensible option, rather than an all-out push to make 40 miles a day with the wind against you.

Fishing in these flooded, silty waters is unpredictable. Smallmouth bass spawn late March-April and may strike aggressively. Bear in mind that during an ODFW study of bass eating habits in April, their stomachs contained 44% crawfish, but another 44% were empty! The rest of their diet was 12% unidentified, so keep trying different lures until you find one that works. Then don't lose it!

Fly fishing is all but impossible, and lures are seldom employed; crank baits, plastic baits with scent, and worms work best. Water may also turn murky after a thunderstorm anytime during the season, altering fish habits. Channel catfish can be caught under any conditions: use cheese or stinky baits, worms, chicken liver or fish guts.

Mid-February to mid-March is reputed to be a good time to catch both bass and salmonids, yet you may encounter wildly high water or push-and wade water, depending mostly on when the snowpack melts, and to a lesser extent, with the amount of rain (it is desert country, but warm rain in snowy mountains can trigger a tsunami towards your part of the canyon). Thunderstorms can also happen anytime during warm weather and may flood the main river or bring down mud from a side canyon. Remember that bass become inactive when the water temperature is below 40 degrees.

Low-Water Season

The John Day River is traditionally listed in guidebooks as "too low to float" below 1,000 cfs. Below 1,500 cfs more rocks begin to show, creating Class III conditions for hard boats and beginners. The main risk is spending all day dragging your boat through the water, which is exhausting and can be dangerous when you are wading in current with a heavy boat.

Extreme low water is 150 to 300 cfs; however, a good boater who can read water well will not spend as much time getting out to push, so the float season never really ends. There are almost always channels to follow, even in the skimpiest rapids, and the long deep pools remain unchanged.

At Homestead Rapid shallows, the best approach is to enter near midstream and then work left to avoid rock wall at bottom. Burnt Ranch Rapid becomes much more technical, worth a scout from the beach on river left. The route is usually down the middle at low water, with your entry depending on how much rock is exposed at the top; the cliff wall at the end is seldom troublesome in reduced current. There are about 20 places where the river separates into shallow and more shallow channels around islands and gravel bars. Choose wisely.

In low water, putting in at Twickenham instead of Service Creek gets you into the Big Bend canyon more easily. To avoid bumping through Homestead Rapid, launch further downstream at Priest Hole; consider taking out above the Clarno Bridge (Clarno East is BLM public access/camping about 4 miles before the bridge). From Cathedral Rock downstream to Clarno is almost all flat water and private land; with a headwind, it's a tough pull. Be sure your shuttle driver knows your takeout site, and that you know your takeout site, too.

Headwinds, slow currents and dragging craft over shallows can cause considerable delays; plan extra time to allow for these slow-downs.

Clear, almost blue waters make both fish and old farming equipment visible on the bottom of the river. I once scraped a foam-floored, self-bailing inflatable kayak over a sharp edge on a metal shard that appeared to be several inches below the surface at a water level of 290 cfs. (no damage to the tough Hypalon floor). The water becomes warm and having to walk your boat through a tricky stretch of rocks is not unpleasant in July or even October most years. The calm pools reflect spectacular rock formations just like a mirror, begging to be photographed in vertical format.

Fishing

Low water is a good time to fly-fish for smallmouth bass, and is also good for lures. Even a mouse pattern, tugged across the surface, will excite bass. Terrestrials include grasshoppers, dragon- and damselflies, and crickets. Attractive bass lures in low waters include traditional trout lures such as the Roostertail, minnow-imitators like

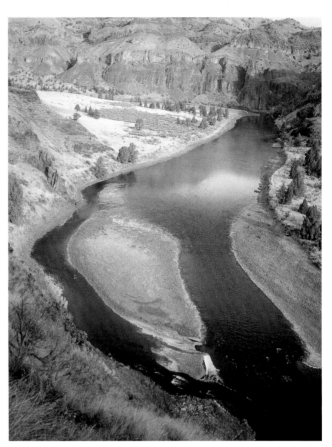

The river offers up an island here when water levels are optimum. Fish where the two currents rejoin at the tail end of the island. Also try tossing lures or flies in the slow, smaller channel.

the Rapala, and even steelhead spoons (Steelies). Poppers, buggers, and even some crappie lures work on bass here. Using Topwater WoodPlugs (Luhr-Jensen) on bass waters is often described as "addictive". Don't be afraid to experiment.

Fishing depends on water clarity, speed of current you're fishing, and depth of water. Big bass hide in shallow weed beds near grassy banks, often unseen and not fished out. They also are found in deep pools. Craig Campbell of Fin 'n Feather uses a crawdad to lure these giants. "They just smash it," he said.

The best steelheading is September through December, when water levels vary from low to flood stage, and peaks in February and March. Steelhead arrive in different areas at different times; news reports are useful. Watch for reports of fish moving above the Cottonwood Bridge. Although managed for wild steelhead, hatchery fin-clipped steelhead are often in the river. Hot Shots, plugs, Steelies and other spoons, plus bait such as nightcrawlers with Corkies are used. Both bank plunking and plugging from the boat are effective. When the water is clear and fish are active (mid to late fall), the old standbys of Purple Perils and Woolly Worms work for fly-anglers.

Managing Agency

Bureau of Land Management, 3050 NE 3rd St., Prineville OR 97754. Source for list of authorized outfitters, river maps (get one that shows private land), and current conditions (fire closures, mandatory equipment). Updates on shuttle drivers.

Shuttles/Services

Service Creek Store (541/468-3331; also rents cat-yaks a.k.a. "bi-yak", inflatable kayaks, rafts), basic services also.
Shamrock Shuttles (541/763-4896 or 763-2236).
J & Z Shuttle Service (541/468-2182 or 468-2447).
Donna's John Day River Shuttles (541/763-4884).

Most shuttles are based in Fossil. In Spray, call the Lone Elk Market (541/468-2443).

Nestled deep in ancient canyons of the John Day River, Service Creek Stage Stop is a travelers' oasis. With a key to the past, they offer rest for the weary traveler and a haven for the intrepid explorer. The house, once a 1920s boarding house, is located on twenty-six acres across Service Creek from the old livery barn. It is now a six-room, four-bath, bed and breakfast catering to individuals, families, and groups. The store, restaurant, and raft rental businesses are next door on the site of the original Service Creek post office. The store carries groceries, beverages, camping and fishing supplies, and rafting accessories. The restaurant features a full menu with hand-cut New York steaks, hamburgers, locally grown produce, homemade soups and desserts.

The raft-rental business provides you with a variety of watercraft for your adventures on the river. For your convenience, they will shuttle your vehicle from your put-in spot to your take-out destination. Guided fishing and eco-tour trips are also available. Email: oregonfishing @servicecreekstagestop.com

Trip Mileage And Landmarks

Mile 0: River mile 157. Service Creek Boat Ramp. New and improved ramp in what was formerly a rough gravel bar. Acceptable for camping the night before the trip. Services at nearby Service Creek Store.

Service Creek is the name of a post office near the junction of Service Creek and the John Day. Established on May 23, 1918, the post office was called Sarviscreek at first, then changed to Servicecreek on December 4, 1918. The name split to two words in 1929. (Service or sarvis berries are a bland berry growing on bushes, an important Native food used in pemmican.) By 1980, the post office was no longer operating.

The Service Creek Bridge, just downstream, has two pillars to avoid. The Service Creek Gauging Station is located just below the bridge. This is where readings of water levels are taken to be reported at the River Forecast Center in Portland, as well as various websites.

Salmon were once snared here in fish traps, outlawed in 1905 due to declining runs.

Shell Rock Mountain, named for ancient shell fossils, is the high peak on river left.

3.4: Old Peters place, homestead shack, river left. BLM public lands on both sides of the river for the next two miles.

6.7: Russo Rapid, Class II+: River mile 150. River dumps hard into left cliff wall, cheat to inside (river right) to avoid collision. There is a nice beach at the bottom of the rapid on river right. This is public land, although an occasional landowner puts up "No Trespassing"

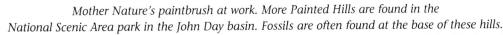

Mother Nature's paintbrush at work. More Painted Hills are found in the National Scenic Area park in the John Day basin. Fossils are often found at the base of these hills.

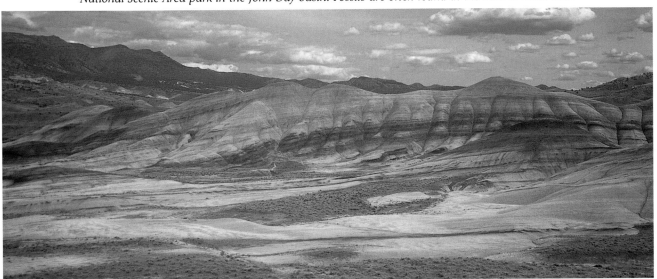

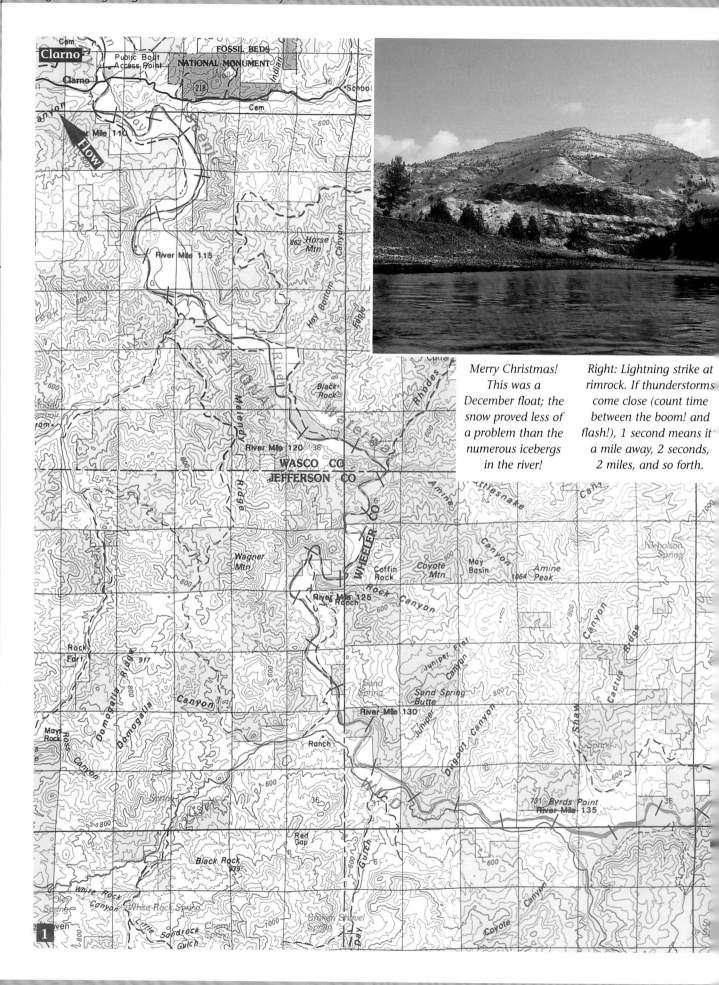

Merry Christmas! This was a December float; the snow proved less of a problem than the numerous icebergs in the river!

Right: Lightning strike at rimrock. If thunderstorms come close (count time between the boom! and flash!), 1 second means it a mile away, 2 seconds, 2 miles, and so forth.

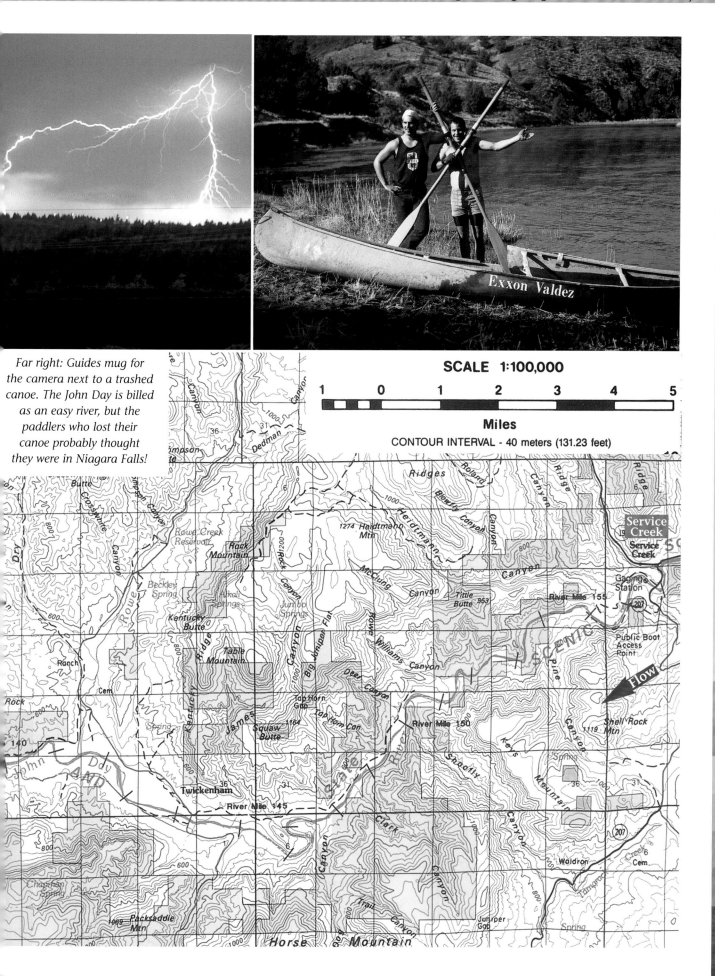

Far right: Guides mug for the camera next to a trashed canoe. The John Day is billed as an easy river, but the paddlers who lost their canoe probably thought they were in Niagara Falls!

SCALE 1:100,000

CONTOUR INTERVAL - 40 meters (131.23 feet)

John Day River Watersheds

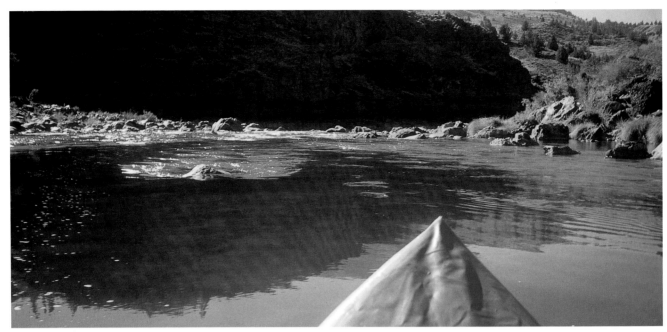

Facing Burnt Ranch Rapid, I point the bow of my inflatable kayak towards my destination (roughly river center) and begin windmilling the feathered blades.

signs to intimidate the public. "It's big country," explained one BLM official; "we take the signs down all the time, but they just pop up again." This rapid is also known as Shoofly after the creek and canyon entering on river left.

8.6: Tap Horn Canyon, named after an early settler, enters river right. There is a ranch on river right and minor rapids followed by an island. A small piece of public land is on river left, the last public land before Twickenham. A Class II rapid is followed by islands with multiple channels in low water.

11.6: Begin broad S-curve. Horse Mountain looms high on left hillside. The neck of land on your right as you loop the first curve is Goose Point. Private lands begin.

13.9: Twickenham, a tiny outpost of several ranches first established in 1896, is easily identified by its bridge over the John Day. Alternate launch/takeout site, river left. Private land extends for 3 miles on river right. This settlement was named after Twickenham, England; previous names were Contention as neighbors contended their own homestead rules, and Big Bottom, probably due to the large bowl shape of the canyon here rather than an obese pioneer.

"Twickenham the Beautiful" is a poem by E.R. Jackman, penned in 1957, intended to be serious, but inviting silly imitations. Instead of "The coyotes howl for Twickenham/the bobcats prowl in Twickenham" boaters come up with "There is no jam in Twickenham/you eat only Spam in Twickenham", and so forth.

Bear in mind that the Twickenham public access is granted by landowners, and abide by use restrictions. Camp downstream at Priest Hole or Homestead and not on the edge of farmlands. Fire is a serious concern for landowners, as well, so obey fire restrictions.

15.4: River bends to the right and then straightens. There is often a large island that forms here.

Public lands on river right for next five miles. Red Rock Mountain is high to the right. After 2 miles, public land is on river left for 3.6 miles.

18.8: Liberty Bottom on river right, thought to be named during Centennial year of 1876. Public lands begin on both sides of the river here, with several established camps, but the best sites are below the rapid.

19.7: Homestead Rapid, Class II+: Landmark: large bluff on river right extends down to river's edge. The current dumps into this bluff at the bottom. Cheat to river left. Entering the rapid at left center is best at optimum water levels. If in doubt, stop to scout. This rapid converts to a washboard at low water; most boats will hang up at the top or middle. When pushing, be ready to jump in fast as the current takes off quickly to crash against the rock wall at the end.

There are several good campsites on river left just below the rapid, and good fishing in the big eddy below this drop. Also a good swimming hole.

20.6: River bends sharp right. Painted Hills are visible high on river right. Black and gray colors are caused by a layer of volcanic ash, while red is tinted by iron oxide in the soil. The hills are sandwich-layered with ash, iron oxide, and clay from old sediment deposits.

Public lands continue on river right for approximately 1.7 miles.

19.7: Landmark: Bridge Creek enters, river left. This creek was spanned by a juniper log in 1862 by gold prospectors headed for Canyon City. A post office was run out of a ranch here from 1868-1882. Private lands for the next 2.2 miles on both banks.

20.3: River mile 135. Byrds Point, elevation 731 feet. Landmark: boulder in mid-channel.

The old homestead of Burnt Ranch is on river left, built about 1900. In 1865, the original ranch was ransacked and burned to the ground by Indians trying to drive off settlers.

Bits of the Old Dalles Military Road, built in 1868, remain in this area.

22.3: Landmarks for Burnt Ranch Rapid include a Class II riffle, a rock on river right.

23.0: Burnt Ranch Rapid: (Schuss Rapid), Class II+ to III. Large beach forms on river left at head of rapid, good camping. This is public land despite some landowners who try to chase campers off. There is a very large, strong river-wide eddy that slows boats down (also good catfishing). Scouting from river left is recommended. At higher levels, cheat the rapid by staying to the inside of the bend (right). The left current dumps into a bluff at the base of the rapid. In low water, pick your way through the center. Lining boats may be necessary, but you cannot line the entire rapid due to sheer walls on right at top and left at bottom. Boats can be waded through at very low waters if you are careful of the current and slippery rocks.

An access road and ramp below this rapid are under construction by the BLM; call the Prineville office for updates. Overall plans call for more public road access on the upper run, while maintaining the longer lower run as a more isolated section, with very little public access from shore or roads.

There are more Class I-II rapids below the main drop with little camping or public access for almost 2 miles.

25.8: Hungry Rock, named by author Arthur Campbell (*John Day River Drift and Historical Guide*). On river right, a large rock composed of conglomerate material appears to be grasping a small boulder (seen about half way up on the rock's left face). The rock-laden waters around this area are good producers of bass. Toss into the eddy water behind rocks and also the tailouts.

Cherry Creek, river left. Two islands form here at optimum river levels. The next 2 miles are private land.

28.3: As river swings left and then right in a gentle bend, Wagner Mountain (elevation 3,333') is seen high on the left. The Wagners settled the John Day area in the 1880s and used a private ferry to cross the river.

Watch high to the right for a large rock formation (2,000' elevation) flat on top, except for a "head" on the left and two "feet" on the right, creating the illusion of a giant rock person laying atop a coffin. This is Campbell's Coffin Rock and a landmark signaling the Big Bend canyon is close (excellent camping and spectacular scenery).

29.1: Enter a sharp loop to the right. This is the entrance to Big Bend Canyon. Immediately on the end of the loop is a large beach on river right which is good camping. The eddy here is good fishing and swimming.

30.3: River mile 125. The river straightens, then bends sharply first right and then left. There is a good camp on river left, the inside of the bend and a high bench site further downstream, also river right. Fishing around this bend and in any arms of the river is very good. There are several camps located on both sides of the river past the second bend.

The second bend, a tight "S" (or zigzag) sharply left, leads to a nice camp on river left, then the river drops into a Class II swirly eddy (more noticeable at low water) far left. As the river turns right and straightens again, there are numerous camps on left and right. A camp on river right with a large slab rock on the left bank is sometimes referred to as Whistling Bird Camp because this rock formation resembles the one found at the rapid on the lower Owyhee River.

31.3: River splits around large island. Good fishing and hiking in this area. This is one of the few islands on the John Day that actually has trees (junipers). The tail end has a landing spot with campsite.

Back on BLM lands, there is a large camp on river right past a twist in the river, then one small and one large on river right at the next right-hand bend. Hiking in this part of the canyon is excellent, with great views of the river and the photogenic Big Bend Canyon. Here the river winds nearly 2.4 miles with the many camps and interesting rock walls. If you got out at river mile 126 at the beginning of Big Bend and went straight as the crow flies, the distance to the end of this loop, at approximately river mile 124.4, would be only about 2/3 of a mile.

33.3: Three Canyons landmark. Amine, Rattlesnake and Rhodes canyons converge with the John Day here on river right (river mile 122, crossing from Jefferson County into Wasco County).

The river runs long, straight and slow at this point, good for trolling. The 3101' butte way up on river right is Sheep Mountain. For the next 2.76 miles, there is private land on both banks and minimal camping.

35.4: Black Rock can be seen high on river right. A sharp bend to the left marks the last large section of public land for camping before the takeout at Clarno, just over 9 miles downstream. There are three larger sites here. Clarno East (river mile 113.5) is the last possible camp before the takeout (and is also a boat ramp).

As the river curves to the right (north) again, there is a large columnar basalt formation on the left bank, an impressive solid rock cliff that extends down to the water's edge. This was named Cathedral Rock by Arthur Campbell, an appropriate title for the monolith, as it does inspire awe. The basalt columns formed from cooling lava twisted, so they are on a slant (most columnar basalt formations are so perfectly vertical that it seems they must have been chiseled by some mysterious ancient peoples).

Fishing around these cliff walls and nearby boulders in the river is excellent. The water is deep, even at 200 cfs, and harbors many large bass. Linger here as long as you can, for once this landmark rock is passed, the canyon opens up and ranch lands signal that civilization, and the end of your float fishing adventure, is all too near.

35.7: On river right, there is a ranch; just past this land is an overhang on the cliff wall. The underside is marked with centuries-old pictographs (Native American rock paintings; petroglyphs are carvings, not paintings). Look for the road that leads up a hill between two small bluffs. Land before this point. There is one landing at a rocky, gravely site with a crude trail up to the road; quartz rocks and crystals can be found along the trail. Other sites require more scrambling over boulders.

Beware of rattlesnakes; you may want to take a paddle or stick to thrust ahead of you into the brush. Once on the road, walk back upstream to the overhang. The pictographs are amazing mostly for their longevity (most pictographs are washed away after hundreds of years). The arid climate has helped to preserve these; also, the location under a protective rock overhang kept the paintings safe from rainstorms.

Treat this site with respect. The pictographs are very fragile. Do not touch them and most importantly, do not deface the wall or add your own drawings or initials. A flash camera (even a disposable one) or fast film (400-800 ASA) will make wonderful memories of this art without harming it. Red ochre or iron oxides were considered sacred by many ancient peoples and were used in the Old World as far back as 50,000 years. Red color represented blood, life and power.

This right side road parallels the river and connects to Highway 218 near the Clarno Bridge. The road is listed as open to the public.

38.7: Power lines cross the river, and Big Muddy Creek enters river left.

The Big Muddy Ranch was a large chunk of land, 100 square miles, that cut a swath from this bank of the upper John Day towards the towns of Antelope and Madras. In 1981, this remote cattle ranch was purchased for $6 million by a group from India planning to set up a commune in the remote outback of north-central Oregon. Their leader was Bhagwan Shree Rajneesh, and the quiet ranch became a bustling town, called Rajneeshpuram.

The Bhagwan was famous for cruising the open country roads in one of his many (up to 80!) Rolls Royces, soliciting followers from all over the world, who turned over their worldly goods to become followers of this charismatic guru. Members wore the "colors of the sunrise": orange, red and yellow. What began as a benevolent religious community quicky metamorphosed into a bizarre cult. The Bhagwan's aides carried assault rifles, bussed in homeless people to add to their voting population in the sparsely occupied Wasco County, plotted to kill the state's attorney general, then began the United State's first real encounter with germ warfare on home soil when they poisoned a salad bar in The Dalles with salmonella organisms.

Finally, the cult imploded, partly due to infighting among the people in power, mostly due to criminal investigations by law officials, that began with immigration laws and eventually revealed stockpiles of arms and cultures of germs, secret plots against the Bhagwan by insiders, and other plots against Oregon officials and townspeople. Top aide Ma Anand Sheila, among others, were found out, arrested, and deported. The Bhagwan died in India in 1990, years after his deportation.

Eventually, in 1998, the ranch was purchased by a billionaire who donated the land to Young Life, a non-denominational Christian ministry. The ranch is now Wildhorse Canyon, where up to 17,000 young people a year camp during desert retreat sessions.

The days of floating by 10-foot-high electric fences topped with barbed wire, patrolled by gun-toting, brightly-dressed fanatics (who were said to sometimes fire "warning shots" over the heads of passing floaters) are, fortunately, over for good.

After passing around an island (both sides are usually runnable, but in low water, use your river-reading skills to pick the deeper channel), caves are seen, high on river left. There will be a half-dozen islands (at optimum or low water) requiring good judgment to avoid dragging your boat.

39.5: Dry Creek, river left. House-sized boulder then appears on river left. Fishing around this boulder, especially in the quiet water behind it, is often good.

40.3: Irrigation equipment (pipes and pumps) on river left. High above this is a shallow cave, excellent for taking a photo from the interior with the river "framed" by the cave walls. Power lines cross the river. (Private land here meets BLM land past the river bend; please respect property rights and abide by any "keep out" signs.)

40.8: Power lines cross the river again and ranches begin to dominate the scenery as you approach Clarno. To your right is Iron Mountain, elevation 3995 feet.

Just past the steep face of this mountain, beyond a ranch on river right, is Clarno East, a tiny bit of public land, for landing a boat avoiding the rest of the Clarno Pool, and possible emergency camping (the only public site since Black Rock).

44.1: Power lines again cross the river. Pine Creek, river right, just beyond, was reportedly the site of a humongous flash flood in 1935, with waves cresting at 30 feet. No lives except cattle were lost, but buildings and fences were swept into the river. This site serves as a somber reminder that, although Oregon deserts flood far less often than those in the Southwest, even a tiny creek or dry riverbed demands respect, as does the power of fast-moving water.

43.7: The river takes a sharp bend to the right, then swings back left as Clarno, the takeout site, is under two miles away. Exploration for natural gas and oil was undertaken in the late 1920s but only small amounts were found and the drilling ceased.

The old Clarno school, built in 1913, sits on high ground, river left. The land is now private.

45.7: River mile 109 Clarno Bridge marks the takeout, located just below the bridge on river right. The takeout has recently been improved, with a wider ramp replacing the scramble through bushes that was often enlivened by rattlesnake encounters. (A 5-foot-long Great Basin rattlesnake was seen here in 2001.)

Clarno, which is just a bridge with several ranches, was named for pioneer homesteader Andrew Clarno. There was a post office established in 1894 (many small towns were named and established only upon the arrival of the post office; even the closure of most of them doesn't change the history). A hotel and ferry boat crossing were also present in the old days.

According to *Oregon Geographic Names* (by Lewis A. McArthur), Clarno discovered that a friend moved in about 20 miles east, near the present town of Fossil. Supposedly, Clarno rode the 20 miles over on horseback and said, "Bill, don't you think you're crowding me a little?"

Lower John Day River

Clarno to Cottonwood

Location
To reach from the west, take Highway 97 (north of Madras) to cutoff at Highway 218, follow this curving road to Clarno. Or approach from Interstate 84, south from Biggs Junction and Wasco on Highway 97 to Shaniko, then south on 218 to Antelope and east on 218 to Clarno. Or take Highway 19 south from Arlington off I-84, through Condon, then west on 218 to reach Clarno. From Prineville, head east on Highway 26 to Mitchell, then north on 207 to junction with 218, finally west to Clarno.

Personality
Desert canyon, very remote area with few ranches, extremely limited public road access to inner canyon. The two main entry roads, Butte Creek and 30-Mile, are closed to public use (although Butte Creek can be

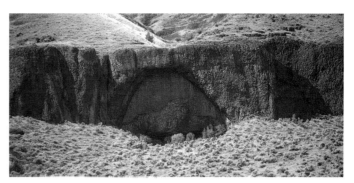

Basalt arch, located high on the hills near the Great Basalt Canyon.

accessed by licensed John Day River outfitters for a fee). The Great Basalt Canyon and Hoot Owl Rock areas are isolated and spectacular, with plentiful camps; great for fishing and exploring. This section of the river curves in great loops such as Horseshoe Bend, the Gooseneck, and The Narrows. There are petroglyphs (carved Native American symbols) at Potlatch Canyon. Photography subjects are endless.

Wildlife is the same as the upper river, except that bighorn sheep have been re-introduced. They are often seen on cliff walls near the river, especially in October. Many geese rest in this canyon, as well, and you might even spot some seagulls. Fishing is even better than the upper section, with more and bigger fish, as the ODFW-BLMs to continue to limit public access while improving the river's status as a trophy smallmouth bass fishery.

Difficulty
Class II+ overall, with Basalt Rapids II+ to III, Clarno Rapid Class III to IV, and several Class IIs plus occasional rocks to dodge, boulders in river, side channels that run dry. This run is considered more difficult for canoes and small craft because of faster current, more and larger rocks in the channels, and greater isolation.

Again, avoid private lands; most of the lower river bank is public land except for the last three miles. Most roads are private.

Gradient
11 feet per mile.

Mileage/Days
Clarno to Cottonwood, 69 miles, 4-7+ days

Average Float Levels/Seasons
Optimum floating conditions occur at 2,000 c.f.s. to 6,000 cfs in April and May, sometimes early June.

High-Water Season
Late November through April. In early spring, the river can approach 30,000 cfs. With a big snowpack and warm weather bringing it down quickly, water levels can rise to 10,000 cfs very quickly. Clarno Rapid's secret is big boul-

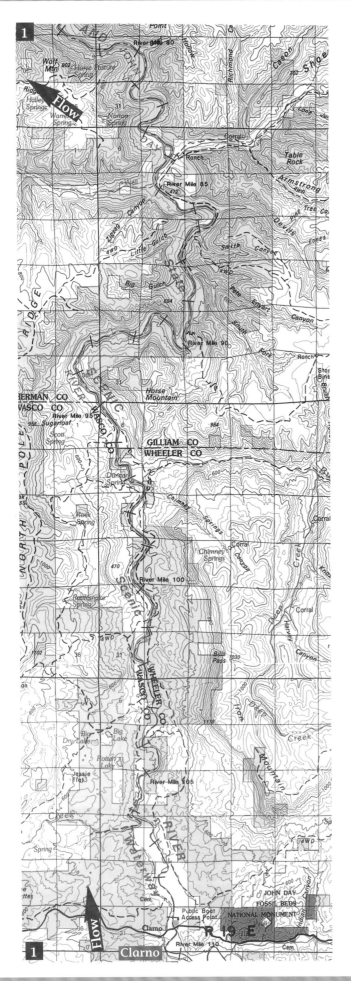

ders hidden in the river bed, which at high water create large reversals and waves, especially in the second drop. The water will be very murky and fast-moving. Canoes and driftboats will probably want to line lower Clarno, and use caution around the Basalt Rapids. Class II waves may appear in places where rapids don't usually form. The greater speed in high water allows for a faster trip. Fishing is variable; with the water cold and murky, bass usually respond to crankbaits and worms.

Low-Water Season

Below 1,000 cfs, Clarno Rapid is very rocky, easily a Class IV. There are big boulders in mid-stream with a tight slot between them that a very skilled boater can make. Beginners should not attempt this run. The upper Clarno and "around the bend" third drop are also very rocky but mostly just make your boat get stuck. Lining your boat past trouble spots is possible; wear your life vest and use caution around ropes and slippery rocks.

There are many dead-end side channels; in areas where the John Day was one wide channel at optimum flows, the river may morph into four channels and you have to take an educated guess as to which route is best, or do a lot of jumping out of the boat to scout ahead. I have run this stretch at 290 cfs in a 12-foot cataraft with little difficulty, but you do need a tough boat as there will be plenty of scraping over shallows and bumping of rocks. Some guides wrench a 16-foot cargo raft down-stream at these lower levels (putting in on private lands to avoid Clarno Rapid); this is sheer determination and not even crowbars and Vaseline could make it easier.

As with the upper river, the chief reason people float in very low waters—from late June to October in an average year—is for the incredibly hot smallmouth bass fishing. There are few boaters, if any, so solitude offers another argument in favor of this low-water insanity. Throw in hunting season for chukar, mule deer and bighorn sheep (once in a lifetime for Oregon hunts), and you can do a "cast and blast" trip. Follow the tips given in the upper John Day description, above, for reading low water flows.

Craft

All craft float this stretch, but canoeists should be experts and travel in groups. Driftboats may have trouble at Clarno (any water level) and Basalt Rapids. Rafts over 14 feet and catarafts can take any higher flows. Small boats such as inflatable kayaks, Cat-yaks and rafts 13 feet and shorter can handle most conditions at average or low water levels, but should avoid high water trips (or have an escort boat, with small-boaters dressed for a dunking in cold water).

Permits

Self-issuing at most put-ins; required for commercial boaters. Note that fire season begins June 1 and lasts into October.

Hazards

Clarno Rapid is rated as Class III in optimum conditions; as Class IV, especially the second drop, in low or high water. Canoes and driftboats should consider lining the second drop; scout from high on the left, and look at both drops before making a decision.

The Great Basalt Rapids are Class II+, with occasional side channels and rock dodging beyond them to keep things interesting for most of the float. The gradient is faster than the upper section, meaning that obstacles come at you faster, so you have less time to react. Parties in inferior craft such as folding kayaks have had to beg a ride out of the canyon from ranchers, once their boats are torn by unexpected rocks or gravel bars.

Rattlesnakes, ticks, and black widow spiders are also found here. A Great Basin rattlesnake about five feet long and very aggressive has been seen at the Clarno launch site, but most rattlesnakes are smaller and more timid.

As with the upper run, weather is unpredictable. Prepare for heat and cold, wind blowing upstream, water levels rising quickly overnight, thunder or wind storms launching your tent or boat into orbit, and so forth. Bear in mind the remoteness of this canyon. Be prepared to take care of your own emergencies.

Fishing

This is a fantastic smallmouth bass fishery, with catches in the state record books—6- to 8-pound fish are in the river, but are crafty. Lots of action with occasional double fish (two bass on one treble hook, or two bass landed to the same boat at the same time). The lower section seems to produce bigger bass. Hoot Owl Canyon is particularly productive. Both sections of the John Day are good for bass fishing from March through the end of October. Fishing gear and technique are similar to the upper run.

The John Day also boasts a great fall-winter steelhead run. Access by river floating may be difficult due to icebergs, below freezing temperatures, and other winter conditions.

Trout are present in the river, as are channel catfish, which can be caught in deep pools near camps and are great for youngsters.

Managing Agency

Bureau of Land Management, 3050 NE 3rd St., Prineville OR 97754. Source for list of authorized outfitters, river maps (get one that shows private land), and current conditions (fire closures).

Shuttles/Services

Service Creek Store (541/468-3331; also rents

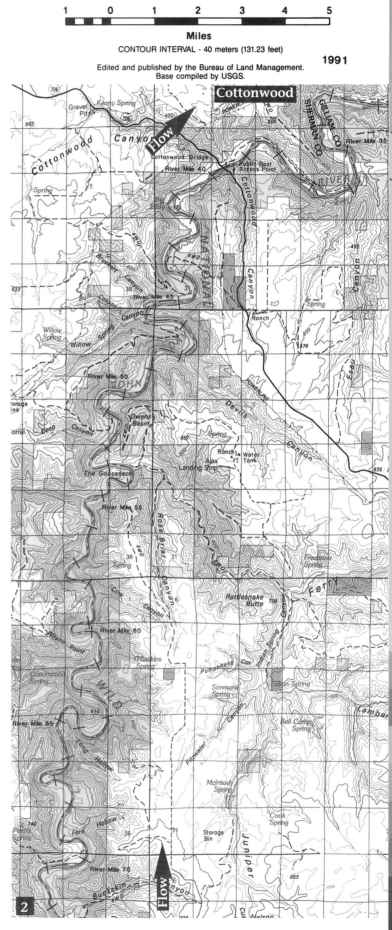

SCALE 1:100,000

Miles

CONTOUR INTERVAL - 40 meters (131.23 feet)

1991

Edited and published by the Bureau of Land Management. Base compiled by USGS.

Cat-yaks, inflatable kayaks), sells gear and supplies.
Shamrock Shuttles 541/763-4896 or 763-2236).
J & Z Shuttle Service (541/468-2182 or 468-2447).
Donna's John Day River Shuttles (541/763-4884).
Most are based in Fossil.

Mileage and Landmark Log

0: River mile 109. Clarno bridge. The steamboat *John Day Queen* sank here.

0.9: The original Andrew Clarno Ranch, river left, near the old Clarno Schoolhouse.

2.5: Large island, once covered by willow trees, is now mostly open. Buildings are below island, river right.

3.8: Island at low water. Rocky shoals and channel picking required.

4.7: Sorefoot Canyon, river left. Site of original school, the Rose Briar School built around 1870.

4.8: Red bluffs, colored by iron oxides, and painted hills formations with some green (mostly from copper).

5.1: Small riffle.

5.6: Clarno Rapid: Class III to IV. Clarno forms around a right turn, dropping in a pair (sometimes a trio) of rapids, both with islands, lots of rocks, and waves. In high water, reversals form, so you may want to cheat on the inside. In very low water, the channel appears blocked until a careful study is conducted. Dead center offers a good line to follow, but you must be ready to pivot and get the right angle, then pull away from the boulders. Scouting from the easy trail high above the river is highly recommended. Many canoes trash here; many more choose to line (lead the boat with two ropes, one person pulling it along, the other feeding out line and keeping its stern straight.)

Be sure to look at all drops. Some boaters see only one big rapid and forget about others. These are shallow and rocky when the river is low. Numerous sleeper rocks lurk just under the surface. The greatest danger, though, is the big drop with strong hydraulics at high water, and big boulders in midstream during minimal levels. The two smaller rapids have only sleepers, no giant boulders in the current, so the technique of deliberately grounding your boat may be used to slow your speed in the current. Most boats slip off with a bit of wiggling or weight shifting.

Many homesteaders flocked to the John Day region during the 1850-1940 years. Farquer McRay built a a six-bedroom house in this region during 1876 (a very large house for those times).

Some of the best fishing for wild steelhead is encountered below Clarno Rapid early in the season. Clarno can swell to an amazing 30-foot drop in very high flows, which the steelhead nevertheless manage to swim through on their way to spawning beds on tributary creeks, such as those off the North Fork of the John Day.

6.7: Mulberry Camp, river right. Parts from pioneer days linger here; some believe this was McRay's first home-site before a flood destroyed it in 1894. Take a walking tour of the old orchard here: walnut, peach, plum and mulberry trees announce that humans once lived here. Last camping for over six miles.

Several sets of riffles, rocks in the river, and narrow channels plague low-water boaters during the next 3 miles.

8.3: Power lines cross the river as it begins a right turn with several islands. Channels are tight and rocky at low waters.

8.8: Old Bill's homestead site, circa 1889, river left. Believed to be the spot he picked to rebuild after losing his original homestead to the flood.

9.5: Yet another McRay place, remodeled several times since 1890.

Power lines cross the river. The river bends left, then meanders back around a soft right turn. Two islands in midstream force low-water channels to change, while a third arrives as the river resumes its northward passage. These islands are tricky at low water. At higher water levels, they disappear.

Another version of the McRay place was built on river left, in 1900. Many of these historical sites are being damaged by winter storms after surviving for centuries. We can only hope that the BLM will allow volunteers to reconstruct these places of interest for future generations to enjoy. (Don't forget to be watchful for rattlesnakes and black widow spiders around old buildings.)

11.5: Power lines cross the river again.

12.2: River mile 97. Butte Creek enters, right bank. This road is through private land. So far, the people who own Stanley Ranch property are allowing only authorized John Day outfitters on the road for boat launching. This is a good time saver, as well as making trips safer in low water (no dodging the bullet in Clarno Rapid!). The Stanleys also charge a fee of about $50 per client for this service.

Butte Creek is a major tributary on the lower John Day, flowing through a steep canyon. At 2,947 feet, Horse Mountain towers over the creek's mouth, its volcanic base straddling four counties: Sherman, Wasco, Gilliam and Wheeler.

14.5: Large island at lower water levels; old buildings on river right.

16.8: Three Rocks. As you pass another island (low waters split the already-thin current into smaller threads), you begin to enter the Great Basalt Canyon, an enormous cliff wall of red-tinted basalt rock. These walls are up to 2,000 feet high. This is one of the most spectacular vistas in the lower canyon. Fishing here, around the rocks, shoals and weeds, is often good. There are eight beautiful camps in two miles of river,

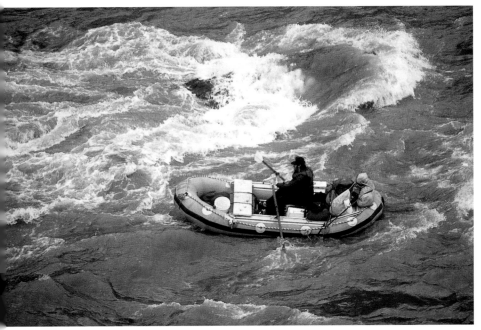

Maneuvering in Clarno Rapid at high water (over 12,000 cfs). Note the large reversal combined with a boulder located right side of the raft.

but right at the base of the left-sided red walls is the most spectacular, a sandy spot on river right.

Beaches abound for easy camp setup and for walking barefoot to the bank for a swim. Rest up for the next set of rapids in the morning.

18.5: This is mostly sagebrush country, but on this isolated island, sizeable trees have taken root. The tail end has a good landing area. The right-side channel often dries up in low water, creating a "side arm" extension of the river that teems with bass, dragonflies, water boatman bugs and other aquatic life.

Red Wall Camp is just past the island on river right, a good beach (until winter floods wash it away), plus a sagebrush flat to spread out a group.

19.2: The river swings wide around to the right, then begins a hairpin turn back left. As you enter this turn, look up high on river right to view the Arch Rocks (volcanic rock curved into graceful arches). Here the John Day twists into a "U" turn.

20.8: Islands that can be tricky at most water levels; they lead into the **Basalt Rapids (Class II+)**. These are followed by an island shaped like a diamond which is flat and mostly gravel. High water wipes these islands off the map. Several canoes have "crashed and burned" in this drop, so use caution.

21: River mile 88. Once the river is back on its due north path, watch for Big Gulch, river left, with small islands once again dividing the flow of the river into narrow channels.

24: Another U-bend to the right, with Devil's Canyon entering at the curved "tip" of the U. As you come back out of the loop heading northwest, there is the Lazy

Rock (it leans over) on river right. Several boulders in the channel and wind often make this passage difficult. A U.S. Geological Survey plaque is on the right bank.

25.7: Zigzag Canyon, river left. The large ridge above it is called North Pole Ridge. Local legend states that a Scottish sheepherder named Finlayson compared the weather in winter here to the North Pole.

25.8: Pipeline, built in 1963, crosses the river. It transports natural gas.

26.7: River mile 84. Major landmark, 30 Mile Creek, river right. The channel here is clogged with islands, gravel bars, rocks and shallows during the low-flow season; usually the right channel is best. The name may derive from early settlers' beliefs that the creek's headwaters are about 30 miles from its confluence with the John Day. There are ranch houses visible on river right.

A private road enters here, but in an emergency, the ranchers may be able to evacuate you.

32.7: River turns left in another U-turn. On river left, an impressive example of columnar basalt forms a large wall straight down to the water's edge. On river right is a large flat suitable for camping. Indeed, the next seven miles are all BLM property. If you poke around on the camping flat, you will see a tiny sheepherder's cabin, which was used from 1899 or so up until 1926.

A large eddy invites swimmers, plus both bass and catfish can be caught here.

33: The river abruptly widens, with another big eddy on river right. Cliff walls reach to the water's edge and below, river right, providing the structure that smallmouth bass prefer to hang out in. Land below this barrier to view the remains of covered wagons (mostly metal rims as this area was struck by lightning, igniting the decades-old dry wood).

In 1928, director Denver Dixon filmed parts of his movie, "The Old Oregon Trail", in this area, leaving the wagon wheels behind. In the movie, three cowboys rescue a wagon train from Indians.

Bear in mind that any item of historical interest (over 50 years old) is considered an artifact by the BLM, part of the public trust. Removing artifacts from their natural environment is illegal, besides being unethical. Thieves don't care about the next floaters who enjoy seeing artifacts in their native environment. (However, your discarded cans and bottles will never be considered artifacts, so take only pictures; leave only footprints.)

John Day River Watersheds

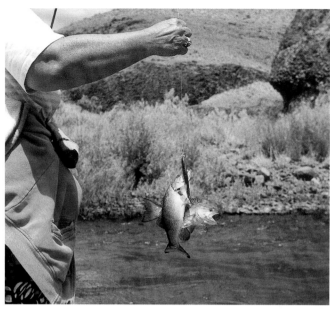

Two small bass fight over one lure.

Usually the better current is far left, and rowing upstream at an angle to cross the wide eddy is necessary. Once you are safely in the main current again, the river snakes right and then left through Horseshoe Bend.

Only 100 yards separates the "Saddle" between the narrow tip of this striking U-bend. Bluffs on both sides of the river range from 1,000 to 2,400 feet high. Most boats take 40 minutes to float what would be a 15-minute dash across the Saddle. As you emerge from the Horseshoe, several islands split the channels; usually the right is deeper.

37.5: Potlatch Canyon, river right. After the river completes its course through Horseshoe Canyon, an SUV road can be seen on river right, at the base of a cliff. Land in the big, slow eddy and walk up to the road, where you will see an overhanging cliff. There are prehistoric Native American petroglyphs—rock carvings—chipped into the basalt walls. One carving resembles a bug with antennae.

Native Americans consider such sites sacred, as do historians. Remember it's illegal as well as uncouth to add your own drawings or try to chip the designs loose as a trophy. Rubbings, once a common way of taking a memory of petroglyph home, have fallen into disfavor since some tourists abuse the process, leaving chalk marks behind, or by having their preservation spray blown to the side of their rubbing paper, which leaves an indelible mark behind.

In the Northwest, the potlatch was an important ceremony, especially with coastal and large-river tribes. With a rich abundance of game, migratory fish such as salmon, berries and roots to gather, the potlatch became more than just a feast, it was an opportunity to show off the wealth of the hosting tribe. More than food was exchanged: beads, mother-of-pearl from shells, "ivory" from antlers and horns, carefully crafted flint tools and arrowheads, buckskins soft as chamois; many things had value.

37.9: Buckskin Canyon, river right. Only about 1 mile on either side of the river here is public land. Sandy beaches in the area make good low-impact camps.

Several springs on river left provide safe drinking water, if they can be reached safely by your group. Be sure to collect from the spring's source rather than its flow; open waters are often contaminated by roaming cattle. Penny Spring is located off a rough SUV path on river left, which can be accessed just past a right turn, before the river completes another U-bend, or from the overgrown trail at the "bottom" of the U. Penny is about a mile uphill. A hike could be continued to the top of the canyon, Adobe Point.

40.3: A large island divides the river (watch for shallow channels in low water). Right after you pass the island is Cave Bluff, located river right, where you can paddle underneath the cliff wall into a small cave. At lower water levels, there is a little beach at the back of the cave. During one trip, I surprised a family of beaver here. River otter and Canada geese also use this cave for shelter, so do not linger very long. Photographs taken from inside, using the opening of the cave to frame the shot, provide an unusual souvenir of your trip.

44: Fern Hollow, river right.

42.8: Several islands. In low water, these impede progress by creating a maze of channels, almost like the braided channels found in glacial rivers of Alaska and Canada. Campbell terms the steep rock formation ahead on river right Stair Step Palisades due to ridges that resemble stairs.

43.6: U-bend begins, first left and then right. As you start out of the U, there is a large island, again troublesome in low water (the left channel usually has more water). This island has a higher elevation than most other John Day islands, safe for camping except during extremely high water levels. Fishing around the island structure is productive for bass. Camping beaches and benches on river right as well.

45: A Class II rapid leads into a false island on river left. This island's left channel may be dry except in high water. Now the river completes another horseshoe bend, passing the small canyons of Pearson and Shell Rock, both on river right.

48.3: Jack Knife Canyon enters on river left. This is a green canyon with lots of plants thriving. The peak ahead on river left is Wilson Point, while downstream and higher up on river right is Rattlesnake Butte. (One autumn day in the late 1860s, Z. Donnell lost his jack knife near this canyon. He found the knife the following spring and named the canyon after his good fortune.)

49: Large boulders are scattered across the river here, creating tight spots during low-water drifts.

The next bend is very constricted, creating a rectangular shape as as the river bends back on itself amid a perpendicular canyon.

Campbell's Hoot Owl Rock is on river right as you enter the bend, with his Citadel Rock at the tip of the U. There are several nice camps here, plus excellent bass fishing. In the flats, chukar, doves and quail make their presence known with distinctive clucks or cooing noises.

Here, the author encountered a large, 20+-pound porcupine that had been chased up a juniper tree by her 90-pound Rottweiler. The porky would have won that battle, most likely, by stabbing barbed quills into the dog's sensitive muzzle. Quills must be plucked quickly (use pliers) or they will work deeper into a dog's skin and become infected.

51.1: River mile 68. Cow Canyon, river right.

51.2: Lon Eakin Flat, river left. Named for a 1900s pioneer. A long island in the channel may be challenging as the river level drops. Stay alert.

This was sheepherder country in the 1860s to the 1940s. The shepherd's lot was a rough one, although many enjoyed the peaceful solitude, spectacular scenery, and independence that herding sheep brought. Campbell quotes a poem from shepherd Diego Varanus:

"On John Day breaks so high and steep
Full many a day I've herded sheep;
I've herded sheep upon those breaks
And killed the lively rattlesnakes...
If I can make enough in time
To take me out of this cold clime;
You bet your life I'll stomp away
From Oregon and the John Day."

I wonder what Veranos would have thought about modern adventure travelers who float this canyon for fun and fish. Maybe he wouldn't have been so eager to ditch the John Day for "warmer climates far away" if only he'd learned to fly-fish!

53.2: River mile 54.53. Little Ferry Canyon, river left. Two low islands are just downstream. Watch for dead channels in low water.

55.8: Entering the Gooseneck, a tight bend to the right, then abruptly left.

56.5: Here you are at the "bottom" of this U-shape, where Ferry Canyon enters on river right (it's actually due east right as the river begins to bend back west into yet another bend).

Ferry Canyon was named for an old ferry boat that carried men, horses and their goods across the John Day. By using the power of the river current, ferry operators were able to move the boat without artificial power—instead, they used cables.

The ferry boat was hooked onto the cable, then the

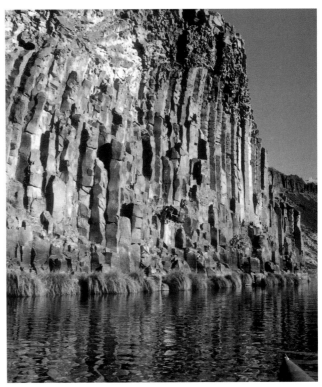

Great columns of basalt reflect upon a good bass area. Structure to hide in, a grassy area where bugs fall in the river, what more does a bass need?

river current slid the boat across the river. The action of "ferrying" a boat across a river is still used in modern whitewater terminology for maneuvering a boat at an angle across the current, using the power of the current to help move the boat.

Remains of the ferry boat operation can be seen in this area. The canyon was first occupied by three brothers named Owens. The remains of George's place are up the canyon along with a stone corral. A rough track leads to the site of Bert Owen's residence high on the hillside, near a spring. Charlie lived just downstream of Ferry Canyon's mouth, on river right. The open space here is named Owens Basin.

Campbell describes an amusing anecdote when Charlie Owens had guests, who noticed his slovenly housekeeping. Before sampling his meal, they asked if the plates were clean. Charlie replied the plates were "as clean as soap and water could get them." At the end of the meal, Charlie put his plate on the floor and yelled "Soap n' Water!" His old hound dog came running to the table, promptly licking the plate clean. This was the first automatic dishwasher in Central Oregon!

60.8: Four or more islands clog the river here, depending on water levels. This spot is a labyrinth of confusing channels at very low water levels. Fishing below islands is usually good.

61.4: Island, watch for shallow channels at less than optimum flows. The river begins a leisurely bend to the right, then wanders back left.

62.8: Site of Charles McCaleb cabin, river left; Devil's Canyon comes in on river right. McCaleb went missing after a goose hunt and his clothes were found on the bank, but there was no body. He was presumed drowned in 1904, according to Anderson.

62.5: At the bottom of this U are two or more islands, with the center channel usually best. Red hills are on right, on river left you can make out a faint road track that is the Taylor Pack Grade. Ravines were filled in to allow for passage of a wagon and team of horses.

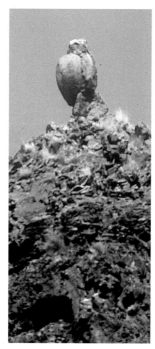

The "Hoot Owl" at dusk looks remarkably like a real owl.

This spot, with a landmark of Willow Spring Canyon coming into the John Day at the U bend of the next loop, is about 7 miles from Cottonwood; private lands begin to emerge along the river, making campsites more difficult to find.

64.6: Multiple islands, including one large island that may be a peninsula in low water. From here power lines are visible high on river left, signaling that civilization is not far. Bruckett Canyon joins on river left at the bottom of the large island.

65.8: Ruggles Pack Grade, a jeep trail, enters the canyon on the peninsula of land at the next U-bend to the right. The land from the big island, around this bend and to River Mile 43, on both river banks is BLM/public. BLM land is on the left a little further, the last two campsites, which are beaches at some levels (and also depending on whether spring floods bring or take sand).

68: River mile 41. Big Eddy. Avoid it unless you like merry-go-rounds. A large island splits the river, but a side channel often runs dry at low water. Sometimes a much smaller island forms just below the big one.

70.6: Cottonwood Bridge and Highway 206 span the river; Cottonwood Canyon enters on river left. This canyon was named for the ubitquois cottonwood trees that live mostly along rivers—even desert rivers—and dump fluff on boaters during early spring. These trees have a distinctive aroma when in bloom that seems to whisper "Spring's here!" into your ear.

The takeout is on river right, a public boat landing with outhouse and information signs.

Can I Continue To Float Downstream To The Columbia?

I have never attempted this segment of the John Day as the river continues its ponderous journey to empty into the mighty Columbia. This stretch is seldom run, for many reasons.

First, there is a mandatory portage at Tumwater Falls and possibly the Narrows. Much of the land is private, so camping and portaging are illegal along most of the river banks. The wind seems to blow harder in this segment, which is just short of 40 miles (hard to do on a day trip, especially when fishing).

The first 22 miles are reportedly mostly Class I-II without much current (at lower water levels). This upper segment is sometimes floated during steelhead season, with take-out access at Klondike-John Day River Road (off Highway 206, Grass Valley), or Rock Creek Road/Hay Canyon Road on river right (east bank). Check with Prineville BLM to confirm public entry.

The next section, about 7 miles, begins to pick up speed. There are numerous boulder gardens at lower levels, potential hydraulics at high water. When the John Day's repeated loops stop, Tumwater Falls is near.

Tumwater Falls and the Narrows are at River Mile 10.2 to 9.8. These may be rated up to Class IV-V depending on your craft and skill, plus the water level. Always scout first. Cliffs block river right, a rocky island guards the middle, and some rock faces are on river left, making portaging/lining more difficult. There is a portage path on river right, but bear in mind the BLM map depicts all private property.

Also, the last 9.8 miles are "Lake Umatilla", better known as the John Day Pool, slackwater backed up from the dammed Columbia. Motorboaters use this dead section of the John Day for accessing smallmouth, steelhead, salmon, shad and even squawfish (or, to be politically correct, the northern pike minnow), which ODFW pays a bounty on, as these trash fish feed on young salmon and steelhead smolts. Most powerboaters have no clue that an extensive, mostly wilderness canyon exists further upstream. A park near I-84 and the mouth of the John Day allows for boat launching, and there is a park upstream on "river" right.

There is some argument that one is not trespassing when using a portage trail, as these were usually established before statehood, and also that all river bars, beaches and other features below the high-water line are open to the public, as according to the Oregon Constitution, all waters belong to the public. Additionally, another point of contention is the issue of whether the John Day River constitutes a "navigable" river. State law defines this as a river with "commerce", which originally meant the transportation of logs, the use of boats to move people and gear, ferries, etc. In modern times, many argue that the floating of the John Day by commercial outfitters constitutes "commerce" and thus confers navigability status to the river. In any case, you should submit a letter to the State Marine Board urging them to formally name the John Day a navigable river, which leaves it open for float fishing.

North Fork John Day River

Probably the least-floated multi-day-trip river in Oregon, the 112 miles of the North Fork of the John Day joins the main stem at Monument, opening possibilities to float hundreds of miles in spring, beginning high in the thick-forested Blue Mountains at Dale and finishing in open desert at either Cottonwood Bridge or the Columbia itself.

Although seen as a minor fork of the larger main stem, the North Fork actually carries twice the water of the John Day, with an annual discharge of 892,600 cfs at Monument. This includes the North Fork, the Middle Fork, Wall Creek, and many other tributaries from the high country that furnish important water resources for spawning fish, in addition to irrigation of crop lands.

The North Fork John Day Wilderness is located above the traditional float starting point at Dale, and that upper portion is considered unnavigable (low water, boulders, no way to get to a put-in site due to roadless wilderness). However, the float beyond the Wilderness Area is mostly wild and primitive, marred only by a few rough roads and some ranches. The river above Dale was once an old placer mining area and has been explored recently by kayakers looking for a new experience, but few other boaters or anglers venture above Dale.

Additionally, the river corridor and surrounding country provide a major migration route for Rocky Mountain elk, mule deer, and other big game. Cougar, bobcat, coyote, and black bear follow the game trails, too. Birds of prey are commonly seen soaring above the river canyon.

In early times, Umatilla Indians used the region for hunting and fishing, digging roots and berry picking. The Gold Rush of the 1860s brought miners into the remote canyons in search of riches. Evidence of their presence—old cabins, mines, implements, etc.—still exists. Modern river travelers take a detour to Ritter, where a nice hot-spring resort awaits.

Dale (Camas Creek) to Monument or Kimberly

Monument was named for a nearby rock formation that resembles a pulpit. The Kimberlys were a pioneer family homesteading in that area.

A shorter, easier run can be made from Wall Creek to Monument (6 miles, 1 day) or from Monument to Kimberly (15 miles, 1-2 days). These are good options for novices, and for winter steelheading in less-remote condi-

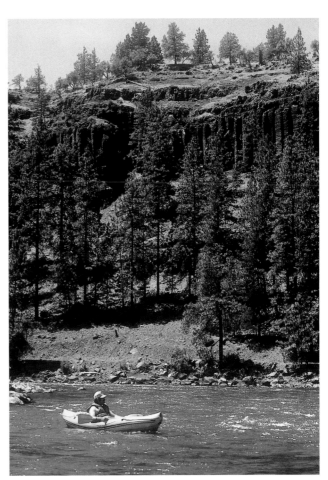

Running current, Class I rapids, in an inexpensive inflatable kayak.

tions. Fly-fishing here is good, as well, in summer, with fewer rocks to dodge. But the excitement of running the entire upper run is worth the necessary training.

Location

From Arlington (I-84), take Highway 19 south to Service Creek. Take Highway 207 east to Kimberly, continue east to Monument and then Long Creek, then take Highway 395 to Dale. From Prineville, take Highway 26 east to Highway 19; proceed north to Kimberly. Follow Highway 207 east along the North Fork to Monument and then to Long Creek. Turn north on Highway 395 to Dale.

Put-in sites are at Tollgate Forest Service Campground (north of Dale) or at the Camas Creek Bridge, and at several river accesses along Highway 395. The campground is about a mile above the town (River Mile 60.5).

Personality

The North Fork of the John Day is a high-country stream, marking the transition from mountainous terrain at the 2,770-foot elevation put-in, through Ponderosa pine forests and down a thousand feet in a dramatic change to open desert, spotted with an occasional juniper tree as the main stem John Day is reached. There are some

John Day River Watersheds

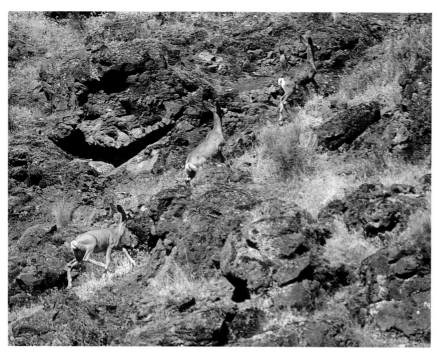

Mule deer are a common sight along this little-used waterway.

Mileage/Days

40 miles, 2-4 days. Add 16 miles and 1+ days if continuing on to Kimberly on the main stem John Day.

Average Float Levels/Seasons

1,500 to 3,500 cfs is the recommended level for floating; these levels occur late April through early June most seasons. The optimal flow is 2,500 cfs. Rises are almost all from snowmelt. There is no official gauge, but the flow at Monument may be estimated by taking 70% of the flow of the main stem John Day at the Service Creek gauge.

High-Water Season

4,000+ cfs may occur early April into May, or during times of hot weather and heavy snow in the mountains, any time late May through June. Soils in the North Fork drainage absorb little water, which means the river can rise very quickly during snowmelt or heavy rainstorms. Even a flow of 3,500 cfs may challenge intermediate level boaters not expecting long, fast rapids with big waves and tricky hydraulics.

High-water boaters should be prepared for occasional big waves, long wave trains, strainers and reversals, in addition to being dressed for dunking. Currents gain speed and finding eddies to stop in may be difficult. Rapids come at a more rapid pace, so boaters may have to scout from the boat if there isn't time to land. Boaters need experience in fast, technical water. Fishing from the boat will be difficult through the upper reaches. The river will slow down and be less technical once closer to Monument.

meadows with good wildflower displays in late spring, besides some interesting columnar basalt formations and "stacked" mountains. Public easements on river right for the first 20 miles allow for camping and river access. Although a dirt road follows the river on the upper stretch, and there are a few houses, the wilderness feel of this run is not interrupted. The river is an intermediate level, "technical" run (fast current with many rocks to dodge).

Difficulty

Class III (III+ at low/high water). This run is faster, rockier and colder—overall more difficult—than the main stem John Day, boated by far fewer people. Very cold water, isolation, and unexpected high water contribute to the degree of difficulty. Weather during the runoff period can include snow flurries and frosty nights. There are about 20 Class II rapids, mostly on the first 2/3 of the run, plus some Class IIIs. The river definitely takes on a Class IV character with mostly high water, due to its "busy" nature and a Class III+ at lower levels, with more shallows but somewhat slower current.

Gradient

21 fpm; rapids are fairly continuous for most of the run. The high elevation of the put-in combined with the smooth river channel combine to create a relatively fast river for an Oregon multi-day trip. This trip should be trained for on steep gradient day trips such as the upper Clackamas and McKenzie, and the high reaches of the North Umpqua.

Low-Water Season

500 cfs to 1,500 cfs (500 is listed for hardshell kayaks as the minimum in the book *Soggy Sneakers*).

As the river drops below 1,500 cfs, rapids become rockier. The current slows a bit, so there is a little more time to pick a route. Without the main stem's long pools, there is more rock dodging, boat dragging and scraping over gravel bars. Wading a boat is more dangerous than on the main stem due to the fast current, as is lining.

Boaters running low water should have smaller, lighter craft that are sturdy enough to survive both grinding over gravel bars and bashing rocks. Carry lighter loads.

Low water gets serious at 1,000 and under; 500 cfs is generally given as the lowest level for kayakers, but a very skilled inflatable kayaker could possibly run lower levels. The river is moderately fast and rocky like the McKenzie above Paradise at a low flow of 1,000 that I once ran.

Soils along the North Fork yield little groundwater needed to maintain minimal floatable flows in the summer. 500 cfs has been done; lower levels await the challenge by skilled boaters in small craft. (Low water is more easily challenged on the sections roadside, a good place to test your abilities in low water craft.)

Craft

Mostly kayaks, some rafts and catarafts; driftboats/canoes possible with skilled boaters at optimum level. In low water, catarafts, smaller rafts, inflatable kayaks and Catyak are practical but boaters should have experience in these small craft on busy rivers before attempting this stream. The river often drops to 500 cfs by June.

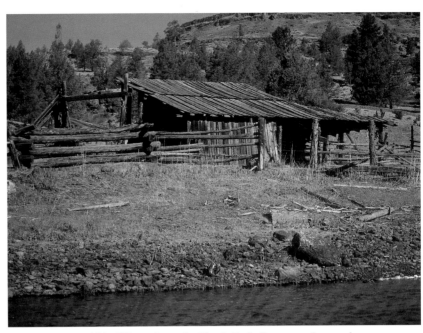

Old building along the North Fork. Because of rugged winters, not many chose to homestead in this area.

Permits

No permits are required to run the North Fork John Day at this time except for commercial outfitters. No new commercial boating permits are being issued.

Hazards

Fast current, busy river with many rapids, plus some big waves and reversals (especially in the first 10 miles—if the first 4 miles are too challenging, walk out), very cold water (snowmelt direct from mountains), isolated run.

The high elevation can bring cold or even frosty/snowy nights, sudden unpredictable storms, including snowstorms in June, and wildly fluctuating flows (optimum one day, flood the next, after a heat wave melts too much snow for the soil to absorb).

Wind is usually not a problem given the strong current. In cold weather, carry survival gear on your person (waterproof matches, fire starter, hand warmers, high-energy food, etc.). Compared to the mainstem John Day, this section gets less attention from boaters, particularly after spring melt is over, so don't expect help from another float party. Avoid private lands.

Fishing

Rainbow trout, bull trout (possibly redside and/or redband trout), salmon, steelhead.

Bass may approach from the main stem John Day when river drops and warms in July. A chemical spill from a truck on Highway 395 killed thousands of fish and ruined fishing for many years, but the fish are on the comeback trail. (Unfortunately, the offending company paid a mere $5,000 fine for this disaster.)

As the John Day is the last undammed major river basin in Oregon, the North Fork and its tributaries support the largest populations of anadromous fish—wild spring chinook and summer steelhead—in the Columbia Basin, fish that must swim up most of Oregon's Columbia, climb Tumwater Falls, then continue another hundred miles to their spawning areas.

Steelhead enter the North Fork peaking in March, when the river is usually too cold and the roads too snowbound for floating. The season ends in April. This is important spawning habitat, so catch and release is usually mandated for wild steelhead (hatchery fish are not released but occasionally find their way upstream; release any wild steelhead carefully).

Most steelhead fishing is done from boat or shore in easier reaches, where the river starts to pool, below the confluence with the Middle Fork. Keep in mind that on the slower reaches of the easier section, during winter steelheading, the river may have mini-icebergs or freeze over in extreme conditions. A good time to fish is when the river drops low after a rise, allowing fish better migrating conditions, but these conditions also produce ice.

Salmon fishing is closed to protect spawning grounds (check with ODFW). Bull trout, found in deeper pools, must be released unharmed. Wild redband trout and mountain whitefish may be caught on upper reaches, but with young steelhead in the river, all trout should be released. Whitefish are good sport, especially when fishing in late spring to early summer with flies. In addition, they are not endangered and provide tasty meals (fillet as you would a catfish or bass, then fry in batter).

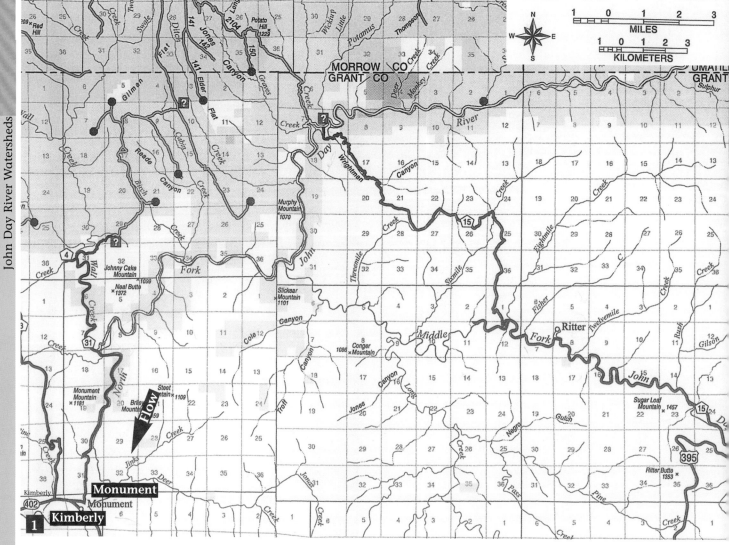

Overall, much of the upper river is to be enjoyed for the experience of wilderness, scenery, wildlife, viewing protected/restored riparian habitat, and running some challenging technical water; while saving heavy fishing for the lower sections.

Managing Agency

Bureau of Land Management, Prineville District; 3050 NE 3rd St., Prineville OR 97754; 541/416-6700.

Shuttles/Services

Boyers Cash Store, Monument, OR 541/934-2290. Services as well as shuttles.

Dale Store, Dale, OR, 541/421-3484

Barbara McCormack, Dale, OR 541/421-3416

Check in at Monument restaurants, gas station, etc. for a last-minute shuttle, or contact the Prineville BLM for updates and commercial outfitters.

Mileage & Highlights

(Note: mileages will differ slightly depending on where you launch.)

0: Tollgate Campground, boat-launch site. Deep forest. Elevation near 3,000 feet. If you put-in at Camas Creek, the mileage is much the same. (Camas is a brilliant blue wildflower that covers the meadows with color every spring; an important Native food. The bulbs were cooked in rock ovens. White camas was usually avoided as it resembles death camas, a poisonous plant.)

0.5: Begin 3.5 miles of busy water, consider aborting the trip if the rapids are too much for your skill level or craft. There are 3 major rapids in the next 10 miles, including long rock gardens (mazes of rocks and waves).

2: Dearborn Creek, river right.

2.5: Jericho Creek, river right.

3: **Class II+**, left bend of the river, long and rocky. Hunter Creek, river right.

6.5: **Grandstand Rapid, Class III.** Scout river right. The river begins a curve to the left, land on inside of curve river right to scout. This is a straight, fast drop ending with a curve to the right as waves crash and roll off cliff wall river left.

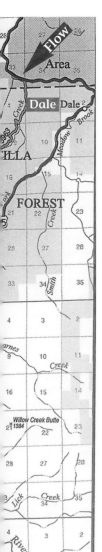

(Note: North Fork rapid names were given by the book *Soggy Sneakers* which features many first descents by kayakers, who are then allowed to name the rapids they encounter. This run was written up for that book by Rob Blickensderfer.)

7.0: House on river right.

7.3: Class II rapid.

7.5: Cabin, river right.

8: **Surprise Rapid, Class III.** Does not look like much from upstream, thus the name. Short drop with big waves at bottom, avoid hole river left.

9.5: **Chainsaw Rapid, Class III.** "Eddy out" (land in eddy to stop boat) on river right to scout. Large standing waves squeezing through narrow, steep river banks. A cabin may be seen on river right.

Part 2 of Chainsaw is a 500'-long but straightforward Class II+.

10: House, river right.

13.5: **Zipper Rapid, Class III.** Scout from either side. Begins with an S-turn, with the main drop at the end of the S.

15.5: Stony Creek, river right.

17.3: **Upper Bridge Rapid, Class III.** A 1000-foot-long boulder garden, fast moving rapid. Landmark: Wrightman wooden bridge. Wrightman Canyon to river left. Possible evacuation site.

18: **Lower Bridge Rapid, Class II+.** Almost as long as the upper run.

Wrightman Canyon marks the end of the river right road, and the beginning of the North Fork's southwesterly turn, which exposes the canyon to the arid climate as the forest gives way to desert. The change occurs surprisingly quickly.

20: Old homestead, with log house on river right.

21.5: Potamus Creek, river right.

22: Concrete bridge spans river.

22.5: Mallory Creek, river right.

24.5: Ditch Creek, river right.

26.5: **Class II+ Rapid,** begins with curve to left.

28: Confluence with Middle Fork John Day, river left, often muddy. The river volume increases as much as 25% with this stem's addition. Campsites in this area are some of the last on public land. Fishing improves, with more and deeper pools.

30.5: Right hill, Johnny Cake Mountain, 1099-foot elevation, named for its layers of basalt that resemble stacked pancakes, or johnny cakes. The smaller hill is Neal Butte.

32: Cabin Creek, river right.

34.5: **Class II+ Rapid,** narrow basalt channel.

35: Left hillside, Briley Mountain, 1159 feet.

35.5: Two Cabin Creek, river right.

36.5: Right hill, Monument Mountain, 1181 feet.

37.5: Barn, cabins, house on river right.

37.7: Wall Creek, river right. A major tributary of the North Fork John Day. The main river becomes larger and pools up even more.

Last campsites close to Monument. Road 31 now follows river. From here, the river flows due south to Monument.

39.2: Cliff walls, river left, signal that Monument is near. Private lands now dominate both sides of river.

40: Bridge over John Day. The new boat landing is just beyond the bridge on river right. The old take-out was located on a gravel bar above the bridge.

From here, the North Fork continues to flow mostly due west to the town of Kimberly, a distance of 16 miles. This segment isn't often floated for its wilderness value, due to slow speed, nominal scenery, agricultural diversion dams, and the paved road that follows it. However, the bass fishing is good beginning in spring, it's good training, plus it's possible to float approximately 20 more miles to Service Creek, the launch site for the upper John Day. Floating all the way from Dale to the Columbia is possible in theory, with the right boat and skills, and at a good water level.

As the river drops quickly from high-country mountains to high desert, forests of fir give way to pine and finally to juniper. The river broadens and becomes slower. And fishing gets easier, in addition to becoming more productive.

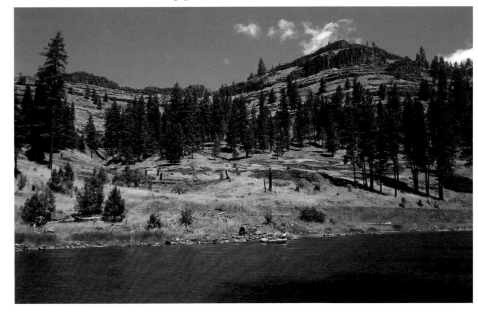

Upper Grande Ronde River & Wallowa River

CHAPTER 5

Upper Grande Ronde River & Wallowa River

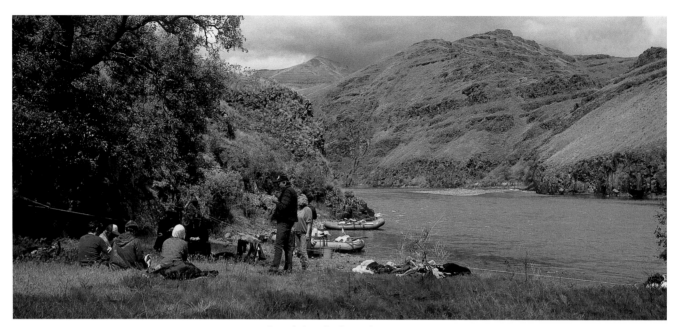

Lunch break along the river.

FRENCH FUR TRAPPERS CALLED THIS RIVER THE "Great Round-About" or Riviere de Grande Ronde for its many twisting turns, most of which are long, lazy loops on the slower section of the river in the La Grande area.

This description also applies to a "great, round" valley where La Grande is located. (Grande is often misspelled as Grand). Another, earlier name was "Glaise" or "Clay" River for the clay-colored appearance the river assumes as it concludes its meandering in the valley and descends

Homer elk live in the canyon year round, most elk migrate into the Grande Ronde Canyon in late fall, when the snow in high mountains becomes too deep to forage food.

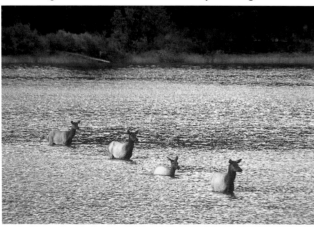

into the great, 2,500-foot-deep canyon (which, if measured from the mountaintops, ranks among the deepest gorges in the nation).

The river straightens as it meets the Wallowa River at "Rondowa" (a combination of "Ronde" and "Wallowa" invented by railroad officials). Floats here actually begin on the Wallowa, at the conjunction of the Wallowa and Minam rivers in the hamlet of Minam (train track, small motel and store, shuttle service, state park with camping). Active train tracks follow the Wallowa from Minam to Rondowa, where vehicle access is halted by a collapsed bridge.

The nearby Wallowa Mountains, named after Native American fish traps used in the Wallowa River, are sometimes called "Oregon's Alps" as they do resemble the European alpine range. They are a geological oddity in Oregon, being granite rather than of volcanic origin. Remember to pronounce this name "Wah-LOW-ah" (LOW rhyming with COW) and never "wallow-ah" as in "what pigs do in the mud."

In its upper section, the great canyon of the Grande Ronde is very steep, ruggedly forested and spotted with basalt rock outcrops (hoodoos); hard for hiking. Boating allows far easier access to this mostly-roadless portion. Most fishermen work the river from road or rail access, meaning very rewarding fishing in the wilderness portion of the canyon.

Combining the upper and lower Grande Ronde floats requires a minimum of five days (unless water levels are above 6,000 cfs or so) to appreciate this unique canyon, with an elevation drop from 2,530 feet at Minam to 820 feet at the mouth... from high-country fir forest to the bottom of stark, barren Hell's Canyon. This is a three-state tour (Oregon, Washington and Idaho).

The great trio of canyons in this region—Grande Ronde, Snake, and Idaho Salmon—were home to the Nez Perce, a Native American tribe famous both for their peaceful co-existence with homesteaders and for their fierce fight against the U.S. Army, which tried to move them out of their spectacular homelands and onto a bleak reservation. Chief Joseph surrendered after a bloody battle in order to save his people. Legend says he was born in a cave located deep within Joseph Canyon, a deep gorge named for him. Joseph Creek joins the Grande Ronde near its mouth.

Another local legend was Spot, a wily bighorn ram whose horns took on Paul Bunyan proportions when described by empty-handed big game hunters. This myth became reality when a hiker found Spot's head and horns intact, the sheep apparently dead from ripe old age. Many record bighorns still come from Joseph Canyon, mostly from private land access. The Oregon Department of Fish and Wildlife auctions a bighorn sheep tag for the Joseph Canyon area, which often produces bids of $50,000 or more. The proceeds go to fund re-population of bighorns in Oregon.

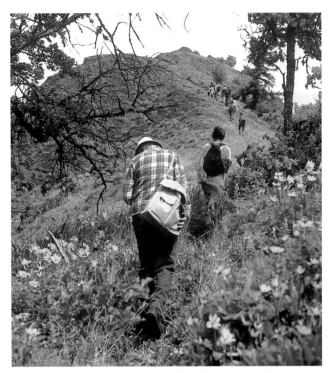

Hikers trek ankle-deep in yellow balsamroot flowers along a rugged elk-made trail to a high vista.

on Interstate 5, then take Interstate 84, traveling in an inverted "L" pattern across the state. Heading directly cross-country from Prineville or Bend means many miles of slow, curvy mountain roads (scenic, but a long and exhausting drive).

Willowa River/Upper Grande Ronde

Minam to Powwatka Bridge, Mud Creek or Troy (Upper Grande Ronde)

Location

Northeast Oregon. From Portland, take Interstate 84 to La Grande. Then take Highway 82 to Minam (14 miles past Elgin). From the south, it's best to head north to Portland

Personality

The Wallowa/upper Grande Ronde float offers the fastest wilderness waters in Oregon that are suitable for intermediate-level boaters. The fishing is also exciting as you try to cast at the top of rapids or in the middle of whitewater while the boat is moving along at 8 mph or more. Wildlife is plentiful, especially in the off-season, as wintering bald eagles and Rocky Mountain elk winter in this canyon. This canyon is one of the few places in Oregon where eastern whitetail deer may be seen; native mule deer

More Homer elk living year-round along the Grande Ronde.
There are large private estates here that prohibit hunting, which is where they all disappear to during elk season.

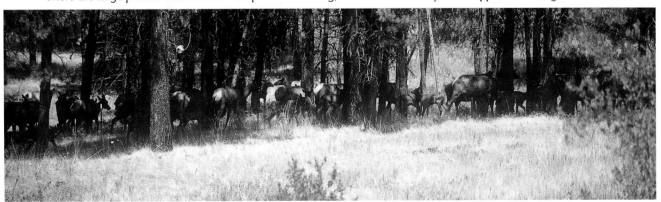

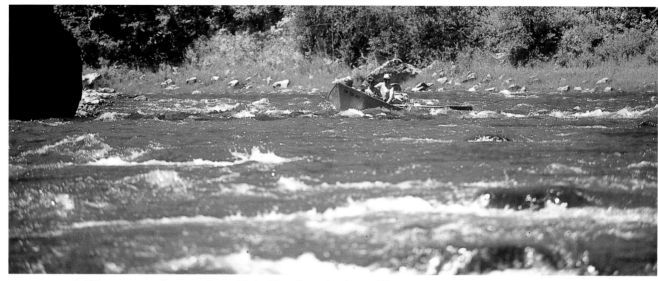

Driftboat approaches a rocky rapid, looking for rocks that will bury a hardshell boat. One skilled person can help others by leading them through each rapid's slots and away from sleeper rocks.

also browse the open meadows. Black bear, bobcat, lynx, cougar, and bighorn sheep are found here, along with hawks and owls, grouse, and river otter. Along with songbirds, an array of colorful butterflies inhabit the canyon.

Even if your fishing is washed out by high waters, you'll not only see wildlife, you'll enjoy the wildflower displays. The big bushes with white blossoms are known as "mock orange" for their heady fragrance. Yellow balsamroot (or mules' ears) cover the open hillsides like fields of miniature sunflowers, while the woods are full of delicate flowers waiting to be discovered.

There are few sandy beaches here; the current is too fast (sand on the bottom of the river indicates a slower section). Most camps are somewhat hidden on terraces above rough landing spots at gravel bars. Look carefully for flat areas in the trees.

Difficulty

Class II+ at optimum flows (some Class III-III+ high water/low water)

Gradient

21 fpm

Mileage/Days

Minam to Powwatka Bridge, 38.2 miles, 2-4+ days

Minam to Troy, 45.5 miles, 3-5+ days

Average Float Levels/Seasons

1,500 to 5,000 cfs; March to July, Troy gauge. Trout fishing is best after high water is past, usually late June, or when the river is 3,000 cfs or lower (Troy gauge).

Minam Roller about to "Maytag" (tumble around in water, as in the brand name of the washing machine) a heavily-loaded 14-foot boat.

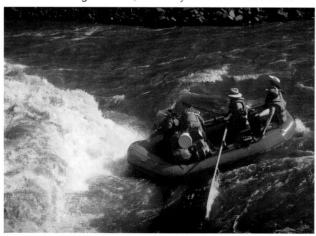

Flip City! They didn't get enough momentum to "push" through this hydraulic, and were overcome by its powerful upstream currents.

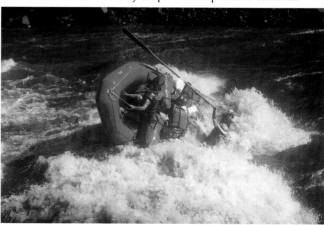

The level of the Wallowa from Minam to Rondowa is about half the Troy reading. Especially in low-water conditions, this is the most serious stretch of fast, shallow, and rocky water. (It's also the best fly-fishing, although landing and/or holding boats in current is always difficult.)

This float starts at Minam, rather than on the Grande Ronde, because the Wallowa River provides up to 90% of the flow at Rondowa, where the two rivers meet. Irrigation depletes part of the Grande Ronde flow in the growing season, while the Wallowa runs unfettered, with more melt-off late in summer than the Grande Ronde, due to its high-elevation snowpack. Above Rondowa, the Grande Ronde itself is very difficult due to shallows and rocks. Also, this area gets a lot of pressure from bank

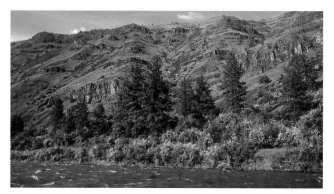

Fragrant "mock orange" blooms proficiently in late spring.

anglers, some of whom walk several miles to a spot. Almost no one walks into the Grande Ronde between Rondowa and the Powwatka Bridge, as the gorge is steep and rugged.

High-Water Season

Levels of 8,000 to 14,000+ cfs may be encountered mid-May to early June depending on weather and snowpack.

As a high-elevation snowpack with little dam control, the Wallowa and Grande Ronde big waters arrive later in the season than other Oregon rivers. A combination of

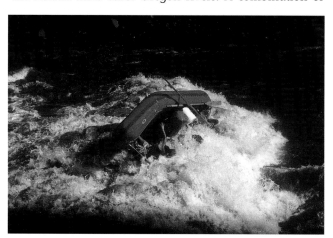

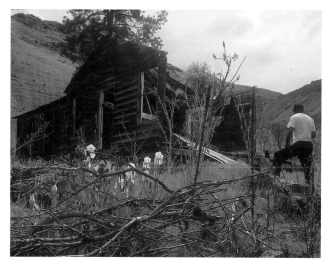

Old homesteads are scattered throughout the canyon. Many still have living reminders that people once lived there, such as these wild iris.

heavy winter snowpack and hot spring weather can surprise boaters with the river up to the trees in their camps. The highest water ever recorded was in February, 1996, a flow of 51,800 cfs. At that level, you could float from Minam to Lewiston, Idaho in a day!

Hazards of high water include the Minam Roller (avoid by putting in at Minam State Park rather than at launch sites in Minam, or cheat river right). This is a big Class III+ hydraulic that can and has flipped heavily loaded 14-foot rafts. The speed of the Wallowa River may increase to as much as 15-20 miles per hour, making eddies vanish and landing nearly impossible. Rescue of flipped boats and overboard personnel is difficult at such speeds.

Rapids have big waves and take on a definite Class III character; eddies on the Grande Ronde itself transform into turbulent and unpredictable whirlpools. The entire 90-mile run to the river's mouth has reportedly been done in a single day by a determined kayaker at high-water levels. Fishing is usually very poor at levels above 6,000 due to off-color or outright muddy water and cold river

This crew had an interesting time. Even though they flipped on a hot day in June, the river was ice-cold from glacial run-off. The river was nearly 14,000 cfs at this point, running at a speed of at least 10 mph. This raft was the last of their group, since none of the other boats had stayed behind to make sure they made it. They were already 10 minutes ahead at the time of the flip. The swimmers abandoned the raft and headed for shore to get out of the icy river. However, the raft was taken by the speeding current downstream. I sometimes wonder how those last boaters got themselves downriver, since the boat was going too fast to recapture it. I can just imagine the expressions of horror on the faces of the others when the empty boat caught up to them.

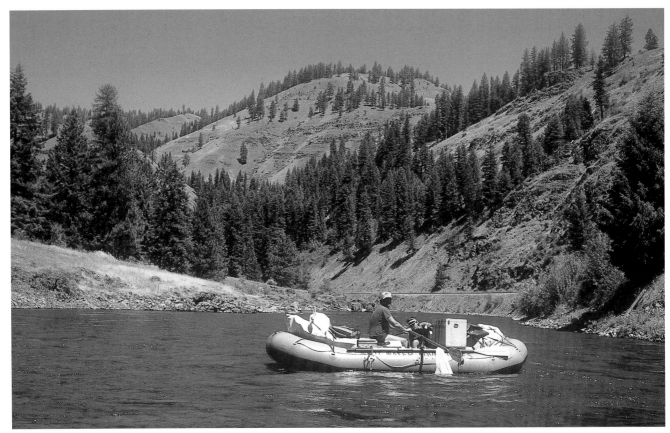

Thick forests gradually give way to patches of open meadows, then to arid desert below Troy.

temperatures; the only good spots will be at the mouths of clear-running creeks.

Although air temperatures may be in the 90s during high-water surges, the Wallowa comes straight from the mountains and will be ice cold. A dunking without protective gear can lead to hypothermia.

In the late 1930s, Buzz Holdstrom, a pioneering whitewater boatman from the Oregon Coast—the first person to run infamous large rapids such as Lava Falls and Separation on the Colorado through Grand Canyon, in a heavy hand-made wooden boat, no less—was hired by the government to float men and their gear through this wild canyon to survey it. Reportedly, Holdstrom was disturbed by the fast, churning waters of the Grande Ronde/Wallowa confluence at flood stage. Before the expedition could resume its downstream journey, Holdstrom was found dead of a gunshot to the head. Accusations flew, but the official cause of death was listed as suicide. Holdstrom had supposedly gone off by himself to shoot camp meat—mule deer or grouse—and when he did not return, search parties found him dead with a gun alongside.

Low-Water Season

Flows below 1,500 cfs occur late July through February during an average snowpack year. Flows of 500 cfs become more practical in late October and early November, when irrigation water is released, bringing the river back up to 800 cfs or higher.

Below 1,000 (Troy gauge), the Wallowa becomes especially shallow and rocky; luckily, the fast speed of the current moves boats off rocks. Use caution when wading and/or pushing boats (stay upstream). Blind Falls is a solid Class III at low water and may trash canoes or driftboats. The low-water route is down the middle; at lower levels, this requires going over mid-stream rocks. Even at 500 cfs the river is boatable by veterans; good water-reading skills

Sun on an iced-in canyon; looks like the ice age has returned.

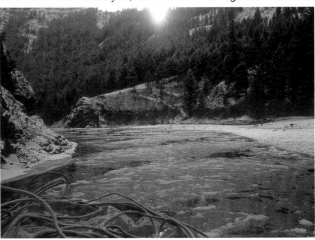

are required to miss sleeper rocks and avoid shoals. This segment is an easier low-water run than the North Fork John Day, even with its fast current.

At Rondowa, conditions improve with the addition of the Grande Ronde (when two rivers merge, they are named as the larger of the two rivers; however, the Wallowa provides as much as 90% of the combined flow here.) Downstream, the river continues to deepen with the addition of numerous creeks and the Wenaha River. The river also often rises in late fall as irrigation water funneled off to fields is returned to the river; just in time for fall steelhead runs and elk hunting season. If you float in November, a pair of hip boots or neoprene waders are a must for the person who has to jump out and push the boat.

Some boaters float in November for elk hunting as well as steelheading. There is almost always very low water. In extreme winters, the river may actually freeze solid in places, requiring boaters to pull their craft over an ice sheet. The risk of breaking through the ice is great. Slush forms, creating rowing conditions that have been described as "trying to row through a Slurpee." One late elk season, boat hunters had to evacuate via train from Rondowa, returning on snowmobiles later (after the hunting season road closures were opened) to fetch their boating gear.

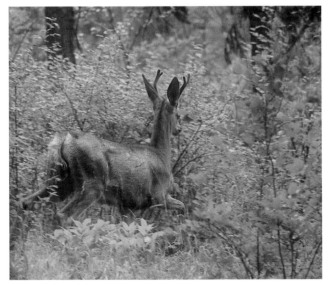

A small muley buck bolts between fir trees.

Obviously, late-season boaters must be prepared with lots of extra clothing (wool and fleece in particular), a supply of dry, split wood for emergency campfires (plus a good fire starter), and camp gear designed for 4-season use (no summer-weight sleeping bags). Chemical hand warmers, propane heaters, and the like are highly recommended. In severe conditions, though, the trip is worthwhile, as thousands of elk and deer wintering in the canyon may be seen, in addition to bald eagles and families of otter. On one cold trip, a hissing sound that

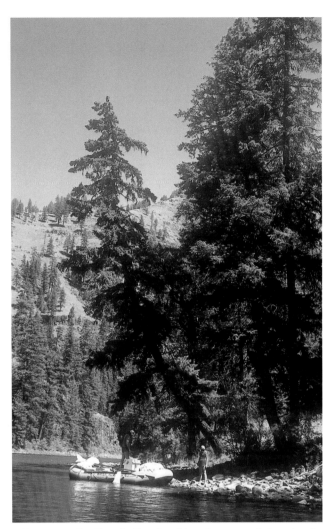

Camps on the Grande Ronde seldom have an obvious landing spot or flat spots for tents and kitchen—sometimes you have to stop and check sites for usability.

sounded ominously like a major leak in the raft turned out to be the dominant otter in a group of five, sounding a threat to the passing craft. Bobcat and cougar are more likely to be visible then, as well. Winter steelheading can be fantastic.

Craft

At optimum levels of 3-4000 cfs, all whitewater boats are suitable. Canoes and driftboats are vulnerable below 1,500 cfs and require good handling to dodge rocks in swift currents at levels between 1,500 and 3,000 cfs. Rafts of all sizes can tackle levels up to 7,000; at high water, you'll want at least a 14-foot raft or cataraft; Cat-yaks, IKs, and other low-water craft do well at levels from 800 cfs to 4,000 cfs.

Permits

Self-issuing permits available at launch sites are required of all boaters. Commercial outfitters must have a permit from the Walla Walla Ranger Station.

Upper Grande Ronde River & Wallowa River

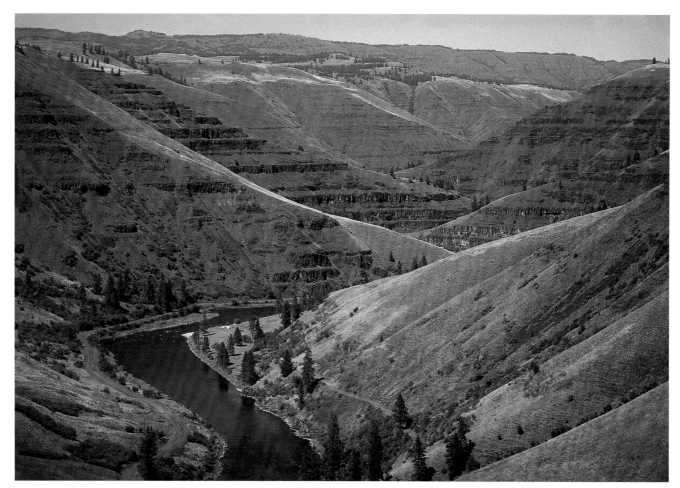

Views on the shuttle run may be as impressive as those on the river.

Hazards

Cold water in spring, rattlesnakes and ticks, tripping over rocks (in and out of the river, "rock bars" make for difficult footing), sudden rises in water levels, fast currents, rugged isolated canyon (very steep if climbing out is necessary, and cell phones don't work unless you are on high ground). The faster current makes this river much more difficult than the John Day, even though the rapids are rated much the same. The rapids take on a more continuous nature, especially at levels greater than 4,000 cfs. Boaters need to develop endurance to handle the constant maneuvering that is required.

The first nine miles on the Wallowa River are always swift and rocky with some good wave action; beginners or those in unforgiving craft such as canoes may be overwhelmed. Strainers are always a risk, especially along this narrower stream. The run gets easier at Rondowa.

Blind or Vincent Falls is always troublesome for canoes; scout first and consider lining. House, or Red Rock, Rapid has big waves at higher water levels and an undercut at other levels; watch for strainers pinned here. Martin's Misery is fairly straightforward at low to medium levels. Sheep Creek is fairly long for a Class II+ rapid. Many rocks, both large and small, seem to jump in front of your boat if you are not experienced in reading and maneuvering rocky rivers, or not paying attention.

Fishing

Excellent for trout from mid-June into fall; good steelhead runs in fall and winter. The best compromise between weather and water conditions for trout fishing usually occur in early to mid July, with low-water, low-competition floats suitable into September and October. Trout from 14 to 18 inches are often caught. Trout hit on all popular flies (provided the water is clear, which may not happen until July), standard lures such as the Roostertail and spinners, and bait (check fishing regulations). Wet nymph imitations work wonders when conditions are right. Only clipped-fin fish may be kept.

Some of the best fly-fishing is found on the Wallowa portion of this run, the nine miles between Minam and Rondowa; however, landing your craft or slowing it down for multiple casts is difficult. Grasshopper and caddis-fly imitations are best for trout in summer. Earlier, match the hatches of evening mayfly and golden stonefly. The Wallowa is considered by some to be the better trout fishery, with flows out of Wallowa Lake that keep the river at a constant temperature—colder water and more oxygen for the trout. The Grande Ronde above Rondowa and below Troy is warmer and the bass start to take over during hot afternoons.

Trout here snap up Simulators, Elk Hair Caddis, hoppers and standard nymphs. A local favorite is the Zug Bug. Prince Nymphs and the Gold-Ribbed Hare's Nymph are also used.

Continuing your float downstream from Powwatka Bridge to Troy multiplies your opportunities for trout fishing. Many fish strike along this stretch, even though it is accessible by gravel road on river left. There are large deep eddies and good pocket water among the rock gardens. This float can be done in one day if you don't mind the long drive to Troy. The drive from Flora, a former ghost town with interesting old buildings, down the hairpin turns to Troy is breathtaking. Mud Creek offers an alternative put-in to Powwatka bridge for about an 8-mile float.

The Troy area also has smallmouth bass (active June-September) and large whitefish (winter). It's not unusual for a trophy bighorn or herd of elk to cross the gravel access roads here, as these game animals seek protection in ranchers' pastures. Fly-anglers with clear-water conditions can toss poppers or Woolly Buggers into bass habitat, on the lower section.

Steelhead arrive in September and stay until April (the season usually closes for summer; check current regs). Wet flies are popular early, when the waters are still low. As the water cools down, the fish become sluggish and anglers usually shift to casting spinners, drifting worms or drifting Corkies with eggs or shrimp. Very few anglers actually float at this time, so there are long stretches of suitable water below Rondowa you can claim as your own. There's always a technique that will produce a hit: back-bouncing, floating bait with a bobber, trolling plugs or "holding up" with plugs (where the rower holds the boat in a likely current, while anglers put their plugs out and move them from side to side, letting the current do the work; no casting involved beyond the initial cast).

In fall, fly-fishing takes presedence, with most anglers using wet flies. Purple Perils, Green Butt Skunks, and Black Leech patterns are used by some local guides. Steelhead may also strike Muddlers, dragonflies, and other traditional steelhead flies.

Bull trout and chinook salmon ply the waters of the Grande Ronde, but fishing for these endangered species is not allowed.

Managing Agency

Walla-Walla Ranger District, 1415 W. Rose St., Walla Walla WA 99362; 509/522-6290. List of authorized outfitters available.

Shuttles/Services

Minam Store and Motel, Minam OR. (541-437-1111). Shuttles, plus last minute supplies of food, flies, worms, and other fishing gear. Also rents boats.
Jenkins Shuttles, (541-962-0366).

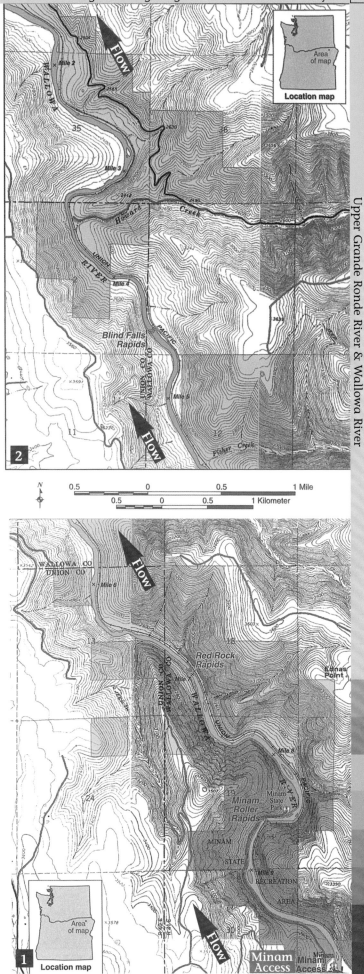

Upper Grande Ronde River & Wallowa River

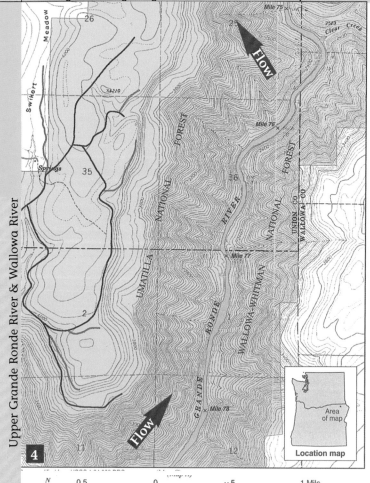

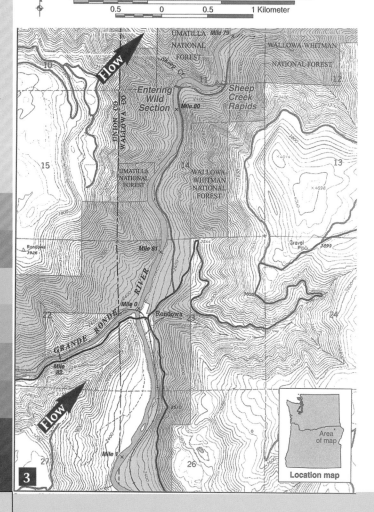

Upper Grande Ronde River & Wallowa River

River Mileage And Highlights

Mile   Landmark

0: Minam Launch Site (Wallowa River, meets the mouth of Minam River). "Minam" derives from Native American "E-mi-ne-mah", a valley where edible roots were gathered. Camping options: one public and one private (the latter open to shuttlers using the Minam Store for shuttles).

1.6: Minam Roller, large reversal at high water (over 7,000 cfs). Avoid by staying far right.

2: Minam State Park (rugged launch site, fee camping)

4.5: House Rock Rapid (a.k.a. Red Rock), **Class II+.** Big boulder midstream, "S" turn required. The high spot on river right is "Edna's Point". Below, watch for "#43" on railroad track, power lines cross the river.

5.8: Blind Falls (a.k.a. Vincent Falls) **Class II+.** Blind drop over ledge, very rocky at lower levels. Usually run midstream. Scout from boat; canoeists scout from shore.

6.8: Schitzo Rapid, Class II, boulder splits river into two channels, both runnable at most water levels, usually the left channel is easier.

7: Howard Creek enters river right, under railroad trestle. Good elk-viewing area.

9: Old homestead, left bank. There are wildflowers and domestic plants gone wild here.

10: Train bridge marks the confluence of Grande Ronde and Wallowa at Rondowa (two buildings, right bank). Last road/train access (the vehicle bridge was removed in 1991, only pillars remain). Watch for logs pinned against the pillars. One boater was killed here when he became pinned between his raft and a bridge pillar.

11.4: Sheep Creek, left bank. Wild sheep are sometimes glimpsed on rock cliffs above left bank. Sheep Creek Camp, right bank, has old logging road that leads back to Rondowa. Beginning of Wild River designation and motorized boat closure. Last easy evacuation area.

   Sheep Creek Rapid begins. This **Class II+** drop is a long series of waves and rocks as the river turns in an S-curve.

13: Small creek enters, right, next to cliffs.

13.4: Camp right bank, big lone pine.

14.1: Camp left, burnt pine, steep cliffs.

14.7: Camp left, small beach.

16: Several small camps on left before Clear Creek is seen entering on river right.

16.7: Elk Ridge camps, river right. This is a large gravel bar with flat, sandy tent sites on the terrace above the gravel. A rugged hike up an elk trail leads to a scenic overlook of the Clear Creek drainage.

18.4: Meadow Creek enters on left. Good camps 1/2 mile past the creek on right bank as river curves, then 2 sites on left bank.

19: Alder Creek enters on left. Camp at mouth. Good open ridge for hiking.

20.5: Martin's Misery Rapid, Class II+. Large standing waves, some hidden rocks at lower flows. From Alder Creek, the river takes strong turn left, then back right; Martin's begins as the river straightens. There are many camps in this area.

23.3: Bear Creek enters left, with three camps at its mouth, plus three just downstream on left (Digs Bar).

25.5: Elbow Creek, left. Good wildflower displays on hillsides above. Four camps, left bank. Watch for Barnes Spring on right, fresh water. More reddish rocks like House Rock begin to appear, most are smaller sleepers, with their brighter color making them easier to spot.

26: Cabin Creek, right, large flat area for camping.

26.7: Grossman Creek, right. Large stream in open canyon. Camps directly across, on left bank. Mr. Grossman was a pioneer trapper who passed away near Rondowa.

27.2: Boundary, end National Forest, begin BLM land.

27.8: Lost Bar, left. Huge gravel bar, good camping, with an island at the end of the bar.

28.8: Three camps on bench or terrace, right bank, above gravel landing sites.

As the river swings to the right, there are more camps on river right, on a large flat area. Fishing on river left is excellent; take your boat across to access this area.

29.8: Island, left channel is usually deeper. More camps on river left.

32: Island splits river, Class II; the left channel usually better. There are rocks and gravel bars to dodge.

32.5: Sickfoot Creek, river right. A huge flat area, site of old homestead. Large catalpa tree at river's edge, old apple and other fruit trees in the meadow. Excellent fishing on left bank, and an old roadbed to hike to scenic vistas. Named after David Rochester, resident on the creek with a clubfoot (Native Americans referred to him as "Sickfoot").

33.3: Begin Rattlesnake Bar on right, a large flat camp with grassy landing area. Named during a trip when two rattlesnakes were ousted from camp, with a third found in a guide's life jacket! Watch your step. The inviting grassy areas near the bank serve as prime rattlesnake habitat. Fishing on the deeper left side continues to be good.

Private land begins on right bank. Left bank is Wenaha State Wildlife Area.

Small island, with reddish cliffs on left, marks site of small camp. The left channel around an island is narrow but fun for boats that fit, otherwise take right channel.

35: Ward Canyon enters on right. The burned area on river right is the Ward Canyon fire, a good place to see wildlife and birds.

Just beyond is the Troy Fire, where wildfire jumped the Grande Ronde and burned the left (north) bank. Last BLM stretch for camping.

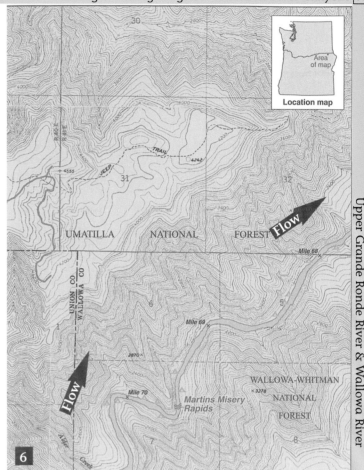

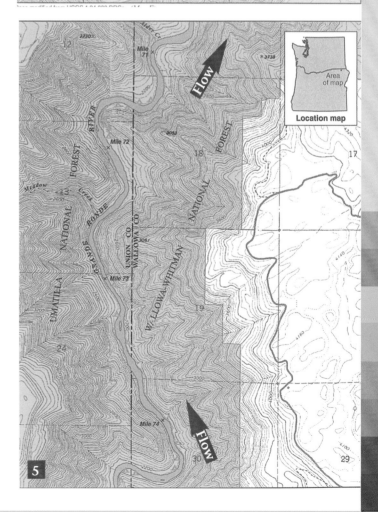

Upper Grande Ronde River & Wallowa River

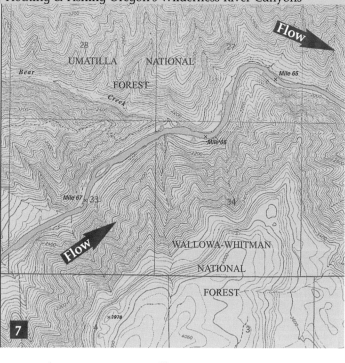

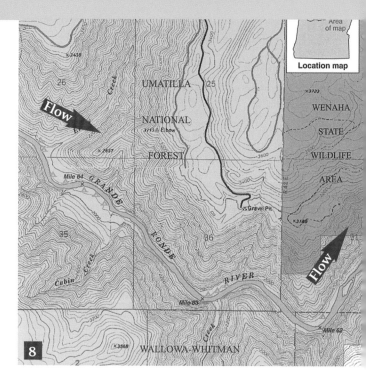

37.5: Mouth of Wildcat Creek, river right. End of Wild River designation; begin stretch of Grande Ronde with a gravel road paralleling downstream to Boggan's Oasis in Washington. Wildcat Creek is private land. Just before the bridge is good fishing through a rocky rapid.

38.2: Powwatka Bridge, takeout river right. Taking out here or at Mud Creek access (1/2 mile downstream) cuts off almost 7 miles of slow floating. The river downstream to Troy and beyond is, however, great for trout fishing.

At the old fish hatchery (on left bank), stay right. Pocket water behind numerous rocks in Class II+ rock gardens here is very productive for anglers who can cast quickly as the boat speeds by in fast currents.

43.9: Double Eddy, strong S-curve causes swirly eddies. This turbulence is stronger in high waters and at any water level, intimidating for hardshell boaters.

44: Wenaha River enters on river left. Once known as the "Salmon" River, the name was changed to Native American, derived from tribe name Wenak-ha, land governed by Chief Wenak. The Northwest didn't need another "Salmon" River, what with the Cal-Salmon, White Salmon and Idaho Salmon (plus a Salmon River already in Oregon near Mt. Hood).

44.1: Town of Troy, Oregon. Take-out site is located on river left below the Troy Bridge. There is a bar/restaurant here with limited supplies available, and a Shilo Inn. Shilo owns a large estate up Powwatka Ridge which is prime elk territory. The post office and town were named after pioneer son Troy Grinstead (not the famous lost city described by Homer).

Lower Grande Ronde River
Troy to Boggan's Oasis or Snake River Confluence (Heller Bar).

Location

Northeast Oregon, southwest Washington, middle Idaho (small stretch along Snake before takeout, right bank).

The lower section of the Grande Ronde flows mostly through Washington State. From the Portland area, take I-84 to Pendleton, then I-80 to LaGrande and Hwy. 82 to Enterprise. Take Highway 3 north to the cutoff to Flora, a small town with a ghost town feel to it; worth some exploration. Flora began as a post office in October 1890, named for the daughter of the first postmaster. From here, the road switchbacks down steep hillsides to the river and access to Troy. Follow the road downstream to put-in at Boggan's Oasis.

The return shuttle is a similarly sinuous gravel road up the canyon to Anatone on Highway 129 in Washington. Leave an extra set of keys with the shuttle driver so your rig can be moved in case the rivers rise (in 1982, my Ford van, parked at Heller Bar, sat in river water up to its doors for three days while the Snake screamed by at over 150,000 cfs).

Personality

A gravel road follows the section between Troy and Boggan's Oasis; the canyon beyond is mostly wilderness except for occasional off-putting "No Trespassing" signs posted on juniper trees.

This lower canyon quickly becomes an arid, open desert with grass and prickly pear cacti, plus some interesting rock formations (arches, window rocks, columnar basalt).

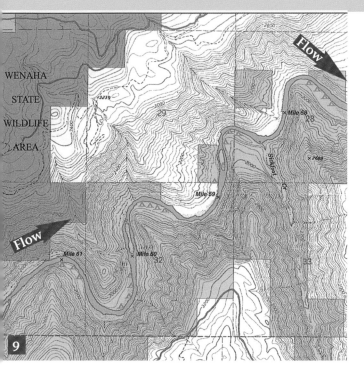

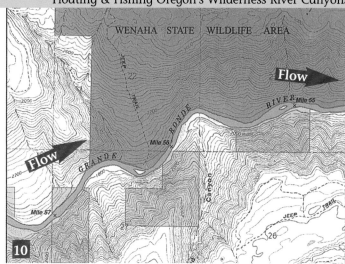

Considerably less popular with whitewater boaters than the upper run, the lower run offers some quiet stretches as well as better fishing early in the season. Considered excellent steelheading as fish are fresher closer to the mouth. Be sure to get a Washington State fishing license before drift fishing. Bighorn sheep are a common sight along the canyon walls and near the occasional ranch. Many boaters combine this run with the upper for a 5- to 8-day trip.

Difficulty
Class II+ with one Class III-IV (The Narrows)

Gradient
17 fpm

Mileage/Days
19 miles (1-2 days) from Troy to Boggan's Oasis.
26 miles (2-3 days) from Boggan's Oasis to Heller Bar (Snake River Confluence).
45 miles (2-4 days) from Troy to Heller Bar.

Average Float Levels/Seasons
1,000 to 6,000 cfs at the Troy gauge. There are fewer shallows and rocks along these stretches of the Grande Ronde, so late-summer and fall/winter floating is easier.

High-Water Season
8,000 cfs and up; in very high water, take a good scout of The Narrows before running, watch the clearance at bridge crossings, and double-tie your boats at night. High water is usually early June.

Low-Water Season
Due to tributary waters, the flow of the Grande Ronde on this section is higher than the level given at the Troy gauge. Low waters slow drift time, but seldom pose much difficulty.

Craft
All whitewater craft. Because there are fewer rocks and shallows to contend with, and the current is slower, canoes are better suited here than the upper. Driftboats are also used. However, The Narrows may have to be lined by boaters in these craft, depending on water levels and the skill of the individual boater.

Permits
No permits are required at this time except for commercial outfitters.

Hazards
Some isolated, rugged canyons are below Boggan's Oasis; The Narrows Rapids; rattlesnakes more common. Consult a map to avoid camping on private lands. Few campsites are available on public land, especially for large groups. Washington State access sites are available if you can't find anything else.

Fishing
Trout fishing spring to fall, excellent for fall and winter steelhead. Use the same techniques as the upper Grande Ronde and John Day steelhead, but be sure you have your Washington State fishing license with you. This is one of the Northwest's top-producing steelhead areas, plus there is more water to float during the September to April season.

Steelhead are more numerous on this stretch, as it is closer to the mouth and the Snake River. Steelhead must travel from the ocean up the length of the Columbia and part of the Snake, dodging dam intakes and finding fish ladders, before reaching the Grande Ronde. The best fishing is from Cottonwood Creek to the Snake. Fish are more heavily concentrated in this lower stretch.

Many anglers use poppers and Woolly Buggers to bring up a bass from the depths of the lower river. Bass begin to hit somewhere below Troy, depending on water

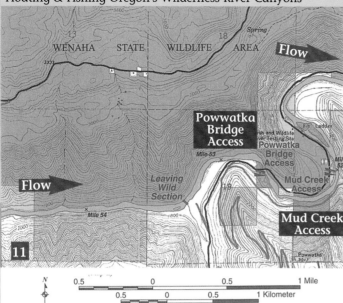

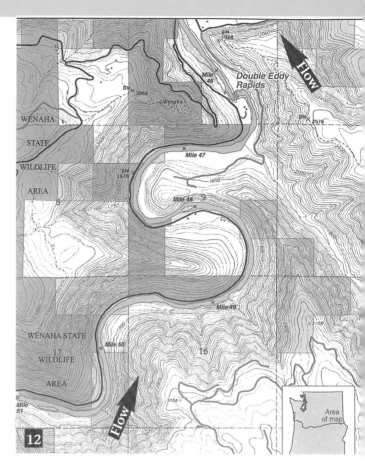

temperatures (they don't survive in the glacial melt of the Minam or Wallowa rivers).

Managing Agency

Walla Walla Ranger District, 1415 W. Rose, Walla Walla WA 99362. 509/522-6290. List of outfitters available.

Shuttles/Services

Minam Store and Motel, Minam, OR. (541-437-1111). Last minute supplies of food, flies, worms, and other fishing gear, too. Also rents boats.

Jenkins Shuttles, (541-962-0366).

Boggans Oasis, Anatone, WA (509-256-3372). Heller Bar on the Snake is in a remote area, and has limited services; Asotin, WA is closest town.

Mileage from Minam
mileage from Troy indicated in ( ).

44.1: Troy, Oregon (Mile 0 starting at Troy).

44.2: Bear Creek enters, river left. Wenaha State Wildlife Area, left bank; right bank, BLM. (0.1).

43.6: Mallory Bridge, Redmond grade road crosses here; end public lands (0.5).

40.2: Grouse Creek, river left (3.9). BLM lands on left and right banks here and downstream about .5 mile.

38.9: Oregon/Washington state line, time to change fishing licenses! End of Oregon State Scenic Waterway and federal Wild & Scenic River classifications (5.2). End public land, river left.

37.3: Horseshoe Bend (6.8). Camping on river right at Brooks Draw. Cow Camp river left only on beach area (ask BLM first).

Sharp bend where river crosses state line twice, use both fishing licenses! (Horseshoe Bend is a statewide feature of Oregon rivers; besides the Grande Ronde, the John Day and Rogue rivers each have one. You can almost "meet yourself coming back" around the sharp turns.)

36.8: Oregon/Washington state line, motorized craft prohibited upstream to mile 79.7 (7.3). BLM lands at end of Horseshoe, river right.

35.9: Menatchee Creek, river left (8.2). McNeil Island is about 2.7 miles downstream.

30.7: Cougar Creek, river left (13.4). Washington State Dept. of Wildlife (WDW) has an established fishing access on river left, the site of an old river ferry crossing. Flat, open, area; hot with little shade. BLM land is just past on river right, Bear Creek and Coyote Canyon.

28.6: Cottonwood Creek, river left (15.5). WDW fishing access, river left. Land to river right just above island and below creek is BLM, on river right.

27.4: WDW Fishing access, river left (16.7) is a large flat area, with little shade. End public access for camping.

26.2: Boggan's Oasis river right (17.9), access to State Hwy. 129, highway crosses river over bridge. Walk uphill from fishing access just upstream of bridge to the Oasis which has mostly cold drinks and ice for hot boaters.

25.7: Buford Creek, river right (18.4).

24: Rock Arch, located high on river left (20.1). Below island on bend to right are campsites, BLM land both sides of river for .75 miles.

23.5: Window Rock (20.6). Halfway up the canyon, the sky passes through open space in rocky canyon wall much like a skylight or window. BLM land continues after brief interruption, both sides. Camps river left downstream.

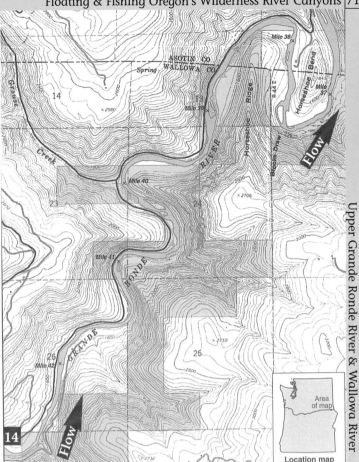

19.3: Deer Creek, river right (24.8). Old homestead here with roses and other domestics gone wild. BLM restrictions apply on leaving artifacts where you find them. Often posted as private property but is on BLM land with camps just upstream and downstream on this narrow U-bend.

18.7: Hole-in-the-Wall (25.4) is a hand-carved tunnel on river left, old ferry site for original highway crossing, access from Montgomery Ridge Road/Shumaker Road Access.

17.7: Shumaker Road Access (26.4), river left. Public lands for a brief distance.

15.8: Shumaker Creek, river left (28.3). Private lands, road on river left. Wildlife Area begins on both sides just below, and extends on left almost down to mile 10. Camps begin on left bank past Shumaker. The "Valley of Horses" is a big field on river left, high bank above river, suitable for group camping.

13.7: Hackberry Creek, river left (30.4). The Wildlife Area continues on left.

10.0: Slippery Creek, river left (34.1). Private lands. This begins long stretch of private lands, with backcountry ranches, best camping above here. Small bits of BLM lands (see map).

4.7: The Narrows Rapids (Class III-IV), mileage from Troy is 39.4.

Scouting is highly recommended. Look for and use an for old roadbed seen high on river right as river loops to the right. Watch for rattlesnakes near the river, also loose rocks.

The rapid has two big drops, one with big waves leading into a tight chute where basalt ledges constrict the river into a slot as narrow as 8 feet wide in lower water levels.

This is a good spot to play with inflatable kayaks; you can carry them back upstream for repeated rides.

Watch for strong hydraulics here; waves can swamp open canoes. Oars and paddles must be shipped close to boats or feathered (tucked in parallel to boat) to avoid breaking them when river is low.

No camping here.

4.3: Mouth of Joseph Creek (39.8). Named after legendary Chief Joseph of the Nez Perce Native Americans. He was reportedly born in a cave along the creek.

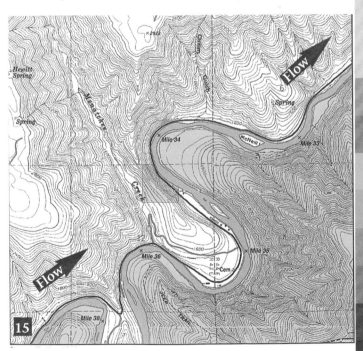

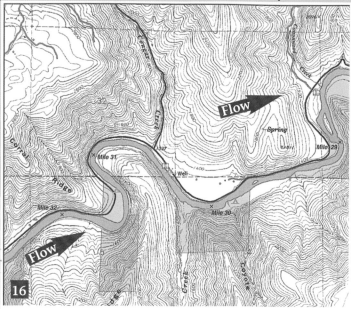

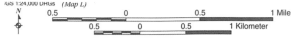

Joseph is remembered as a peacemaker who tried to avoid war with the Calvary and white settlers, but refused to leave the beautiful canyon lands his ancestors had resided in for centuries, provoking a long fight. The Nez Perce waged a brilliant campaign of hide and seek by using their knowledge of the canyons to avoid the Cavalry.

They might have successfully avoided capture by fleeing to Canada, but in winter Calvary horses had grain to sustain the chase by soldiers; the Nez Perce Appaloosa ponies (spotted horses) were strong, but had little forage. In addition, the Calvary was all fighting men, while the Nez Perce was retreating as a tribe, with women and children, which slowed their escape.

Chief Joseph, forced to surrender or have his people slaughtered, made a famous speech, "From here to where the sun sets, I shall fight no more forever," then the proud and independent people were forced to live on a reservation. Many of their magnificent

Appaloosas were destroyed, the Calvary's idea to limit the tribe's migrations and any possible retaliation. Fortunately, like the buffalo, a few of the pretty spotted horses survived to continue the breed into present times, bred surreptiously by whites who could not let the breed die.

Today, Appaloosas are popular trail and pack horses, as sure-footed on steep trails as their ancestors were for the gentle Nez Perce. Many of the most cherished Appaloosas have most blotches and spots on the rear end only; it is said that Joseph's favorite horse featured a spotted pattern on its rump that resembled a hand print, and so was known for its speed and spirit (as if the horse was continuously being slapped on the rump).

Chief Joseph's memory lives on in Joseph Days, a festival every summer in the hamlet of Joseph.

Joseph Creek slashes through a very steep and rugged gorge which may be viewed on top from

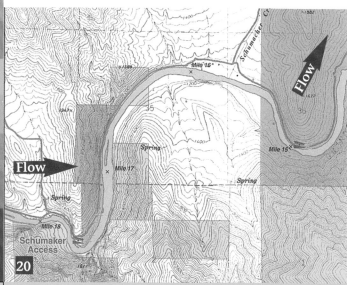

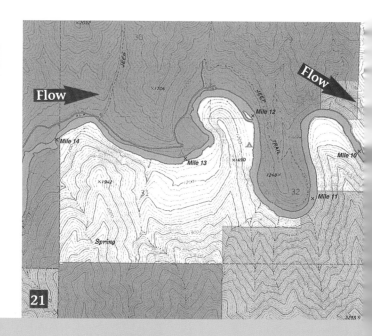

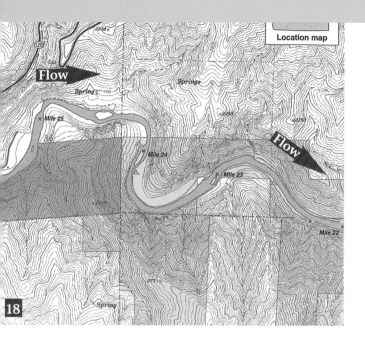

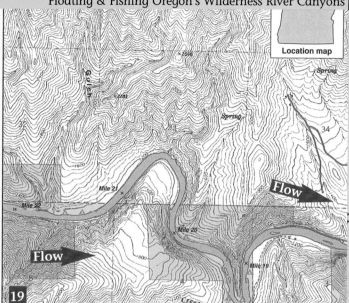

Highway 3 during the shuttle drive. The spirit of the determined leader surely lingers in the winds that sweep the high rimrock.

2.9: Bridge Rapid, Class II-III (41.2) happens just before the county road crosses the river. Large waves and occasionally troublesome turbulence mark the last whitewater on the Grande Ronde River. Both sides of the river here are Wildlife Areas (right bank only .5 mile below).

2.0: WDW Fishing Access (42.1), river left, alternate take-out, camping.

0.0: 45 miles from Troy, the Grande Ronde confluences with the Snake River in Hell's Canyon. Stay near river left to reach Heller Bar, the takeout (limited services available), .25 mile downstream, river left.

The Snake is a big, broad river that is easy to get lost in; be alert. Floaters must also be aware of power boats once on the Snake, watching for wakes, as well as keeping part of the boat ramp clear for launching/loading power boats to avoid "user conflicts". Right bank is now Idaho.

The nearest outpost of civilization is Asotin, Washington, 23 miles north. If you miss the takeout, the next major stop along the river is Lewiston, Idaho.

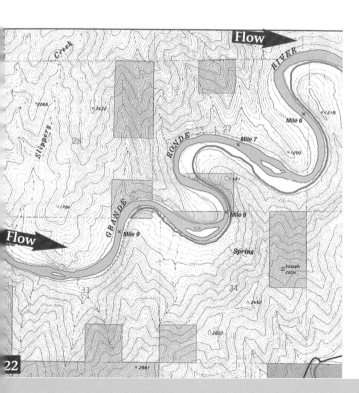

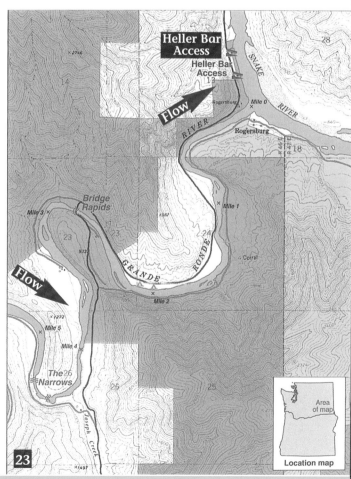

Lower Deschutes River

CHAPTER 6

Lower Deschutes River
100 miles from Pelton Dam to Columbia River

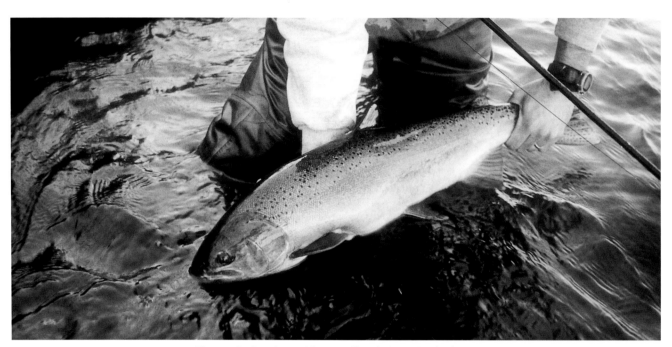

Fly-caught Deschutes River steelhead. Scott Cook photo.

THE DESCHUTES IS A WORLD-CLASS NATIVE TROUT fishery, with many hatches taking place almost year-round.

Additionally, the river and its scenic desert canyon offers a warm, dry refuge to residents of Portland, Seattle and other "wet side of the mountains" dwellers. Bend, a popular tourist destination, is still two hours away from the lower Deschutes (the "upper upper" Deschutes flows through Bend, where much of the river is channeled off into irrigation tracks). The lower Deschutes is fed by Pelton Regulating Dam, but also by natural aquifers, enough water in this volcanic desert land to grow mint and lavish golf courses in addition to trout.

Natives called this great river of the desert "Towornehiooks", with Lewis and Clark recording the name as best they could; on their return trip, they changed the name to Clarks River. Easier to spell, perhaps. Klamath tribes called it the "place of the kolam root", possibly a reference to balsamroot, which is still collected today for the Warm Springs Root Festival, along with wild onion, bitterroot and other desert plants.

As fur trading began, with many French trappers in the area, the river became known as Riviere des Chutes, or "River of the Falls", not for the whitewater of the Deschutes, but for the falls on the Columbia near its mouth (now buried under dam backwaters). Explorer Peter Skene Ogden (Ogden State Park at the Crooked, a major tributary) refers to Deschutes as early as 1826. The name is pronounced "duh-shoots" or sometimes "dee-shoots."

The lower Deschutes is divided into two parts: "Upper" from Warm Springs to Sherars Falls, and "Lower lower" from various put-ins below Sherars/Buckhollow to its confluence with the Columbia. The upper canyon, especially in the Mutton Mountains area, is more varied and colorful, with the lower canyon mostly deeper basalt. The upper is favored for trout fishing, especially by fly-anglers, while the lower's summer and fall steelhead runs are considered superior. Both sections make excellent drifts. (There is no "float fishing" by strict definition here, as angling from a floating device has been prohibited for many years, but often float-in is the only public access to river banks.)

There is little float-in fishing with floatable whitewater on the reaches near Bend, due to the presence of many large waterfalls (Pringle, Big Falls, Steelhead, Dillon, Lava Island), although there are quiet canoeing sections above Bend. Without water in season, the stretch from

Bend downstream to Billy Chinook Reservoir is a shadow of its former self, still good fishing but not pleasant floating, with the constant dragging over rocks (the section gets as low as 100 cfs) and the nerve-racking alertness necessary to avoid being swept over a falls. Also, much land there is private. Maps of float sections above Bend, on public lands, are available from the Deschutes National Forest.

Warm Springs to Maupin or Sandy Beach (Upper section)

Location

Central Oregon, two hours' drive from Portland or Bend. From Portland, take Highway 26 over Mt. Hood to town of Warm Springs.

The launch is located just south of town, upstream of the bridge crossing the Deschutes. From Bend, take Hwy. 97 north to Madras (closest town for gas, other services); at northernmost edge of town, veer left onto Highway 26 which winds down into the Deschutes River Canyon. The launch will be located on your left just before the bridge. Very busy on Friday and Saturday (arrive very early or launch mid-week, trailered boats have priority at the back-in ramp).

No camping is allowed at Warm Springs, but the road to Mecca Camp is on the right (east) side before you cross the bridge over the river (take the upper road).

Personality

The Deschutes is a big, powerful river flowing through the heart of the Central Oregon desert. Unlike most desert rivers, however, waters of the Deschutes are cool and almost always a brilliant blue-green, perfect for fly-fishing, as well as swimming and body-surfing big waves. This stretch of the river runs through a canyon of colorful rhyolite rock formations. Ancient lava flows have left pillars, slabs and rimrock of pure basalt, the gray-black rock that composes most of the canyon.

This portion of the Deschutes has a railroad paralleling the river first on the right bank, then left at North Junction; a private road from Locked Gate near Maupin upstream almost to Whitehorse Rapid; the Warm Springs Indian Reservation on river left downstream nearly to Dant, with roads into the river at Dry Creek and across from Whiskey Dick camp; the scattered homes of ranchers and the Deschutes River Club (cabins used mostly for fishing vacations)—yet, the feeling of being in a wild canyon remains, especially in the Mutton Mountains stretch.

The canyon is now known for its osprey population, which has grown from a single nest when I first floated the river in 1981 to dozens of nests in present day. Nesting platforms were installed and power poles specially roofed to encourage these "fish hawks" to nest in safe areas. They have responded by building elaborate stick nests, some adorned with bright orange flagging tape scavenged from ranches and roadsides. Golden eagles nest high in the rimrock and may be glimpsed soaring overhead, while turkey vultures glide endlessly on thermal currents, waiting for the desert's next victim. Notable bird life also includes the nighthawk, a bat-like bird that swoops over the river in early twilight, making a "whoosh" like a bull-roarer as it snatches insects from the air.

Difficulty

Class III+, advanced intermediate, with Whitehorse Rapid sometimes rated Class IV.

Trout must be stalked carefully on the Deschutes—if you can see them clearly, chances are they can see you. Watch your shadow, as fish are on the lookout for predators such as osprey swooping down from above.

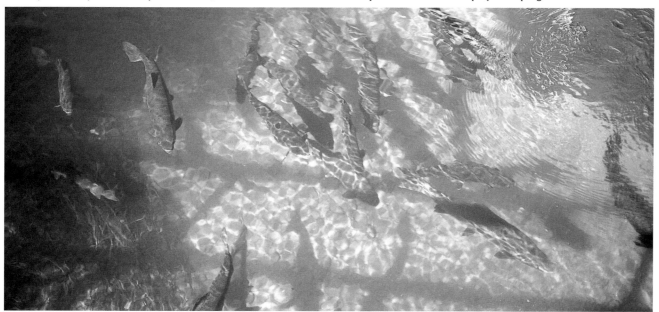

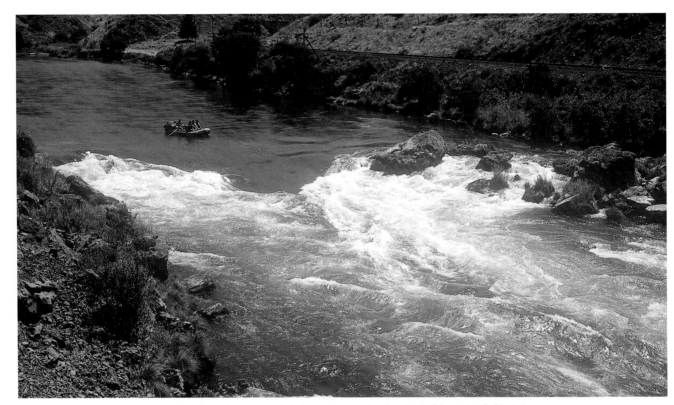

From a high vantage, the V-slick, or tongue, is clearly visible at Buckskin Mary.
The tip of this downstream-V points directly at the safest route.

However, the rapids are very straightforward and as such are often successfully navigated by novices. The rapids are, except for Whitehorse, classic pool and drop, mostly forgiving to beginners. Whitehorse is definitely a IV for driftboats and other craft that don't do well bouncing off rocks.

Gradient

12 fpm. The Deschutes flows at this steady pace for most of the lower 100 miles, so even flat stretches have stronger currents than the novice can discern.

Mileage/Days

Warm Springs to Trout Creek, 1 day, 9 miles. This is a good day trip for fishing, without major whitewater. Class I+ with some minor rocks, riffles, gravel bars and side channels as obstacles.

Novice float-anglers can add an overnight at, say, Frog Springs Camp, to fully appreciate the time needed to fish and appreciate this stretch of prime fishing water. Good hatches along this section.

Warm Springs to Maupin, 2-5 days, 45.5 miles. This is a popular 2- to 3-day float, but for fishing, 4-5 days is better, since fishing from the boat is not allowed. The constant stops and wading, fish-stalking, removing flies from overhanging branches, etc. requires time and patience. The gradient is fairly fast in flat sections for pool and drop, allowing tardy boaters to make good time even against the wind.

Trout Creek to Maupin, 2-5 days, 44.6 miles. You only save an hour's float time launching at Trout Creek, versus the extra time required to drive into Gateway Recreation Site. The South Junction, a former 2-day trip launch site further downstream, is now closed to boat launches (but open for fishing access).

Maupin to Sandy Beach, 6 miles, 1/2 day. Many boaters eager for whitewater add this half of the "Maupin run" to their overnight trips. Eight rapids rated Class II or above (One, Oak Springs, is a Class III+ to IV) attract the splash-and-giggle crowd, but are fun to float.

Unloading cargo is usually easier at the Maupin City Park take-out (fee required) than at Sandy Beach take-out. Commercial driftboat fishing trips disembark at Harpham Flat.

Average Float Levels/Seasons

The 100 miles of the Deschutes below Pelton Regulating Dam boasts a reliable, year-round ideal flow of 3,000 to 6,000 cfs, with a summer average about 3,500 cfs. Water levels are recorded at the Moody gauge.

High-Water Season

Winter storms November to April may bring the river up somewhat, seldom to the extent of the *La Nina* event in February, 1996 (over 70,000 cfs, with outhouses floating down the river and roads under water).

Most high water averages 6,000 to 10,000 cfs with Whitehorse Rapid being much easier to run, its washboard rocks covered over. Both Oak Springs and Boxcar swell to enormous proportions during very high water. A few wave sets that barely rate a Class I+ in moderate conditions gush to haystack size in flooding (particularly in spots where the river is funneled through a narrow slot).

With its excellent summer and fall steelheading, few people bother to attempt the Deschutes in winter or early spring, even though there are hatches year-round. The first big fishing event begins in May, with the giant stonefly hatch.

One thrill of a run on the lower section of Whitehorse when the river is higher, say about 4,500 cfs or greater, is a reversal dubbed The Dungeon as even a large raft disappears into darkness beneath a wall of water (if the hole is hit correctly). This spot is easily avoidable; in fact, most boaters simply float by in mid-stream, unaware of the turbulent drop just a few feet further to their right.

Low-Water Season

Thanks to a fortunate combination of its enormous groundwater reserves—flowing through porous volcanic basalt rock—and the Pelton Regulating Dam, which re-releases water from the reservoir, the Deschutes runs so constant that the river is considered "Mr. Reliable" when other rivers are too high or low or too murky to float and/or fish.

There is almost never a level below 3,000 cfs along the lower 100 miles of river (the record low of 2,400 cfs

was set in December 1957). Flows of 3,000 to 3,500 encountered in August and early September make minor changes in routes; the only two rapids tougher in lower water are Whitehorse (more washboards) and Oak Springs (sharp shelves of basalt below the main drop await like shark teeth, ready to chomp on the helpless legs and arms of boaters tossed overboard). Many boaters consider the Maupin run better in low water, with waves at Wapinita, Surf City, White River and Elevator (both upper and lower) actually delivering more bounce.

Craft

All craft float the Deschutes. Those using open canoes and driftboats must be very experienced to avoid crash-and-burn runs at Whitehorse and Oak Springs. Many boaters, including rank beginners, rent inflatable kayaks or buy discount store "rubber duckies" and run all the rapids, usually gleefully unaware of any risk. Inflatable rafts of the 12- to 14-foot range do exceptionally well, with almost no real flip risks other than Boxcar and Oak Springs, or broadsiding the notorious rock located in the middle of Whitehorse.

Permits

No lottery-type permits are required as yet, although a limited-entry system is being considered (try to launch on days other than Friday-Saturday from Warm Springs and

The best part of the upper Deschutes run: Whitehorse Canyon down to Buckskin Mary camps. Linger as long as you can.

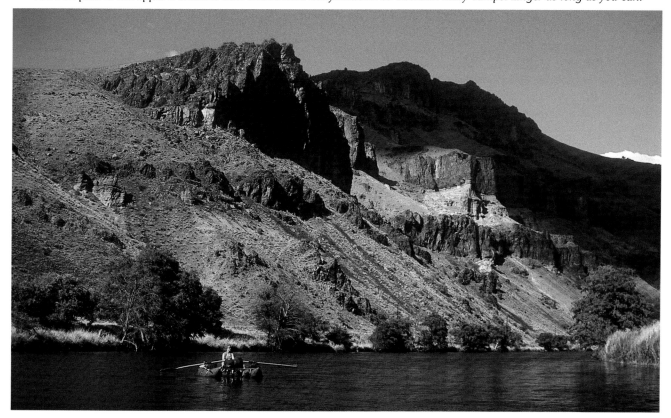

Lower Deschutes River

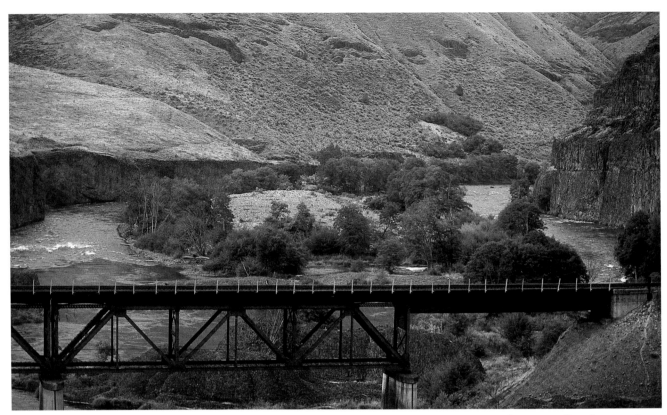

Train trestle over the lower Deschutes crossing from Buckhollow to Macks Canyon. Competition between railroad companies resulted in such "dirty pool" as the two teams tried to slow each other down with unexpected rattlesnake deliveries and arson.

Trout Creek whenever you can, or run the day section from Harpham to Sandy Beach on weekdays, not weekends).

Boater passes are required for all floaters and must be purchased in advance of the trip (available at local stores and on the Internet). These are $2-5 per person per day (more on summer weekends; additionally, the BLM tags boats launching at Harpham Flat on summer weekends). Especially watch for new regulations, and for old rules with big fines if violated (fire season, boating while intoxicated, etc.)

Persons planning to fish or camp on lands belonging to the Confederated Tribes (left bank) need a special permit and location map.

Hazards

Cold water, even on a 100-degree day. Rattlesnakes are common in grassy areas, especially right along the river where anglers must walk to access bank fishing. Ticks are present, especially in spring.

Black widow spiders lurk under rocks and in old buildings, even in outhouses. Scorpions are scary, but yellow jackets, common in late summer or around left-behind trash, kill more people (yet another reason to pack up your trash). Especially watch pop and beer cans, as yellow jackets can crawl inside, unseen, then sting on the mouth or in the throat.

Wildfire is a special risk in Deschutes country. Follow smoking and fire regulations closely. Pick up used butts (besides a fire hazard, these are ugly, can poison wildlife, and never decompose). In case of fire, stay on or near the river. Begin floating downstream as soon as possible; since the Deschutes winds almost always blow upstream, you can out-run the smoke. Strong winds may also limit mileage, especially in the afternoon.

The intense desert sun can cause problems if boaters do not waterfight, swim, jump overboard, or wrap a wet cloth around head/neck. Sunglasses are essential for eye protection from the sun. Polarized glasses help you spot fish and rocks lurking ahead when the sun is blinding. Broad-brimmed hats and neck cloths (like Lawrence of Arabia) blunt the glare and rays (also can be wetted down for additional cooling). Drink water often (but again, not the river unless filtered).

Skunks in camps present a unique hazard. To discourage them, hang garbage high and keep a clean kitchen. Spotted skunks are brazen enough to stroll into camp as twilight settles, as well as staging midnight raids. They have the right of way; keep your distance and don't tease them or throw objects.

Poison hemlock and water hemlock grow lush along the Deschutes. Both plants can kill. They resemble wild carrot or parsnips. Poison oak is present, appearing with leaf tips more pointed, much like Eastern poison ivy. The rash that results from touching it is the same, however. Jimson weed, a large riverside plant with trumpet-shaped flowers, also contains poisonous compounds. Small white flowers that resemble a wild lily might be Death Camas. Rather than risk illness, or deplete the desert of fragile vegetation, eat the foods you bring with you. Nettles may be seen in boggy areas; they sting, but the hurt is short-lived. Many of these poisonous plants are found along other Oregon rivers, too, so learn them.

Trespassing on private land, even unknowingly, is taboo and landowners are likely to prosecute. Especially avoid the Indian Reservation, islands in the reservation area, fishing on the left side of the river without a tribal permit to do so, Deschutes Club land and cabins. Most private lands are marked with yellow signs (Reservation land), BLM markers, or regular "keep out" signs and fencing.

River courtesy is vital to avoid "river rage" (don't intrude on another group, camp at a distance; be very courteous of bank anglers as you float past, etc.).

The rare hummingbird moth looks and acts like a hummingbird as it feeds on "bouncing Betty" wildflowers.

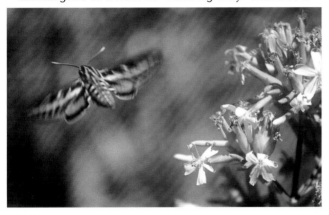

Waterfights, particularly in the Maupin stretch, can become ferocious and a strong stance (whistle, stern voice) is necessary to deter drenchings. It's not uncommon for a novice rafter to float right over the line of a shore fisherman. Try to signal those "uncouth" boaters that you are fishing (without using the middle finger, please). Limit time on boat ramps. Practice good camping ethics; for example, "micro-trash" such as cigarette butts and bread ties left in camps never decompose, serve only as an ugly reminder of the carelessness of others.

Fishing

"It's the best in the West," for fly-fishing trout, says Bend guide Scott Cook. Anglers are drawn to the Deschutes by a strong summer steelhead run, combined with big native redside trout that gorge on giant stoneflies and attack hatches year-round. There is limited walk-in fishing—so floating in opens up much more water for fishing, especially mid-week. Anglers are reminded that fishing from a floating device is illegal. (Consult a current copy of the ODFW regulations before planning your trip;

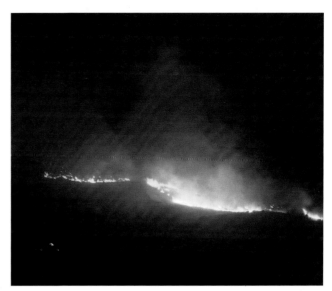

Fire is a constant concern in Deschutes country. Fires have closed portions of the river to floaters in recent years.

note, a handicapped angler may fish from the boat with a special permit.)

Only artificial flies and lures may be used. Practice catch and release for native fish. (To safely release a fish, handle it as little as possible. Wet your hands first. Fish, and trout in particular, need to retain their "slime" coating to be healthy. Don't squeeze, limit use of a net, keep the fish in the water as much as possible, and help the fish recover before you let it go. Never throw a trout back overboard, release it gently at the surface.)

A study of the lower 100 miles of the Deschutes trout fishery made years ago revealed that these measures are working: ODFW estimated there are an average of 2,000 trout over eight inches long for every mile of river!

Another reminder: the Deschutes is a difficult and dangerous river to wade. Fishermen are lost nearly every season to the swift current. Wade with a buddy, wear waders that won't hold you down, and if swept away by current, get into the "lawn chair position" to keep your feet from getting caught under rocks. Wade with extreme caution. Rocks are slippery, and this is a big and powerful river. Besides watching out for your safety, consider that you must cover a lot of water while fishing in order to score fish. Don't let the excitement get to you, and beware of hypothermia, heat stroke, rattlesnakes, exhaustion and other dangers of a coldwater river in the broiling desert. I rate the Deschutes as a Class 4 fishing river (expert) for those on their own; it's easier with a guide.

With Pelton Regulating Dam releasing a steady volume of 50-degree water (which warms to about 65 degrees both downstream and in late summer), the entire river is a tailwater fishery, sustaining a world-famous native trout and steelhead population. Because the most trout are near the colder waters of the dam, fishing from the bank and/or floating from Warm Springs to Trout Creek (1-2 days) are popular.

Fishing for trout is excellent, but wading has limitations. Usually you must scramble among shoreline brush, duck under trees, chase off rattlesnakes or skunks, and then risk getting your fly stuck in an overhanging cottonwood, as this is where the fish are. Deschutes trout sometimes lurk in deep pools, but they prefer the shade under trees and bushes next to shore, which hides them from predators, as well as providing them with a source of bugs to eat. If you can cast behind rocks or sneak up on shallows near gravel bars, these also yield fish. Most anglers fly-fish, but traditional lures are used by some. Those trusty Roostertails have caught many trout on many Oregon rivers. The basic spoon lure hoodwinks trout in addition to steelhead. Hardware works best in deeper pools and currents, the opposite of good for fly-fishing. Several guides recommend using "a lot of black and purple" in the Deschutes canyon.

The Deschutes "redsides" are a large, thick-slabbed version of the rainbow trout. Some anglers compare them to footballs due to their shape. Redsides average 12 to 15 inches with an occasional muscular 18- to 20-incher waiting to tow you and your rod downstream. They tend to stay in their territory, about a mile of river, for their entire lives. Wild trout tend to strike even if not hungry when something is in their territory. If properly handled during release, the same redside can provide thrills for numerous anglers.

The Hook Fly Shop at Sunriver (resort out of Bend) suggests nymphs and dry flies, size 14-16 Hare's Ears, green copper, all caddis imitations, and Parachute Adams'.

The Deschutes is also renowned for its reliable hatches. Hatches occur year-round, with the Deschutes one of the few Oregon rivers where bugs hatch vigorously even in autumn. The easiest way to see what is hatching is to row your boat under an overhanging branch and hit the branch with your oar. Bugs will fall into the boat, where they can be examined up close and identified. Fly shops from Bend to the Columbia Gorge stand ready to sell you classic and modern Deschutes patterns. Not unusual, especially early evening, is what I call a "Bug Tornado" with thousands of hatch bugs swirling in a funnel like a Kansas twister. With hatches of this magnitude, early twilight brings out the bats, swallows and nighthawks for an aerial feeding frenzy.

One popular time to fish is May and June, when the salmonflies (stoneflies) emerge. Before then, an imitation nymph works. Once these big (2- to 4-inch-long) red-orange insects have hatched, the trout engage in a feeding frenzy. Orange caddisflies hatch alongside the stonefly, besides later in summer, and trout love them almost as

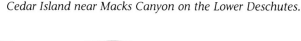

Cedar Island near Macks Canyon on the Lower Deschutes.

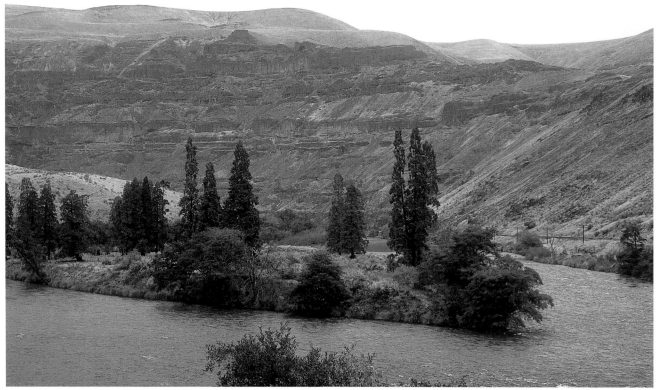

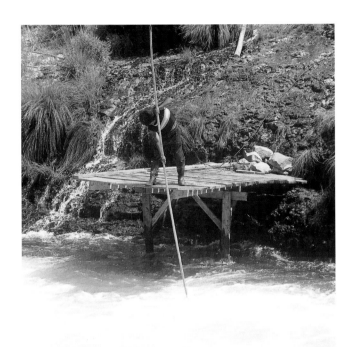

*Natives still dip nets for salmon, as they have
for thousands of years on the Deschutes.*

much as they savor the stonefly. Most caddisfly larva imitations work, too. Work nymphs bumping slowly along the bottom, as real insects crawl. The best hatches happen on the upper run, when the bushes are almost covered with the huge ugly critters. If your fly collection doesn't include a stonefly or stonefly nymph, you can buy these locally or tie one on the spot. Make it big and ugly.

Another stonefly hatch occurs concurrently or later than the big orange "salmonfly": the smaller yellow stonefly. The first weeks of June are when the weather and water conditions combine for fantastic fly-fishing. "The fish (redsides) really bulk up," says Cook. Then, as the last pupae open, "the fish are kind of full, there are fewer bugs, and they tend to not be quite as picky—more willing to come up and take an imitation." Different things trigger a hatch, according to Cook, such as cloud cover and water temperature.

Many other popular dry-fly patterns used on the Deschutes include the March Brown, Elk Hair Caddis, Adams, Dave's Hopper, and the Mac Salmon, as well as other "emerger" imitations. Deschutes trout take midges, damselflies, the pupae of flying insects, and mayflies (sometimes confused with the salmon/stonefly that also emerges in May). "Hare's Ears, Adams', Royal Wulff, and Elk Hair Caddises," suggests Jason Blackman of Numb Butt Fly Company. "There are 200 different patterns." His shop handles specialized Deschutes patterns: the Stimulator, the Rastarman Stone Fly, Kaufman's Stonefly (fished dry or wet), and the Girdle Bug.

However, trout are also opportunists and will take crawfish, grasshoppers (in late summer and early fall),

periwinkles (water snails) and smaller fish. Most trout will not rise to a fly unless there is a hatch happening, unless you fish areas where shoreline vegetation is dumping bugs into the water, although the territorial instinct sometimes kicks in when they see something strange.

Most fly-anglers on the Deschutes cast nymphs on the bottom, cast dry flies upstream, and work caddis pupae downstream. Here your ability to "read" the river to avoid obstacles, to understand what the bottom of the river looks like and how it affects river currents will prove useful in finding fish hangouts. Trout like structure, such as rocky fields on river bottoms, where they can gorge on nymphs while taking a break from fighting the current. Eddies behind rocks are the perfect redside habitat, offering fish the equivalent of a La-Z-Boy chair complete with a bowl of chips (bugs floating through). More insects emerge in August, so check under rocks near shore to find "burrowing" and "clinging" nymphs; also, examine shoreline greenery for evidence of empty pupae and winged adults.

Eddies near shore are good fishing, especially under brush or branches and in the tailouts (end currents). Root wads, downed logs, and other hook-munchers hide trout, too. Look for water of moderate depth (two to six feet) for fly-fishing, so the fish can see your offering.

Approach any sign of fish, or a rise (subtle on the Deschutes, watch for a swirl on the surface or a glimpse of a fin), or water that appears to be good habitat. You may not see any sign of the fish itself, but move towards the water stealthily. Be aware of where your shadow falls, and don't splash around when wading. Deschutes trout are smart due to heavy angling pressure, many of the larger redsides have been caught and released and almost seem to sense a hook or an angler.

At one camp in the Whiskey Dick area, our group stopped to scout available sites downstream. Since I'd sprained an ankle (back in the city), I stayed behind. Also nursing a sore lower back, I waded out and sat in the river up to my waist. (Try this for about 30 minutes, wearing shorts, and you too can become a member of the "Numb Butt Society"). After a few minutes of sitting quietly, a large trout—about 17 inches—cleared the surface. On my next trip a week later, what appeared to be the exact same fish jumped again in the same small eddy. I think that fish knew my rod was buried under the cargo!

Nymphs are best fished on the river bottom, not dangling above it, which does not look real to a redside; weight your line accordingly. Stonefly nymphs are heavy and hard to finesse as one would a delicate nymph imitation. Caddis larvae, the little tubes made of stuck-together bits of rock that house the caddis nymph, can be cast downstream so that they move at an angle to the current. Trout love these so much that when you cut a trout open, a look at the stomach contents will often reveal empty caddis larva cases—pebbles and all!

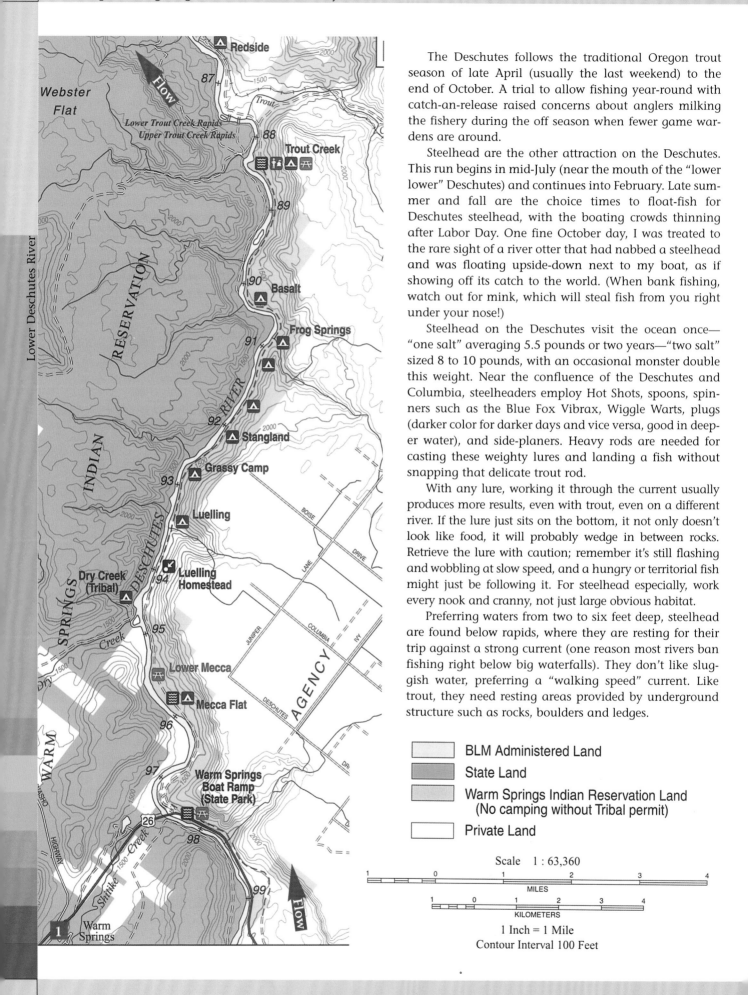

The Deschutes follows the traditional Oregon trout season of late April (usually the last weekend) to the end of October. A trial to allow fishing year-round with catch-an-release raised concerns about anglers milking the fishery during the off season when fewer game wardens are around.

Steelhead are the other attraction on the Deschutes. This run begins in mid-July (near the mouth of the "lower lower" Deschutes) and continues into February. Late summer and fall are the choice times to float-fish for Deschutes steelhead, with the boating crowds thinning after Labor Day. One fine October day, I was treated to the rare sight of a river otter that had nabbed a steelhead and was floating upside-down next to my boat, as if showing off its catch to the world. (When bank fishing, watch out for mink, which will steal fish from you right under your nose!)

Steelhead on the Deschutes visit the ocean once— "one salt" averaging 5.5 pounds or two years—"two salt" sized 8 to 10 pounds, with an occasional monster double this weight. Near the confluence of the Deschutes and Columbia, steelheaders employ Hot Shots, spoons, spinners such as the Blue Fox Vibrax, Wiggle Warts, plugs (darker color for darker days and vice versa, good in deeper water), and side-planers. Heavy rods are needed for casting these weighty lures and landing a fish without snapping that delicate trout rod.

With any lure, working it through the current usually produces more results, even with trout, even on a different river. If the lure just sits on the bottom, it not only doesn't look like food, it will probably wedge in between rocks. Retrieve the lure with caution; remember it's still flashing and wobbling at slow speed, and a hungry or territorial fish might just be following it. For steelhead especially, work every nook and cranny, not just large obvious habitat.

Preferring waters from two to six feet deep, steelhead are found below rapids, where they are resting for their trip against a strong current (one reason most rivers ban fishing right below big waterfalls). They don't like sluggish water, preferring a "walking speed" current. Like trout, they need resting areas provided by underground structure such as rocks, boulders and ledges.

BLM Administered Land

State Land

Warm Springs Indian Reservation Land
    (No camping without Tribal permit)

Private Land

Scale   1 : 63,360

MILES

KILOMETERS

1 Inch = 1 Mile
Contour Interval 100 Feet

Steelhead also favor the "line" that separates fast current from slow, eddy lines and tailouts. You don't have to wade to neck-deep water—sometimes steelhead are right next to shore, under the trees much like trout. Fish like "riffly" water because it's oxygenated. Don't cast to the same spot each time, vary your casts. Try three feet out, thirty feet out, and so forth.

Steelhead must be stalked like a trout, especially by fly-anglers, as their "lure" won't cast as far as a spoon or Hot Shot. Cast your offering from upstream at an angle to the current, so that it floats into the holding water. Let the offering float naturally, don't help. Steelhead may follow a fly before grabbing it, so be patient and don't yank. Most steelhead hook themselves on a fly. Many fishing guides claim their clients land more wild steelhead than hatchery fish, with experts speculating the reason is wild fish, especially steelhead and salmon, are more territorial, attacking anything in their "turf". They may follow your fly and not accept it, so cast each stretch of water thoroughly, even if you don't see signs of fish.

Numb Butts uses nymphs, egg patterns, girdle bugs and stonefly nymphs on Deschutes River steelhead. In the Macks Canyon area (lower lower), they prefer the Green Butt Skunk and Purple Peril.

Salmon fishing is possible on the Deschutes, depending on the season and the size of the season's "run" of fish. Regulations vary, so consult ODFW. Generally, the Warm Springs Confederated Tribes is the only area that allows limited bait fishing a certain distance below Sherars Falls, on property they own. Sherars is worth a look just to see migratory fish jumping at the waterfall and wiggling through the fish ladder (river left), and to contemplate the awesome forces of nature that created this thundering cascade. No floating is allowed here.

"We don't fish for salmon on the Deschutes very often," says Blackman. "The water's all wrong for flies." Salmon prefer the deep pools, which are hard to work with any fly.

When salmon fishing is allowed, anglers use heavy rods, 12-pound-test line, and terminal rigs of salmon eggs or other bait, usually "dressed up" with red wool or Spin N Glos plus a good chunk of lead weight (3 to 5 ounces). Put the rig onto the river bottom and let it bounce, with no slack in the line, so you can feel these giants take. Salmon may mouth bait or lures without the angler feeling anything, perhaps just that the line has stopped.

If you yank and it pulls back, you probably have a salmon. If the line doesn't give, you have a "rock fish" (stuck on a rock, kiss your terminal rig goodbye). Try not to let snagging a "trash" fish ruin your day. Northern pike minnow, or squawfish, are so hated for their destruction of fry that the state offers a cash bounty on these Columbia/tributary water "suckers". Many anglers throw them onto shore to die, where they feed mink, muskrat, turkey vulture, and other scavengers.

Managing Agency

Prineville Bureau of Land Management, 3050 NE 3rd St., Prineville OR 97754. 541/416-6700. List of authorized fishing/float trip outfitters and rental companies. Also: Confederated Tribes of Warm Springs (permits at Warm Springs Market).

Shuttles

Widely available.

The Oasis Resort, Maupin, OR 541/395-2611. Their sister store, **River Central**, is the place to go during the busy summer months for shuttles, boater passes, flies and T-shirts. Guided fishing trips and fly-fishing lessons available. From Portland, pick up a driver in Maupin for a lower fee. Also shuttles lower river.

Linda's Shuttles, Maupin OR 541/225-4632 or 1-877-225-4632. 24-passenger buses available for large groups to avoid carpooling.

Tim Sturgeon "Fish", Madras OR 541/475-6009. Will meet you at Warm Springs Launch so your car doesn't sit there.

Deschutes River U-Boat, Maupin OR 541/395-2503. Raft rentals, delivery, shuttles, store, boater passes.

River Mileage And Landmarks

Mile   Landmark   (RM= river mile from mouth)

0: Warm Springs Boat Ramp (state park). (RM 95) Boat ramp, raft rigging area (no ramp, blocked by boulders), outhouses, garbage service. No camping allowed. Watch gear closely here, keep all your equipment together in one site rather than spread all over. Things disappear when others mistake your stuff for theirs, and thieves sometimes work the area. Many people prefer to have cars shuttled rather than leave them at this site.

When floating under the highway bridge, give the piers a large berth. The current slamming into them is surprisingly strong.

There are several small, enjoyable Class I+ rapids for the next few miles. Avoid floating close to shore on river right over gravel beds, which are spawning beds for steelhead and easily damaged. Also, do not wade or fish the beds (signs informing of the beds are usually present).

1.6: Mecca Flat, river right, campground, vehicle access from the town of Warm Springs (only legal camping in the Warm Springs area, fee required). To access this area, locate gravel roads just west of the Warm Springs launch site (east of the Deschutes bridge). Access for boat launching (unimproved ramp, traction issues for trailered boats), fishing and the 7.6-mile trail to Trout Creek. The trail follows an old railroad bed.

Mecca was a station on the old Oregon Trunk railroad line and had a post office established in 1911. This name probably derived from the fact that this portion of the Deschutes Canyon was considered the worst

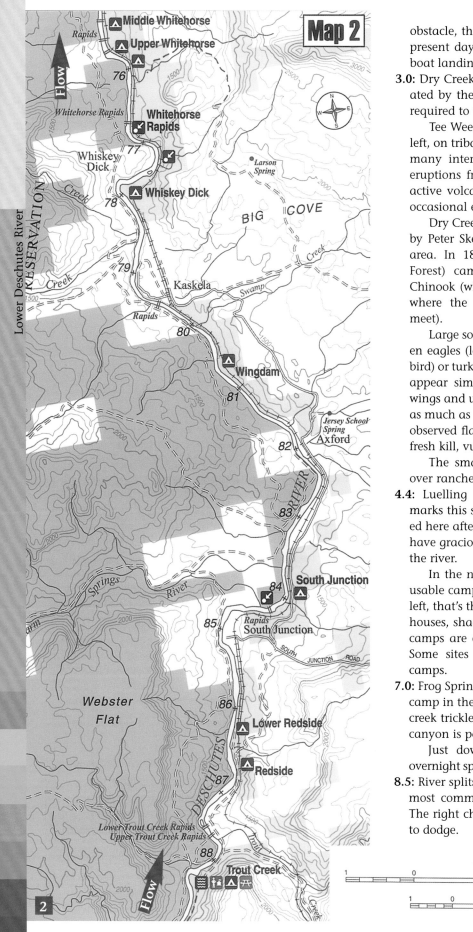

obstacle, thus getting there was the promised land. In present day, Mecca lures many fly-fishermen with its boat landing, camping and walk-in access to the river.

3.0: Dry Creek, river left. This is a fee campground operated by the Warm Springs Tribes. A special permit is required to use this camp.

Tee Wees Butte is the large rock formation on river left, on tribal land. This stretch to Trout Creek contains many interesting volcanic/basalt shapes created by eruptions from nearby Mt. Hood, still considered an active volcano with its steam vents, hot springs and occasional earthquakes.

Dry Creek Flat was the site of several winter fordings by Peter Skene Ogden, the first white explorer in this area. In 1843, John C. Fremont (Fremont National Forest) camped here with his Native guide, Billy Chinook (whose name was later given to the reservoir where the Crooked, Metolius and Deschutes rivers meet).

Large soaring birds seen in this region may be golden eagles (look for the glint of "gold" underneath the bird) or turkey vultures. Both have large wingspans and appear similar, except that golden eagles flap their wings and usually are alone or in a pair. Vultures glide as much as possible to conserve energy and are seldom observed flapping wings. In a good thermal or over a fresh kill, vultures circle in groups of three or more.

The smaller redtail hawk is also seen, especially over ranchers' pastures.

4.4: Luelling Campsite, river right. A seasonal creek marks this small group site. The Luellings homesteaded here after acquiring the land from the railroad and have graciously granted public access from the trail to the river.

In the next 2.3 miles, there are approximately 12 usable campsites on river right (remember, avoid river left, that's the reservation). Sites vary as to having outhouses, shade, good landing areas, and privacy. Most camps are easily located by watching for outhouses. Some sites are close together, counted as separate camps.

7.0: Frog Springs campsite, river right. This is the choicest camp in the area above Trout Creek. A beautiful, clear creek trickles through the site and some hiking up the canyon is possible. Watch for rattlesnakes here.

Just downstream is Basalt camp, another nice overnight spot with towering cliffs behind the open flats.

8.5: River splits around a large island. The left channel is most commonly taken and is fairly straightforward. The right channel is tight with a few interesting rocks to dodge.

Scale   1 : 63,360

MILES

KILOMETERS

9.4: Trout Creek Campground, river right. (RM87) The 2000-foot-deep canyon opens as you approach this large flat. Except for trees near the river, the sun bears down on this graveled site. Picnic tables may be used for setting up lunch, but camping requires a fee. There is also a good boat ramp here (the takeout for one-day trips). A ranger station is manned here during the summer.

There are some strong eddies on both sides of the river here. Veteran boaters often entertain themselves by having their greenhorn passengers take the oars and get "stuck" in these merry-go-rounds. Keep to the center flow to avoid them.

Trout Creek was the site of a fierce battle between Chief Paulina, of the Snake Indians, and the Warm Springs Confederated Tribes, who lived on the reservation. Paulina and his warriors raided the reservation for horses, cattle and food. His killing of both Natives and whites caused him to be despised by both sides. In the years of 1855-1867, the Tribes joined the calvary in the hunt for Paulina.

In 1867, Paulina stole cattle from a ranch owned by Andrew Clarno (John Day River pioneer). Local ranchers then joined the manhunt, including Mr. Howard Maupin, who is credited with killing the renegade. Paulina took two bullets from Maupin's Henry rifle, ending his reign of terror, at the Paulina Cove on Trout Creek. Years later, Maupin and family were buried in a small pioneer graveyard along the edge of the creek. (The Deschutes town of Maupin was named for this cattle rancher, postmaster of Antelope, veteran of the Mexican War and ferry boat operator on the Deschutes at the mouth of Bakeoven Creek.)

A plaque at Trout Creek Campground honors the preservationist Stewart Udall, former Secretary of the Interior: "Future generations will remember us for the roads we don't build."

The main river channel narrows and deepens as you leave this last outpost of civilization. This is a good place to jump overboard to cool off (never dive; always choose deep water for jumping). To your right, Trout Creek is a trickle with algae-slimed rocks. The roar ahead is the first serious whitewater.

10.1: Upper Trout Creek Rapid, Class II. Stay middle or left, dodge small rocks that protrude, and ride the small standing waves at the bottom. This is the warmup for the next drop.

10.3: Trout Creek Rapid, Class II+. River divides around an island. The left side is tempting, but is narrow enough to be blocked by strainers. River right is the safest and most fun route, with nice large haystacks at the bottom. A boulder protrudes at the rapid's head, almost midstream, and a few other rocks pop up in lower water. Once into the drop, keep your boat straight to avoid swamping in the waves.

11.2: Redside camp, river right. Two sites with outhouse. Just below is the lower Redside, one large camp.

Most camps on the Deschutes are easily identified by locating the light-green outhouses, which are visible from a good distance at times, occasionally hidden. Newer outhouses with handicapped access are brown and marked in Braille.

13.9: South Junction, river right below a wave train, is just downstream and across from the mouth of the Warm Springs River. This is a drive-in camp and fishing access (fee required). Boaters once lugged heavy gear up steps and across the train tracks to the river for a shorter 2-day trip, but this launch has been closed.

The Warm Springs River and tribe were named after the hot springs found upstream, where the Kah-Ne-Tah Resort diverts them into a giant outdoor swimming pool. There are other, hidden hot springs that were sacred sites for the Native Americans, as sweat lodges were for other tribes. The river is closed to the public unless escorted by tribal guides (inflatable kayak trips are available at the resort, which also has rental tipis, convention facilities, and a small casino).

At the confluence of the two rivers, fishing is excellent. Nature's best angler, the osprey, knows instinctively that this is the place to build a nest. The former power pole on river left is topped by the first nesting osprey in this area; a manmade platform built on river right in recent years was meant to lure them to a safer spot, but was ignored. New platforms in other territory, though, are now occupied. Young may be seen in this nest and others late May and June, or sitting in trees crying for attention as the adults teach them to fish later in the season.

The sight of an osprey plummeting to the river, actually submerging its body, and emerging with a squirming trout grasped in its talons is a special Deschutes experience. Osprey are said to score fish only once in ten dives, and they are known to rotate the fish in their talons so that its head faces forward, to improve flight aerodynamics. The "teenage" osprey often follow float fishermen downstream, hoping to grab a released cripple. Many trout hatcheries must place netting over rearing ponds to keep the opportunistic birds of prey out of the "free sushi" zone.

Reportedly the ODFW received photos of a large salmon an angler had landed which had an osprey corpse imbedded in its back. Apparently the bird had eyes bigger than its stomach, and once latched onto the oversize fish, could not release its talons before the salmon dove, drowning the osprey. The salmon, determined to spawn, kept swimming upstream, towing the dead bird along until it was mostly bones.

Osprey now nest on many platforms along this stretch as the generations have overcome DDT and other environmental perils. As their numbers grow, new nest sites are built every few miles, providing alert boaters with entertainment.

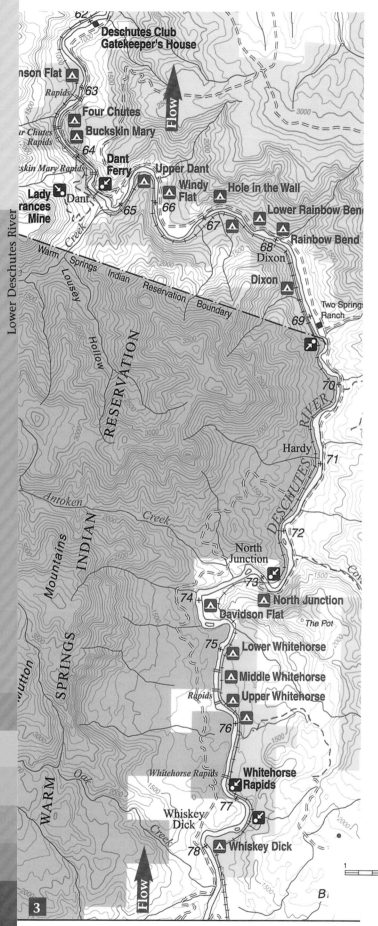

17.3: After several small riffles, Wingdam camp, river right, is reached. This is an open site with an obvious outhouse.

18.8: The "switching station" of Kaskela, now a few houses, is on river right. These houses were once homes for railroad workers, who expected to load logs floated down the Warm Springs River onto the Oregon Trunk, which never happened (the Tribes now have their own sawmill and bring in a good income logging trees on the highlands of their reservation). Kaskela was a Tribal chief. A set of unexpectedly large standing waves, Class II, provides a break from the flat water. Lands are private until the Whiskey Dick "peninsula" is reached.

From here you can see the Mutton Mountains, which make up the most remote section of the upper Deschutes float. They were named for wild mountain sheep that once lived in this area (mutton being the term for sheep meat, as venison is deer meat). References by Ogden in 1825 to "rimrock sheep" probably meant bighorn, which were native to the Deschutes Canyon but wiped out by domestic sheep diseases and over-hunting. Bighorns have been replanted on the lower Deschutes and will probably be re-introduced into the Mutton Mountains, as well. The river carves out a colorful canyon topped by the green-treed mountains beginning in the Whitehorse Rapids area down to North Junction. The Whitehorse drops were formed as the river cut through these unstable rock structures.

There is a rapid with washboard rocks, often laced with strainers, on river right that should be avoided. A prime camp's landing site is precariously tucked inside this danger zone, but a good boater can make the pull. This is the smallest landing site but has good brush shelter from winds. Large redside trout are often seen rising in this area.

As you come around the sharp left to right bend, there is a large rock nearly midstream that snags many a beginner. It resembles a fun wave when viewed at a distance. Weaker boaters should not only get right to avoid this rock, but also to cheat the inside of this bend if they wish to camp here. The left side has a strong current that is difficult to fight.

20.3: Whiskey Dick camp, river right. Four or more parties often jam in here as this is the last overnight spot before Whitehorse, and one of the best camps on a 3-day trip. In 1981, during my first float, we nicknamed this site "Lone Pine" because of the large, solo Ponderosa pine that marks the main, large campsite in

Scale   1 : 63,360

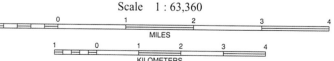

MILES

KILOMETERS

the middle of the flat. Seedling trees, maybe two feet high, were planted years later, with signs encouraging floaters to water them; now these former seedlings tower over humans. The pine is no longer lonely.

Many boaters construct tiny wing dams in the river to stop the water in wading pools (these are just piles of river rocks to build a pool, the river will wash them away in the next flood). The desirable lower camp tends to become a mudflat in summer since the flood of 1996 and may be difficult unloading. The last camps are higher on the bank but may be all that is available on a busy Friday night.

Tip: To find the best campsite for your group, land at the head of the Whiskey Dick flat. The very first camp is usually unoccupied, due to its difficult access across strainers, rocks, and strong currents, but the effort is worthwhile. This first camp is a nice camp for a group of 8 to 12 people, with excellent fishing. This camp also offers some shelter from storms or wind, and a little shade.

From here, tie your boats and walk the flat, checking all the sites, to see which ones are open, where the shade is, which fishing area looks good, the position of the outhouses, and so forth. If the lower camps are taken, you can stay here; if a better one is open, go for it. Old river saying: The last camp is better than the next camp (because you can't go upstream on a river once you've passed an open camp). Keep this in mind when floating other rivers. Also, sometimes you must take a camp that's at hand rather than try for a better one that might be occupied or not as nice as you thought.

The Whiskey Dick area is the best site to view the rare hummingbird moth, a moth that beats its wings and hovers exactly like a hummingbird. It feeds on nectar from flowers growing on this flat. Chasing it with a camera is good exercise.

20. 5: Island. Keep left; many anglers work the slow right arm of the river and will not appreciate an intruding boat. Staying in the left current also lets you warm up for Whitehorse, the most difficult rapid on this run in terms of length, just around the bend.

Landmarks for Whitehorse Rapid are the "warning shelf"—a **Class II+** rapid with rocks and waves, plus a large, orange-colored rock formation on river right. This volcanic outcropping is unstable due to strong pressures during lava flows, and rocks often break loose and tumble to the train tracks below. Wire fences hold back most rocks, while warning devices alert engineers to the presence of rocks on the tracks.

If you see a boulder on river right with "Whitehorse" written in white letters, it's too late to land! The river here sweeps sharply on a right bend, into Class III-IV water with currents lasting over a mile. A long swim after an overturned boat or overboard paddler is possible, and dangerous.

21: Two landing sites on river right allow tie up and scouting of Whitehorse; both are rough scrambles up loose gravel and poison oak. Be sure your boat is tied tight! When scouting, use the trail left of the tracks (walking on the tracks is considered dangerous, and is also considered trespassing).

Whitehorse (RM74.5) should be scouted at the entrance carefully, then checked downstream. I prefer to end a scout with another look at the entrance, because I believe a good entry makes for a good run in whitewater. Look for landmarks, such as a rock with tufts of grass on it, or a "tongue" (a perfect V-shape for entering a rapid) a certain distance from the big tree on shore, and fix these in your mind.

The river spreads very wide here; water does go "far left" but almost everyone runs the "right" side of the river. Divide this right channel into middle (expert route, currents take boats directly into "Oh, Shit!" rock, a notorious wrap/flip site), middle right (slip around rocks or go over the first small hydraulic for a good line, about 30 feet from shore), and far right (safe, the easiest route to be rescued from shore, but too far right deteriorates into a minefield of small rocks. Rafts can usually survive, but hard boats will take a thrashing).

Driftboaters like the middle right channel, where a small slick marks the proper entry. The boater must then maneuver quickly to miss an upcoming rock. This maneuver may be too tight for a large or heavy cargo raft, and for most beginners.

Those in large boats should stand to better see into the drop, as they approach. (Sit down for stability once you have the route identified.) Sideways at an angle to the current is best in rafts and catarafts, to increase vision and set up for pushing and/or pulling into final position.

Once past the entrance, run the big waves head-on, then set up to miss the House Rock at the bottom (or to land in the eddy on river right just above this rock, an expert move to set up for rescue of other boaters).

Besides the notorious "Oh Shit!" boulder, there are several big rocks that demand attention in the first third of this rapid. Any can wreck a boat. Remember your highside technique, and try to hit a rock head-on rather than sideways. The big waves at the bottom of the main drop may swamp open boats.

As you finish to the left of the House Rock, don't celebrate. That was only the first drop (The first drop is 150 yards long; the rapid drops 25 feet in 300 yards, 75 feet in 3 miles, a substantial drop). Whitehorse continues with another maze of rocks and waves to untangle, two sets of Class II+, one just beyond House Rock, the other around the bend. The most dangerous aspect of Whitehorse is its length, a half mile long, which is a cold swim for any overboards.

21.5: Three camps on river right, the lower two are called Upper Whitehorse (two sites for medium groups) and

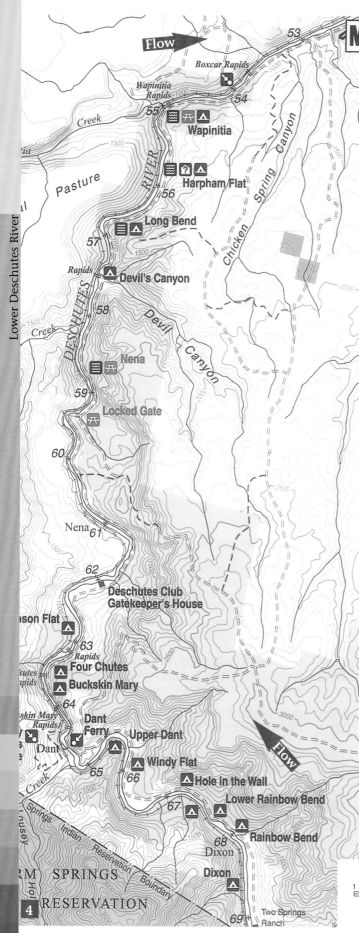

Lower Deschutes River

Middle Whitehorse (two sites for large groups with outhouse). The first camp is small, right at the base of the railroad, but shady with good fishing.

The entire flat at Whitehorse is public land and offers good fishing from the right bank (left is still Reservation).

The river appears to go around an island in the fourth set of rapids. Go far left, left of the big boulder at the bottom of this channel, as the right side is a nightmare of rocks and logs. Much lost gear may be found along the shore. This boulder in the left channel, and several other rocks, are potential wrap sites, so be careful.

As the river swings around, you can see the right channel rejoining, and a narrow slot in midstream that requires quick maneuvering to reach. Just beyond, a camp with landing site is visible river right. This is the landmark for Dungeon, a hole on river right just above the camp. It's more ferocious at higher levels, but a fun drop for inflatables and kayaks only. Avoid it by staying left of center.

22: The river begins a sharp left turn around Davidson Flat, a large flat area on river right. There is camping (five sites) beyond the island and at the end of the U-bend. Much of Davidson Flat is private land, with the public allowed to use it. There is a "jumping rock", a high ledge, near a basalt pillar on river right that the public may use (never dive, just jump, with a PFD).

The right side of the island offers fun Class II waves, then the river goes around a sharp turn to the right. Cheat this turn on the inside bend so you don't get stuck in the river left eddy.

23.25: An almost-identical bend occurs around the bottom of Davidson Flat, more camping with outhouse. Again, cheat to the inside or you may be swept into the strong eddy on river left. There is a dramatic orange-red rock wall here. The eddy on river right comes and goes, along with the patch of sand, but the still waters make for good swimming.

Note: Boaters are not allowed to gather wood from the enormous pile here, much brought in by the 1996 flood—or any wood in the Deschutes corridor—as it encompasses important animal habitat, providing homes, in particular, to needy black widow spiders. You may want to sleep in a tent here.

Another island and a bridge marks North Junction, where train tracks cross the river. The bridge is off-limits, as are the small houses. Another rapid offers fun waves. There is a good lunch spot or camp site just below the bridge on river right. From North Junction, there is about 5 miles of private land on river right

Scale   1 : 63,360

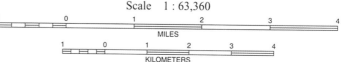

MILES

KILOMETERS

with no camping or stopping. The next campground is Dixon, river left, at River Mile 69.4.

Between 1909 and 1911, two competing railroads each tried to build tracks first on "their" side of the river, but the Reservation forced both sides to cross at North Junction. The federal government passed the Canyon Act that made the companies compromise and share 11 miles of track between North and South junctions.

25.3: Small island, main channel is right. This is the Wire hole, named either for haywire thrown into the river by sheepherders or for early fly-fisher Frank B. Wire.

26.3: Island or gravel bar, stay in middle. Old Hardy railroad building site on river left.

27.6: House, river right, known as Hernando's Hideaway, stay in left channel.

Huge basalt boulders are in the river here. The island with the large pinnacle is Dill Island, named for pioneer fishing guide Don Dill. There is a nice landing spot for lunch on the right side of the island.

Guides once called this Toilet Island after the careless use of the open rock faces as bathrooms. High water cleaned the island. Camping there is now illegal and the proper boater carries a container to remove solid wastes and toilet paper.

24.5: Reservation land ends on river left. Twin Springs Ranch is just below on river right. Technically, the railroad tracks are off limits, but there is a large chunk of BLM land on river left here. Three small camps, Dixon, are about 1/2 mile downstream on river left.

28.9: Dixon, railroad, river left. Across and just downstream on river right is Rainbow Bend, with up to five sites for small and large groups, then Lower Rainbow Bend just downstream. Two camps are on river left.

30.5: Hole in the Wall, camp on river right, small or medium groups, outhouse.

31.25: A long bend of the river leads to Windy Flat, four campsites on river right, outhouse. Strange root formations at the base of some trees are found on river right along this stretch.

Just downstream is Upper Dant, one campsite with outhouse.

31.7: Large stretch of flatwater on river right known as Big Eddy and good area for fishing.

32.6: Perlite Riffle. The large flat on river right is called Clubhouse Flat, and is the start of the Deschutes Club lands, private lands started by the club in 1937. Two anglers were so absorbed in their fishing that they had to be dragged to the business meeting.

In 1945, miner Afford discovered perlite, a type of volcanic glass, at this site and downstream at Dant. Dant and Russell developed the mines, the perlite was used in acoustical tile and plasterboard, as a sound absorber. The Lady Frances mine can be seen from a good distance, high on river left. The mine is no longer active. The houses at Dant were purchased by more fishermen, the Deschutes Homeowners Association.

Watch the thick vegetation on river left in this area, as families of racoons are often seen near the river. Mule deer are common in the backyards of houses on both right and left.

32.9: Dant, river left. Location of Dant Ferry Boat, used to ferry goods and people across to river left. Made from a war surplus lifeboat, the ferry may be a large obstacle if in mid-channel, so be alert. Dant has the only stop sign along this canyon. The train tunnel on river left is the narrowest on that side, and a mine worker was killed in the 1940s when caught in the tunnel with an oncoming train. The gate on river right where cars park to access the ferry was known as the Iron Curtain as it was seemingly always locked.

Dant is followed by a long, quiet, deep pool; water dammed up by the abrupt drop of Buckskin Mary Rapid. There is almost no current, and afternoon winds can bring a boat to a halt.

33.2: Buckskin Mary Rapid, Class II+. (RM65) Note horizon line (edge where river seems to drop off into nowhere) that indicates a steep drop. Steps on river right are for body surfers walking back upstream to float through in their life jackets. To run the rapid, position on the large, obvious V-slick in midstream. Keep your boat straight and in the middle, as there are rocks on both sides. An extra rock rolled off the road on river right several years ago, adding to the excitement, and raising the rapid up from a Class II, and must be avoided by body surfers.

Ride the waves, pushing on oars or paddling hard to keep up momentum. There is a big, backcurling wave at the bottom that can flip very small boats. Steps on river right lead up to the road and upriver to the head of the rapid. Both sets of steps were constructed to lessen erosion on river banks.

Caves are obvious high on river left. These were used to store blasting powder during railroad construction times, around 1900.

33.7: Buckskin Mary campsite. Four sites suitable for medium to large groups, river right. The last camp is most secluded, right at the head of the Four Chutes (and requires good ferrying skills to reach). Watch for skunks in this area, as they are both common and bold. Poison oak is also found growing in camp, on one boulder in particular. The road behind the camp is the private access road for the Deschutes Club, and is accessed by law enforcement officers, as well. Campers may use the road to walk back and forth to bodysurf sites.

Sometime during the night, while you are deep in dreamland, a loud noise and bright light will jolt you back to reality. A train is coming towards your camp! Don't panic; the railroad tracks are on the opposite

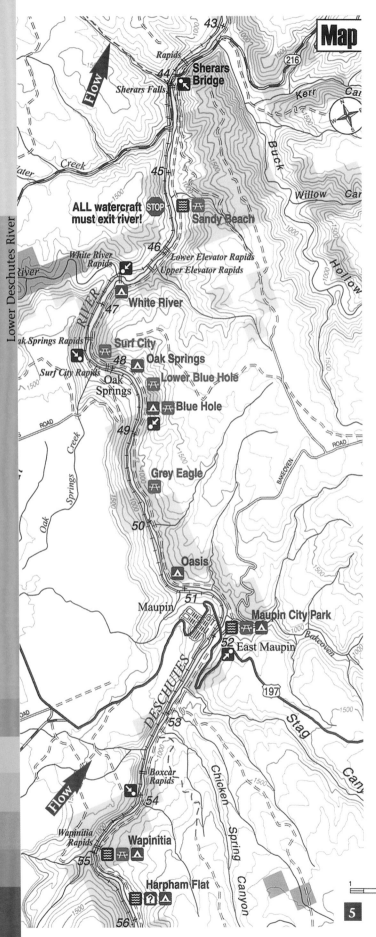

Lower Deschutes River

bank. However, this canyon produces an echo effect that tricks drowsy boaters out of their beds.

Boaters should remember to smoke only while sitting in the boat in the water during fire season, and at any time of the year, to PICK UP their butts. My last trip in 2002 saw dozens of ugly butts in what was to be the kitchen area—not very appetizing.

34.2: First of the "Four Chutes" Rapids, a series of pool-and-drop rapids that are very enjoyable Class II+ runs with fun standing waves. All four have rocks hidden in them, so use caution. On the first chute, always go far left. There is a rocky island in mid-stream and a narrow right chute that eats boats. The left side has a set of straight waves to run, or a little more left, a small reversal that can trash unprepared boaters. Stick to the slick.

The second of the Four Chutes campsites is directly below the first drop, with a nice eddy and sometimes a good landing beach. One must walk back to the Buckskin Mary outhouse along a riverside trail or set up their own.

Another camp is just downstream on river right; no outhouse.

34.4: Second Chute seems to head towards a boulder river left of mid-stream. Ride the waves and watch your oar placement.

34.5: Third Chute is fairly straightforward, watch for reeds and grassy area below on river left; great area for wildlife viewing. Fishing around these rapids and their tailouts, eddies and grassy river banks is good.

34.6: Fourth Chute is a fun ride down waves on river right, which ends with a sneaky oar-munching boulder on left edge. At some water levels, hidden rocks can become reversals for driftboats to avoid.

34.7: Johnson Flat, left bank, has a huge camping area with an outhouse, but no shade. A good fishing camp, but watch for rattlesnakes. Once I stopped here and little signs announced the presence of snake traps for a "rattlesnake survey". Figuring biologists would set up the survey near a large concentration of snakes, I left.

34.9: An old house, river left, used to house sheep-shearing and lambing workers when the hills were covered with herds of sheep. A wood ferry was used to cross the river. The house has been redecorated and is on private land.

The next three miles or so are private land.

Old building and hay field on river right were once Hunt's Hay Ranch.

35.6: Deschutes Club Gatekeeper's House, river right. Emergency radio, drinking water, hiker's check-in station, emergency firetruck parks here in fire season.

Scale   1 : 63,360

MILES

KILOMETERS

5

36.6: Nena, railroad switching station, river left. Private land. "Nena" is a Native word meaning "tall, white cottonwood trees".

Caves on river right were used by early Natives. Mostly they are now "Cow Caves" used for shelter, although good "frame" photos can be taken from inside them. Any artifacts have been looted.

38.2: Locked Gate, river right. This marks the furthest upstream that the general public can drive on the Deschutes Club road before it becomes a private road. There is vehicle access (not a good takeout), outhouse, day parking. Hikers/fishermen are allowed to walk the road upstream to Buckskin Mary.

38.9: Nena picnic site, river right. Day-use site only, fishing access. Private land on river left since Johnson Flat now ends.

Nena Creek enters, river left.

40.1: Devil's Canyon, river right. Fee campsite, vehicle access, outhouse, tables, garbage cans. Whitewater near mouth of canyon has some rocks in it, shallows, standing waves, run the obvious V-slot.

40.5: Long Bend starts, a curve first left, then sharp right. Location of Long Bend launch site (recommended for large groups on day trips), fee campsite, garbage cans, tables, outhouse, boat ramp.

41.4: Harpham Flat, river right. Main launch site for one-day trips out of Maupin. Formerly Dutchman's Flat, land now owned by the Confederated Tribes and managed by the BLM. Very busy site with lots of cars, people and boats on weekends.

Landmark: Identify approach of major whitewater 1.4 miles downstream from this boat ramp by watching for a hillside straight ahead that is covered with juniper trees, the first such tree-covered hill since the Mutton Mountains.

42: Wapinitia campsite, river right. Boat landing, fee campsite, vehicle access, outhouse, tables, garbage cans. Often used as a take-out by driftboat groups to avoid two large rapids.

42.3: Wapinitia Rapids, Class III. Drops in three parts. The first part has a few bouncy waves, then a calm stretch. Immediately move to river right (ten feet from bank) as the next drop comes into view (a strong eddy and boulder on the left as you end this fun set of standing waves must be avoided). Keep right for the third drop, which takes you perilously close to a boulder at the bottom, and a really big wave that tries to dump or wrap the boat against the rock. Cheat a little right of this boulder.

The left side of the third drop is sometimes run but requires crossing an enormously strong current in a short distance, so most boaters enjoy the bouncy "haystacks" (large standing waves) on river right. This is a good site for whitewater photography from shore.

The big wave at the bottom of Wapinitia is fairly recent, caused by a rockfall from the access road. The former wave train was tamer and more of a Class II ride.

A short distance downstream from Wapinitia is Cape Canaveral or Devil's Hole, a drop over a boulder on far river right that looks like nothing from upstream. Avoid this drop at low water unless your crew is gonzo (and it's not for driftboats or canoes). Hit straight on with momentum, having everyone hang on and brace as you enter the drop. Grab any overboards quickly as more rapids are coming up.

43: Boxcar Rapid, Class III+ (IV in high water). This is a blind corner just below the "Cape". Large basalt boulders on river right shore mark the beginning of this legendary rapid; it's not as fearsome as many believe. Scouting from the road on river right is recommended the first time.

To run, set up river left, about ten feet from cliffs, close to the cliffs until you pass a small but sneaky outcrop of rocks on river right. Pull back out of the strongest of the left current and ride it around the bend into the drop. (If the speed of the current concerns you, cheat more inside—river right—into the large eddy, which slows the boat enough that you can not only thoroughly scout standing up, but practically set up a lunch table.)

As you approach the drop at the bottom, the left chute runs over a large submerged boulder into a flip hole. The hydraulics are powerful at higher flows. A diagonal wave, just to the right of this current, is another potential boat-flipper. The center run is clean, and you can push back into the left once past the dropoff ledge to the bottom of the hole, for a splash and a good photo (a photographer from Whitewater Pix in Maupin takes pictures here in summer, and on busy weekends, also at Wapinitia).

The right side has a drop over a rocky shelf, bumpy but not dangerous for larger inflatables. Any swimmers on the left need to be rescued quickly as there is a sharp-edged boulder at bottom middle. More boats flip here than any other place on the Deschutes, due to the large numbers of inexperienced floaters and flimsy small craft that run the day-trip section. However, most overboards end up in the slow eddy waters on river right.

Boxcar Rapid is named for a nasty train wreck of the Oregon Trunk Line in March 1954. As the train came around the corner, the track was blocked by a rockfall, causing twelve boxcars and three locomotives to derail. One boxcar and one locomotive landed in the river. Two men who went into the river died: Fireman Earl Sutton's body was later recovered at Cedar Island on the lower river; Engineer Barton was entombed in the locomotive. Such wrecks are less common today due to sensors (often solar powered) and special fences in unstable rocky areas such as the one at Whitehorse.

Lower Deschutes River

Lower Deschutes River

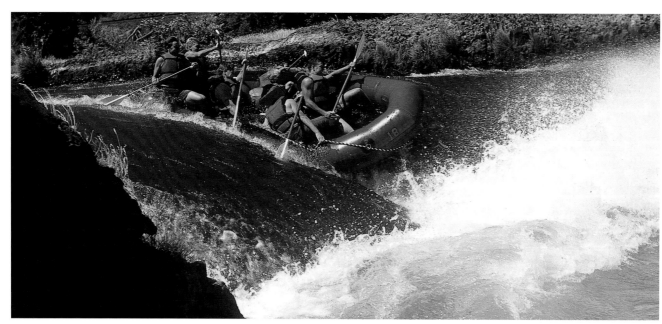

Taking an edge of the hole at Oak Springs is safer, but you need to be a little further to river left than this boat. Scout first time; check out where there is a seam or pillow of water in the current. Stay left of this current. Don't go far right, as boats are often Maytagged in the rough side of the reversal.

Some boaters believe the submerged boxcar created the rapid, but it's caused by the underground boulder. Both train cars were removed from the river. (Guides are known to tell the story and then casually mention that not only is the boxcar still underwater, but the door is open, and overboard passengers sometimes get sucked inside...).

43.3: Class II standing waves begin after a short recovery area. The best run is on the far left.

Several smaller rapids, with minor rock dodging and nice waves, follow. The old Maupin Mill Site can be seen on the rimrock, river left; the mill now produces log cabin homes.

45.6: Tom Allen Riffle, Class I+, named for pioneer of the Fly Fishers Club of Oregon. Pipeline supported by cable crosses the river, and a large waterfall on river left is a large natural spring; fancy houses line the hillside.

45.6: Class I+, Riffle with some nice waves as river bends left, ride current from right of midstream to left, avoiding a rocky ledge on river left mid-way, and pulling away from the rocky left bank at the bottom. Highway 197 bridge crosses just below. Deep water for jumping overboard.

Imperial Rafting (formerly C.J.'s) on river right has private eating area and tourist facilities.

45.8: Maupin City Park, (RM52.1) river right, is a big, green oasis in the desert. Day-use lunch area, boat landing, water, camping with RV hookups or tents, flush toilets, showers, garbage, RV dump station and shuttle parking are available. A fee is charged for launching/landing a boat and for using the park, which is worthwhile if you are unloading overnight gear.

Established in 1880, Maupin was named for Howard Maupin, who came West to Oregon in 1863 (and is remembered for killing Chief Paulina, for whom Paulina Lake was named). Maupin once operated a ferry just downstream at Bakeoven Creek. The town became Hunt's Ferry for a while, but Maupin's Ferry, shortened to Maupin by the Post Office in 1909, stuck.

East Maupin, with the Oasis Resort (cabins, café, T-shirts, etc.), Allstar and Deschutes U-boat (with store), Whitewater Pix (and ice cream store) are all within easy walking distance. The main part of town, including the sole gas station, is "up the hill" (north across the bridge), where Rainbow Tavern and other establishments offer nighttime entertainment.

Bakeoven Road, which connects to the river access road below Maupin, and Bakeoven Creek, which enters north of Maupin, were named for a German baker who was traveling the desert trail alone when Indians stole his horses, leaving him just his wagon and supplies. The enterprising pioneer built ovens from lava rock and clay alongside the trail, then started baking bread. When more Indians arrived, they "broke bread" instead of his head. He also sold bread to gold miners along the trail. The name Bakeoven is also suitable in summer, when the road absorbs the desert heat—no place to walk barefoot!

46.1: Maupin Riffle, run river left. The middle and most of the right are shallow gravel and boats get stuck. Watch for the color change from blue-green waters to brown that indicates a gravel bar. The far right is runnable but not with the fun standing waves.

46.7: Oasis Campground, not to be confused with the resort, is a BLM campsite popular with day-trip boaters. Just finding a place to park here is difficult on Friday night. Fees are charged for this campsite which has outhouses, tables, firepits (usable only in the off season) and a Dumpster.

46.9: Schitzo or Staircase Rapid, Class II. River splits around an island. Wading anglers often occupy the left channel, and it is not as fun as the right channel, which has bigger waves. Enter middle right (getting right early so that you don't get pulled into the island), dodge a rock on far river right, and work back to the middle as the currents converge, riding out the roller-coaster waves.

47.9: Grey Eagle day-use site has outhouse, garbage pick-up, tables, and a nice landing spot. Good shade from trees. Some commercial outfitters set up lunches for clients here.

49: Blue Hole is a fee campground, day-use area, with a wheelchair accessible dock (rebuilt in 1998 after being destroyed by huge flood waters), installed by volunteer efforts. Long, quiet deep water for jumping overboard continues until the river shallows in a Class I riffle. Lower Blue Hole is a day-use site with very good fishing.

Just below is Oak Springs campsite, a BLM fee area with outhouse, tables, garbage service.

Landmark: Notice the hillside ahead of you is covered in lush greenery and there are islands with green grass in the river ahead. This is the warning for Oak Springs. Pay attention to the many shelves of flat, often sharp-edged volcanic flows here as the river begins narrowing; avoid bumping these shelves.

49.6: Surf City is a set of big standing waves favored by kayak surfers, also a parking site on river right. The river begins a bend to the right as the entrance to Oak Springs comes into view.

The Oak Springs Fish Hatchery is seen high on river left, with numerous springs feeding the lush greenery as well as the hatchery ponds where rainbow trout and summer steelhead are raised.

49.9: Oak Springs Rapid, Class IV (risky swim, flip, injury area). Land on gravel island right of middle to scout (wade to shore, walk down paved road to overlook). The main drop is below a small lava island; a larger lava island on far left has a tiny channel and is seldom run on purpose.

There are three main routes: river left, which seldom causes trouble (although the approach to left is over shoals and sharp-edged rocks in late summer). To run, get left early and set up to run the big wave head-on. Next, a diagonal wave is immediately hit, usually no problem.

Once below the main drop, stay left to avoid nasty ledges on river right, and maneuver as necessary around ledges on left and center. This is the best route in low water to miss the ledges, which have injured many boaters. Instruct overboards to get upstream of the boat so they are not mashed between the boat and

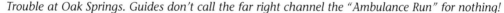

Trouble at Oak Springs. Guides don't call the far right channel the "Ambulance Run" for nothing!

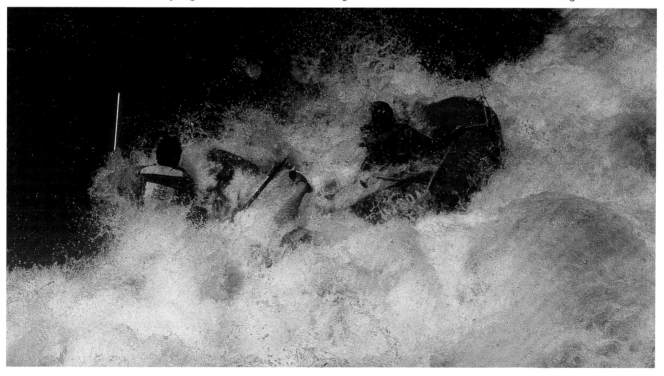

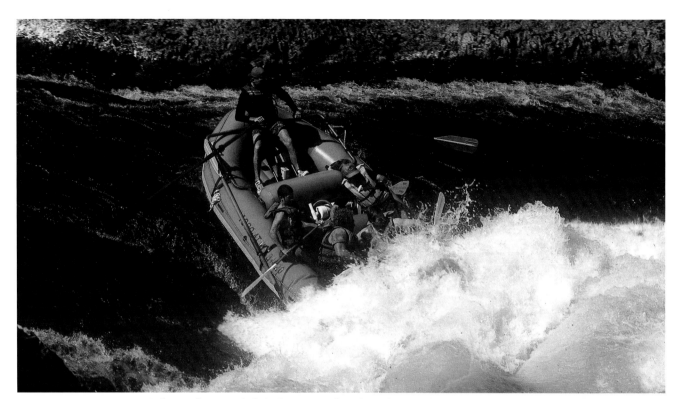

A "gonzo" run at Oak Springs; note that the raft started left of the hole and pushed back into a part of it, rather than take the full hit at far right.

rock. Some outfitters call this the Ambulance Run due to the number of injuries that occur here.

Right-side runs: The safest run of all (best driftboat run) is to ride snug to the rock island, especially for small boats. This smooth tongue carries you safely past the menacing hole on river right. Edge run (large rafts only): As the boat goes over the steep drop, situate about three feet off the right of the island, so that your boat takes the edge of the giant reversal. People can still go overboard, but it's less likely. Running the hole head-on is not recommended due to the possibility of an overboard being trapped under the boat as it "surfs" (gets stuck) in the reversal, as well as the risk of hitting the ledges with boat or body. Many "blooper" films are shot here.

50.7: White River Campground, river right. The landmark for White River Rapid is the often-milky-tinted river mouth, river left, under the railroad bridge. Boaters often pull out of the top of the rapid to land on the sandy beach, walk upstream, and bodysurf the White River chutes. The White River is made white by glacial meltoff full of silt from Mt. Hood. From here or the road, you can see both Mt. Hood and the White; this is the only major river in Oregon where you can see both the headwaters and mouth at the same place.

The fee campsite is owned and operated by the Tribes.

50.8: White River Rapids, Class II+. Enter near midstream, watch for a really big wave in low water that will almost stand a boat on end (keep boat straight and dig oars in for momentum). As the river turns right, there are rocks to dodge and waves to hit. A boulder at the bottom, right of center, attacks inattentive boaters.

51.3: Upper Elevator Rapid, Class II. Aka Upper Roller Coaster Rapid. Large rollercoaster waves are easy to run; stay in center and keep your boat straight.

Many boaters land below this rapid on river left to bodysurf through the waves. Wear lifejacket, shoes, and shorts with good elastic (the wave action has been known to wash loose pants off!). Walk back upstream to a jump-in site on lava rock, jump in, and immediately swim to mid-stream to avoid bumping rocks. Assume the lawnchair position and hold your breath in wave crests; breathe in troughs.

As the wave train ends, promptly turn over to your belly and swim diagonal to the current to get back to shore. Some swimmers are weakened by the cold water and must be rescued (by throwbag line or another swimmer).

The most dangerous part of the bodysurf stop is landing and getting out of the boat/out of the water after a swim. The water is over your head in many places, and the rocky underwater ledges are sharp and slippery. Be careful!

51.5: Lower Elevator Rapid, Class II+. Aka. Lower Roller Coaster Rapid. Most people don't want to bodysurf here as the waves are bigger and trashier. Aim for the largest waves in river center and keep paddling/rowing for momentum. These waves are best in low water.

51.7: Upper Osborne Rapid, Class II. On far left, there is a trashy little reversal that can be run by inflatables and kayaks. Work back mid-stream to hit wave train, which leads into a rock (boats can hit, wrap and even flip, very embarrassing as the takeout is around the corner).

51.8: Sandy Beach. **Mandatory takeout for all boats.** (RM44.5) It is now illegal to run below this takeout, even though Lower Osborne Rapid (Class II+) and The Swirlies as well as the narrowest site on the Deschutes are located in the closed section.

You can observe The Narrows of the Deschutes from the road as you drive north to Sherars Falls, where a massive brickbat basalt flow impeded the river's flow; the depth here at 4-5,000 cfs could be up to 100 feet! Shears Falls was likely caused by a lava flow from Mt. Hood blocking the Deschutes, which then wore a pathway through the hardened rock. The many shelves upstream and downstream of the falls attest to the power of the lava flow in this narrowest spot on the lower Deschutes.

53.5: Sherars Falls, Class IV. Very hazardous—do not attempt! (RM 44.0) The falls plunges 15 feet over a basalt cliff, ending in treacherous reversals that can hold a small floating object for hours. This was a Native camp where the Tribes fished for migratory fish trying to get up the fish ladder on river right. They still fish from platforms, wearing safety lines and wielding long-handled dip nets. Modern fishing is done for cer-emonial and subsistence reasons. The public is some-times allowed to bait fish for salmon near the falls; check with the Tribes to see when it's open.

In 1871, Joseph Sherar bought the bridge for $7,040, linking the major towns of Canyon City on the John Day River with The Dalles on the Columbia. Gold and supplies crossed Sherars Bridge for $3.75 per wagon and $1 per driver. Shears was once supplied with an inn, which burned down in 1940. The Pony Express ran between the two towns, making 225 miles in 28 hours at 50 cents a letter.

Below Sherars Falls, the Upper and Lower Bridge rapids are also closed; the next legal put-in is Buckhollow. The 2.8 miles between Sandy Beach land-ing and Buckhollow landing have been closed to pro-tect migrating fish.

"Lower Lower" Deschutes River

Buckhollow to Columbia River

Location

North Central Oregon. The launch site at Buckhollow is located 8.4 miles downstream from Maupin. To reach Maupin from Portland, take Interstate 84 east to The Dalles and then head south on 197; or take Highway 26 over Mt. Hood, then follow Highway 216 to Maupin. The trip ends near Biggs, 20 miles east from The Dalles on I-84.

The power of Sherars Falls is awesome. This is a good site to watch steelhead and salmon trying to jump the steep slope. A fish ladder on river left helps them along with stairs to climb.

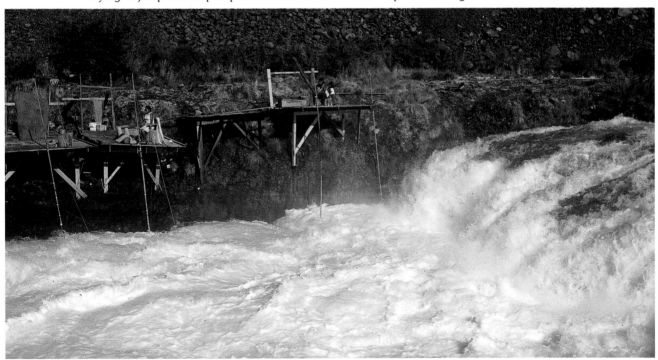

Lower Deschutes River

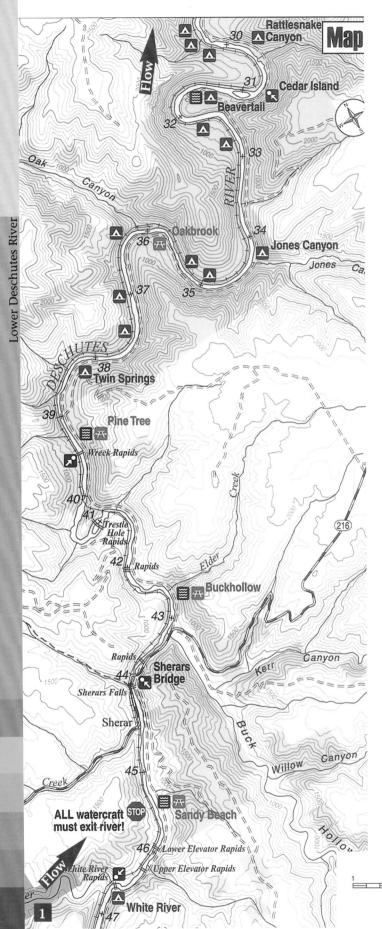

Personality

Much like the upper run, with more severe desert country.

The water seems to feel warmer, the air temperatures hotter, probably due to the rocky canyon. A deep basalt canyon with impressive basalt pillars, columns and boulders has mostly flat water with good current, with some big rapids located near the end of the trip. This segment has more public land due to the purchase of a large private ranch with boater pass fees and donated funds. Bighorn sheep have been reintroduced and golden eagles are common.

Again, the railroad follows the river. Additionally, there is road access along the river right down to Macks Canyon (floating this reach is easier than driving the rough gravel road). Jetboats operate every other week, mostly ferrying fishermen upstream to camps or angling spots.

The lower run is well-known for its big runs of fighting summer steelhead that hit both lures and flies aggressively, so the late summer months and early fall are busy and exciting times for fishermen.

The river continues to be large with powerful currents, and remains a beautiful blue-green color with lush vegetation along the shore.

Difficulty

Mostly Class III (some boaters consider some rapids Class IV but none are as long as Whitehorse on the upper).

Gradient:

12 fpm

Mileage/Days

Buckhollow to Columbia River, 43.4 miles, 2+ days, Class III-III+.

Buckhollow to Pine Tree, Class III, 3.2 Miles, 1/2-1 day (road on right).

Pine Tree to Macks Canyon, 15.25 miles, 1-2+ days, Class II+ (road on right).

Macks Canyon to Columbia River, 24.25 miles, 2+ days, Class III-III+ (roadless).

Average Float Levels/Seasons

The 100 miles of the Deschutes below Pelton Regulating Dam boasts a reliable, year-round ideal flow of 3,000 to 6,000 cfs, with a summer average about 3,500 cfs. Water levels taken at the Moody gauge near the Columbia River.

High-Water Season

See upper section. The flip wave in Colorado actually gets worse at lower levels.

Scale   1 : 63,360

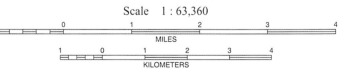

Low-Water Season

See upper section. Again, the lower Deschutes is never too low to float.

Craft

All craft float this last segment of the Deschutes, from "rubber duckies" to driftboats. However, there are big waves, sharp lava rocks, and reversals that can rip or flip many small boats.

Permits

No permit lottery system yet. Boater passes are mandatory and may be purchased at local stores, or on the Internet. Weekday trips are recommended whenever possible, as the more weekend use the Deschutes gets, the sooner a permit system will be imposed.

Hazards

Much the same as the upper: more sharp rocks for swimmers to avoid, rattlesnakes, black widow spiders, ticks (mostly in spring), scorpions, big waves and strong hydraulics, semi-remote country below Macks Canyon, oppressive heat (splash a lot) and sunburn, strong currents for wading anglers to cope with, jetboats when permitted (let them have the middle channel and wait for them to come upstream through a rapid first, as they can't maneuver without power). Remember the wind often blows very hard in the afternoon, and thunderstorms can develop fast late in the day.

Fishing

Native redside trout, native steelhead, hatchery fish, salmon. Same methods as upper but emphasis is on summer and fall steelhead, with runs beginning in July. Trout anglers prefer the upper but may find the lower less populated by other anglers before steelhead season. "Bounty hunting" for Northern pike minnows (suckers) at mouth of Deschutes.

Managing Agency

Prineville Bureau of Land Management, 3050 NE 3rd St., Prineville, OR 97754. 541/416-6700. Check for motorized boat schedule, list of outfitters, current regulations.

Shuttles

Widely available.

The Oasis Resort, Maupin, OR 541/395-2611. Their sister store, Oasis North, is the place to go during the busy summer months for shuttles, boater passes, flies and T-shirts. From Portland, pick up a driver in Maupin for a lower fee.

Linda's Shuttles, Maupin, OR 541/225-4632 or 1-877-225-4632. 24-passenger buses available for large groups to avoid parking hassles.

Tim Sturgeon "Fish", Madras, OR 541/475-6009.

Pat Beida, Maupin, OR, 541/298-4004, lower Deschutes shuttles.

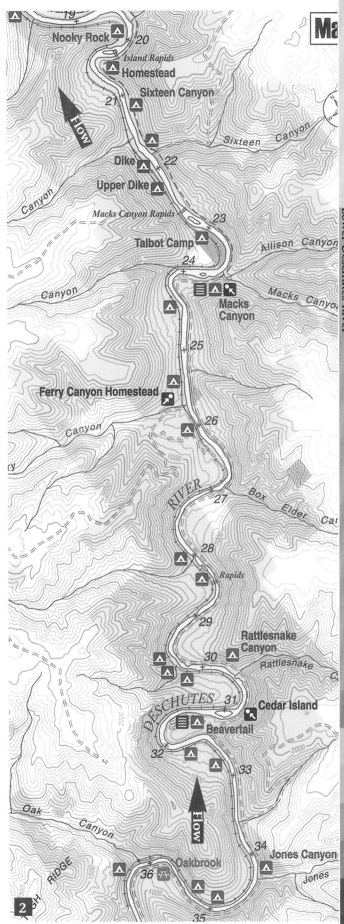

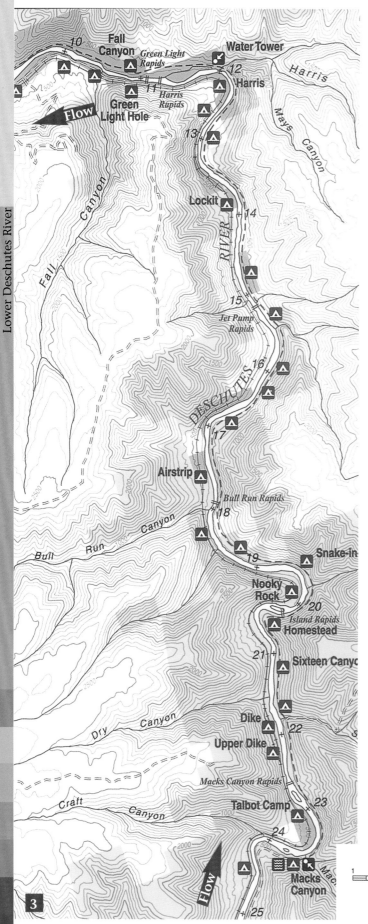

Check out fly shops in nearby Bend (see appendix) for fly selections, guided fishing trips, and fishing tips.

Mileage/Highlights

0: Buckhollow Launch, (RM41.5) river right, day use only, outhouse, boat ramp.

1.5: Class 1+ rapid. Canyon narrows; basalt columns resemble cake layers.

This rapid leads into the Twin Crossings, the only railroad tracks on the lower section found on river right. This crossing isolates a peninsula of basalt rock which the river winds around, beginning with an island. Several rapids keep you on your toes.

In 1909, two companies vied to be the first to complete a railroad through the Deschutes Canyon, an important shipping route before trucks and highways took over. Using laborers armed only with black powder, picks, and shovels, both sides dug impressive tunnels, carved flat areas into hillsides for laying track, and survived pranks from their opponents trying to slow them down. The Twin Crossings were built by H.F. Carleton with 150 Italian workers who were paid double-time wages of $5 per day.

1.8: Trestle Hole Rapid, Class II+. River divided by island. Good kayak playspot. Small waves in left channel, large standing waves in right channel. The right channel develops a hole at high water that is infamous for surfing and trashing kayaks.

Riffles at bottom of island present no problems, but there are two more rapids as you round the U-bend of the Twin Crossings.

River bends hard to the right as it rounds the "peninsula" of basalt. Large standing waves in mid-stream may force boats into cliff walls, so be ready to pull away.

The railroad bridge is visible ahead, about 100 yards before the rapid begins. Left of mid-stream will avoid submerged ledges and rocks.

3.2: Wreck Rapid, Class III. Large standing waves, rocks in current, sometimes develops strong hydraulics. Stay left for an easier run, right to be trashed.

The name "Wreck" derives from a September 1949 head-on collision between two engines, one northbound, one southbound. The engines were to switch over at Oakbrook Station, just downstream, but alas, a miscalculation in timing caused the crash. Three men perished, along with many horses carried on the southbound train. The only surviving horse was taken to Maupin and lived out its natural life as Oregon Trunk.

Remnants of the wreck, from steel rails to horse bones, are still found in the area. In prehistoric times,

Scale 1 : 63,360

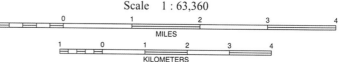

MILES

KILOMETERS

tropical trees such as teak were found, as were mammoth, rhinoceros and other large Ice Age creatures. Fossils and petrified wood are all that remains to tell their stories. Remember to take only pictures, leave only footprints.

Many interesting basalt formations are found along this stretch: silt-and-talus slopes eroded by flash floods (also known as dry waterfalls), columnar basalt in all shapes and sizes, layered rock, pinnacles, and boulders in the river.

3.5: Pine Tree, river right, is a boat landing with outhouse. Many day-trippers add this section from Buckhollow to Pine Tree to their run from Harpham Flat to Sandy Beach. It's best run in the morning to avoid fierce upstream winds.

4.6: Twin Springs campsite. Fee campsite with road access, outhouse, garbage pickup.

Two additional campsites are located on river left (away from the gravel access road) in the next 2 miles. Tygh Ridge is the high ground on river left.

Tygh Ridge and Valley derive from the name of one of the current Confederated Tribes on the reservation. In the 1840s and 50s, railroad and explorer surveys spelled this tribe's name as "Tysch" or "Taih."

7: Oakbrook picnic site, day use only. Has outhouse and tables.

Two camps are found within a mile, both on river left.

8.5: Jones Canyon enters, river right. Campsite at mouth. Fee site with tables, outhouse, tables, garbage service.

After 1.4 miles, three campsites are found on river left, away from the road.

11.4: Beavertail campsite is a road access camp much like Jones Canyon. Just past the camp, you round Cedar Island, which hosts a rare stand of western (incense) cedar trees.

This region was the site of numerous fights between the two "dueling digger" crews of the competing railroad companies. One side rolled a boulder down on an Oregon Trunk work train, and the fight was on. A watchman was posted on the Deschutes Railroad construction site, who discovered a lit fuse leading to a keg of black powder right in camp. He was able to stomp out the fuse in time, but many of his crew left anyway. Such antics as obliterating survey markers along the track routes were common.

12.4: Rattlesnake Canyon campsite. A fee site with the usual amenities, river right.

There are 5 campsites located on river left in the next 2 miles.

15.6: Box Elder Canyon, river right.

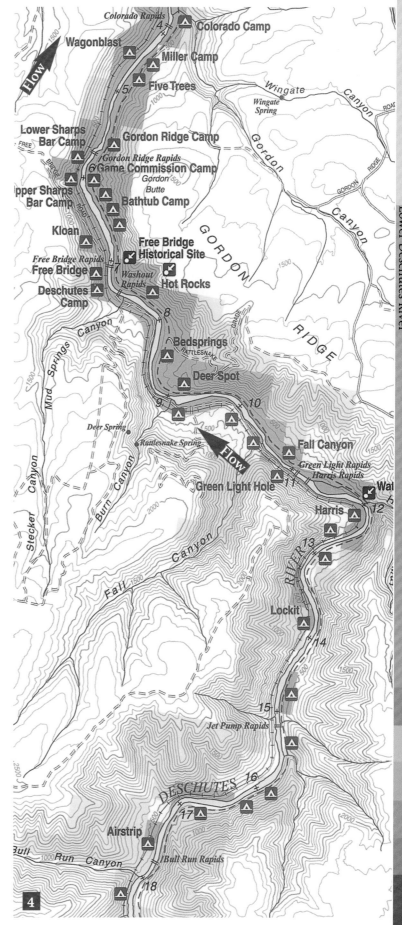

Lower Deschutes River

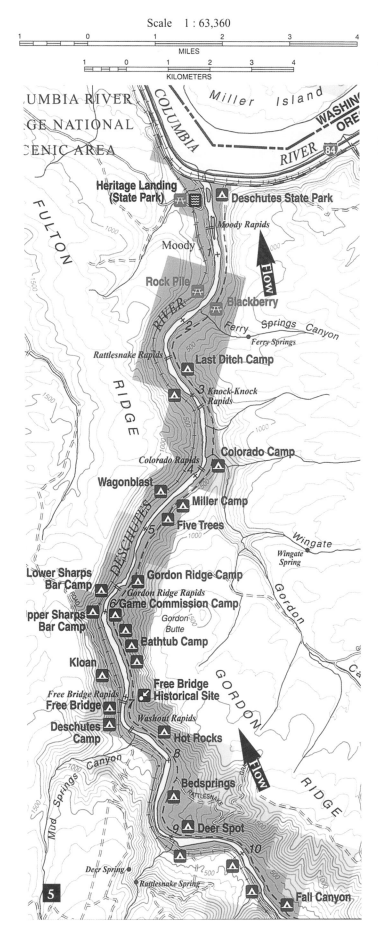

You think your cargo boat is heavy? The railroad workers, over 6,800 strong, ate about 15,000 pounds of fresh beef every day. Part of the competition between the rival companies included stampeding cattle and buying all available hay even though it was not needed or used ... just to delay the rival company.

11.4: Beavertail camp, river right, fee camp.

11.8: Cedar Island splits the Deschutes. Both channels are runnable, with the left having bigger waves (plus some rocks to avoid); river right is smaller but easier, with shallows at the lower end of the island.

Cedar Island got its name from the western (incense) cedars that grow on this largish island, one of few Deschutes islands that can support these water-loving trees. Their isolation has saved them from logging and wildfires.

12.4: Rattlesnake Canyon enters on river right. There is a fee campsite here with amenities. Large standing waves lead into submerged boulders and ledges, so move mid-stream at the bottom to avoid these obstacles. There is a good car camp on the right, followed by 5 camps on river left (away from the road) in the next 2 miles. Watch for a Class II rapid at mile 13.3. Standing waves as the river drops over a shelf. The landmark is several boulders on river left.

15.6: Box Elder Canyon enters, river right. A river left camp is about 1 mile downstream. Elderberry is a tall shrub with bright red or dark blue berries. The blue berries were dried and used dried in pemmican or fermented for wine making. The red berries are reputedly edible but may make some people sick.

16.1: Sinamox, Chinook Indian jargon for the number seven, was used for this railroad station as it was the seventh from the north end of the Oregon Trunk Railway. Good grazing slopes on both river banks led to the area being a major lambing and wool-producing area.

Two camps are found at Ferry Canyon, one .4 miles upstream on river left, the other .2 mile downstream on river left.

17.2: Ferry Canyon & Homestead. The canyon enters on river left. Named for a 1900-era ferry boat crossing, which likely carried loads of sheep across the river. Rock foundations are all that remain of the ferry dock.

This was also the site of a sun-kink that caused yet another train wreck. On a very intensely hot day, the Deschutes desert sun hits the metal rails, causing the rails to expand and buckle or "kink". These warped tracks derailed eleven cars and a caboose.

Up Ferry Canyon is a small homestead, which is now a BLM administrative site. The caretaker is available for emergencies only; otherwise, don't disturb.

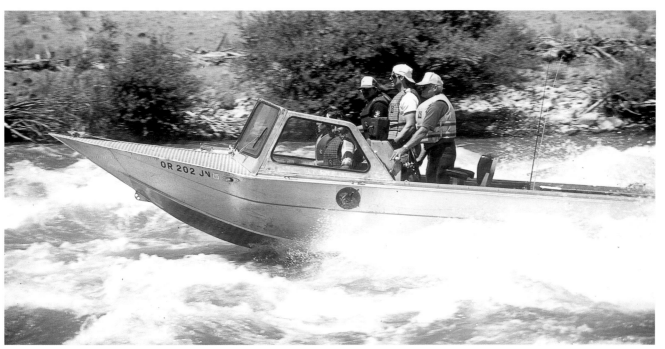

Jet boats are allowed to operate every other week, usually shuttling in anglers who have only a day or two to fish. Floating a river offers a different experience for those who have the time.

Another camp is found on river left at 1.1 miles downstream.

18.9: Macks Canyon, river right. (RM24.7) The river takes a sharp bend to the right and there is a small island near the camp. Macks Canyon and Allison Canyon join at the Deschutes.

This is the last drive-in campsite, with fees charged. From here downstream there are no roads, just a primitive trail that follows the old railroad bed for 23 miles to Deschutes State Park at the mouth.

Thomas Condon, a pastor and paleontologist (dinosaur fossil enthusiast), explored this region in 1860-70, which at that time was so littered by fossils that many early travelers noted their presence in their journals. Along with the John Day fossil beds, this area has contributed much to the understanding of how ancient beasts and plants lived.

Native Americans also used this site as a winter encampment more than 2,000 years ago, known as the Pit House Village for its subterranean pit houses. The Natives hunted bighorn sheep, mule deer, and probably made good use of the river by harvesting freshwater mussels, crayfish, trout, salmon and other critters. This area is fenced off to protect fragile artifacts; please do not disturb the site.

Just downstream is the rock formation of a black powder storage shelter used by the Oregon Trunk. Guards were posted at such shelters to prevent sabotage by the competition. The Deschutes River railroads were the last use of black powder for blasting by the government; since 1910, dynamite or other explosives

replaced the volatile black powder. Steam-powered shovels were also tried to speed up the "pick rocks with hand tools" technique. The equipment was disassembled, lowered into the canyon with ropes, then put back together. Alas, all the work was for naught as the mighty basalt of the Deschutes Canyon could not be broken apart by such tools.

19.7: Talbot Camp, river left is followed by an island.

20.1: Macks Canyon Rapid, Class II. Usually right is the best route.

20.9: Dike, two camps river left. Dike derives from a volcanic formation known as a "volcanic dike"; lava pours into a crack in the ground, assuming its shape, then the ground around it erodes, leaving only the "dike" standing alone.

Sixteen Canyon enters on river right, Dry Canyon on the left. There is a camp at its mouth and two sites (Homestead, 22.3) within the next mile on river right.

22.5: Island Rapid. The river curves in a sharp bend to the right, with the right channel around the island usually the best route.

22.9: Nooky Rock campsite, river left. Nestled on the inside of the U bend, this site has a sandy beach and good shade. Impressive basalt formation on river right.

23.3: Snake-in-the-Box campsite, river right.

Rattlesnakes are sometimes found in dens, consisting of dozens or even hundreds of snakes. According to one story, a railroad crew broke into a rattlesnake den, gathered the snakes into burlap bags, then stealthily rowed them across the river at night. The snakes were then left in the middle of the "enemy" camp of the

Lower Deschutes River

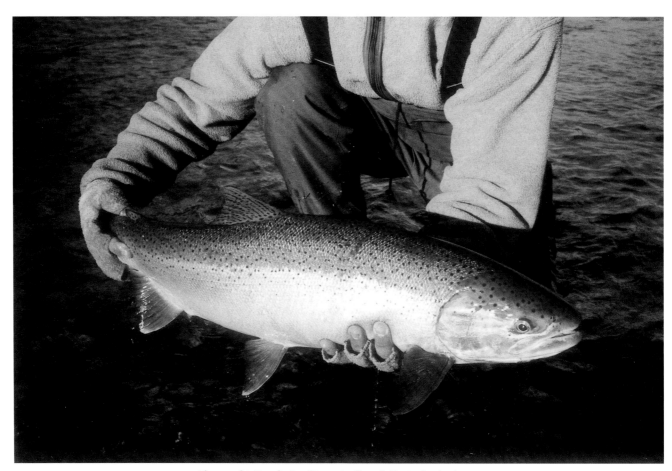

Fly-caught Deschutes River steelhead. Scott Cook photo.

Italian workers. (Cold snakes are sluggish, like all chilled reptiles, easily gathered up at night. Once the sun rose, the rival crew watched the antics of the Italians as they discovered this "gift". Many packed up and left!)

24.8: Bull Run Rapid, Class II. Landmark: Bull Run Canyon enters on river left. Ride the wave train down the center, but watch for a submerged rock at the end.

25.1: Airstrip, river left. Planes once landed in the flat areas here; this is now a campsite.

27.6: Jet Pump Rapid, Class II+. Right is shallow, left rocky. Ride the haystacks down the center. This is a possible bodysurf rapid, but additional flotation (such as an inner tube) is recommended to avoid butt-bumping.

There are four camps on river right in the next 1.7 miles.

29: Lockit (RM13.5) (Chinook jargon for "four"), marks the fourth station from the north terminal of the Oregon Trunk. Several train accidents have occurred around this region.

The camp here, on river left, has a sandy beach, outhouse, and shade. Bodysurfing is possible, but check for rocks first. Just under a mile downstream, a cave is visible high on the left side, carved into the basalt cliffs. There are also two camps, one on each side of the river.

30.8: Water tower, landmark for Harris Canyon. A campsite located near the mouth of Harris Canyon can accommodate two large groups.

The river takes another U-bend as the mouth of Harris Canyon comes into the inside bend. Here the river takes a brief detour to the west, departing from its mostly-northern flow. This region was first homesteaded by John E. Harris, which then went to Frank Barton, whose caretaker built an elaborate irrigation system using wooden water wheels and flumes. Many Native artifacts, such as a storage facility for dried salmon, have been found here. Petroglyphs are also up the canyon, and a burial ground is nearby.

Railroad building began here in 1909. This is the last remaining water tower.

31.4: Harris Rapid, Class II. With shallows on river left and rocks in the right, this rapid is usually run midstream.

31.5: Green Light Rapid, Class II+. Run the large waves head-on, watching for hidden rocks and turbulence. Green, red or yellow lights from the railroad are seen along the river, hence the name.

Fall Canyon on river right and Green Light Hole on river left provide good campsites and fishing just below the rapid. Fall Canyon enters river left.

The next three camps on river left are on private land and use is restricted: no fires, no dogs, no camping when cattle are present.

33.3: Burn Canyon enters on river left. There are two springs located up the canyon. Deer Spot campsite is on river right, with Bedsprings and Hot Rocks just down the river.

Lava turns red due to iron oxides; the east (right) bank displays this color. Burn Canyon was named for the many wildfires in the area, many caused by the activity of the railroads. Sparks from brakes and engines ignited tinder-dry grasses, just as cigarette butts do today. Early-day workers had to chase the fires uphill. Strong, hot afternoon winds not only fanned the flames, but also caused the fires to jump this broad river. The modern adventurer needs to be extra careful with fire, especially during the fire season.

The large rock formation on river right is Gordon Ridge, which means the big rapids are approaching.

35.3: Washout Rapid, Class III to III+. A flash flood through a dry stream bed of Mud Springs Canyon forced boulders into the river in 1996, creating a new rapid. Scout from river right. There are big waves and hydraulics to tackle in this drop. Difficulty varies with the water level, but good boaters may sneak most of the big stuff.

This is one of very few new rapids formed in the Pacific Northwest in recent years (especially since dam controls), which doesn't see many summer rainstorms. Crystal Rapid in Arizona was formed by a flash flood in the 1960s, in much the same manner—water crashing down a dry creek and clogging the river with boulders, which causes waves and holes to form. "Canyoneers" who explore the Southwest have also had trouble with flash floods in summer.

35.6: Free Bridge Historical Site. The original road bridging The Dalles with Moro (a town established in 1868 by Henry Barnam, who ran a trading post) crossed the Deschutes here, and remnants of the road can still be seen on shore. The road was built by Harris of Harris Canyon fame. In an ironic twist, the "free" bridge began as a toll bridge. Wasco County bought the bridge and removed the toll. The bridge was rebuilt in 1905 and collapsed in 1914 under suspicious circumstances. Other roads and bridges took its place.

Motorboaters are not allowed to camp on river left (west) between this site and Sharps Bar, which opens up 5 campsites to float-ins only.

35.7: Free Bridge Rapid, Class II. Ride the small waves head-on, keeping an eye out for rocks in the shallows.

Four camps on river right provide plenty of room for both powerboaters and floaters.

37: Lower Sharps Bar Camp, river left.

37.1: Gordon Ridge Rapid, Class III. The channel here is lengthy and narrow. If you need to scout, use the right bank. Stay right until the river drops over a basalt ledge. To run the ledge, look for the tongue or "V-slick", a smooth, downstream-pointing V-shape that indicates no hidden rocks. Much basalt rock is in the rapid.

There is a camp just below the rapid if you need to rest and recover. Gordon Ridge, Rapid and Canyon were named for the Scottish homesteader.

Three more camps on both sides of the river lead to the next big drop.

38.9: Colorado Rapid, Class III to III+. (RM4) Probably named after the Colorado River, famous for its huge haystack waves and giant hydraulics. A large wave train has a wave at the bottom that, at certain water levels (not flood level), develops into a "backcurler" or a combination of wave-reversal action that can flip a 14-foot raft. This can be cheated on the side.

39.6: Knock-knock Rapid, Class II. Small waves offer a chance to relax after the towering haystacks of Colorado.

40: Last Ditch Camp, river right. This is the last place to camp before reaching the Columbia River.

From here on down, all floaters must observe a pass-through zone, from Rattlesnake Rapid down to Moody. No stopping is allowed in this zone, to permit walk-in fishermen access to the famed Deschutes fishery.

40.2: Rattlesnake Rapid, Class III to III+. Scouting recommended. Rocky ledges narrow this into a tight drop with strong hydraulics. Look for a smooth tongue left of center. The right side drops into a nasty reversal with sharp rocks ready to stab any overboards. Once below the main drop, watch for more rocks in the middle of the river.

The high ground to your left is Fulton Ridge.

42.2: Moody Rapid, Class II+. The Deschutes funnels into a tight slot between basalt rock ledges, forcing a large set of turbulent waves to develop. Check before you commit to this run, making sure no jetboaters or inner tubers are ahead of you in the narrow space. Watch out, too, for the occasional "boogie boarder" who tries to surf a board attached by a rope; this is dangerous for an oncoming boat that may become entangled.

The gauging station that registers the cfs of the Deschutes is located at Moody.

42.6: Heritage Landing, river left. Take-out site, boat ramp, toilet, trailer parking, water.

42.7: Deschutes State Park, river right. Fee campsite, trail head up to Macks Canyon, RV hookups, plus the usual amenities.

You don't actually merge with the Columbia; both parks are about 1/5 mile above the confluence. Nearby Celilo Village is where Natives once netted Columbia salmon and steelhead by the millions before dams were constructed.

CHAPTER 7

Owyhee River
(pronounced "Oh-Why-Hee")
Oregon runs with notes on Idaho and Nevada runs

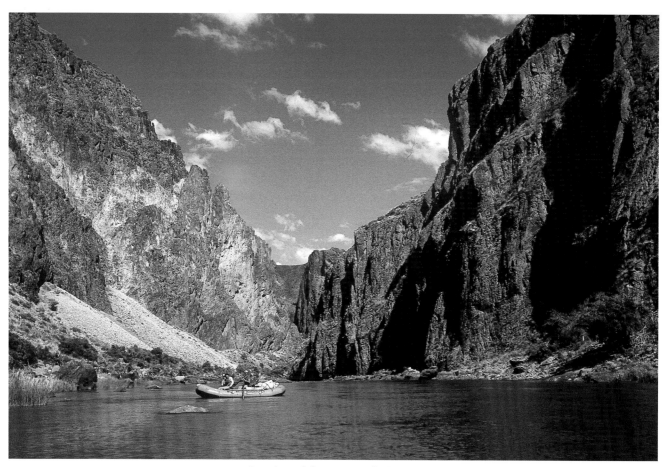

Overview of the canyon closing in.

THIS IS, HANDS DOWN, THE MOST SPECTACULAR OF Oregon's navigable waterways. If the name implies Paradise, that's because the river was named after Hawaii, in a roundabout fashion. Fur trapper Donald McKenzie (of Oregon's McKenzie River) lead an expedition into the Snake River country in 1819, a trip which included two "Owyhees" or Hawaiian natives (such was the old-fashioned spelling). McKenzie sent the Hawaiians up the river to scout for beaver, and they never returned. Believed murdered by the Snake tribe, known for their bad tempers and dislike of intruders, this is probably true.

However, another tale claims the Hawaiians joined a Paiute tribe and left mysterious Hawaiian petroglyphs behind as evidence of their survival. In the early writings of explorer Peter Skene Ogden (Ogden State Park, Crooked River Gorge), he refers to this river as the "Sandwich Island" River, a clear reference to the

first name for Hawaii (after the Earl of Sandwich). Ogden also uses the title "Owyhee River" later in the year 1826.

Headwatering in Nevada's mining country near Elko, the Owyhee flows mostly northwest in two forks into the southwestern corner of Idaho. Here the South Fork and the East Fork offer extremely remote runs through deep basalt canyons, merging just beyond Crutcher Crossing to form the main stem Owyhee. Deep Creek, a major tributary of the East Fork, is runnable early in the season by canoes and kayaks.

Once on the Oregon side, first the West Little Owyhee (Louse Canyon, actually a pretty place) joins at Five Bar (private) and then Antelope Creek (west side) adds its flow. The Owyhee becomes a real river at Three Forks boat landing, accessible by passenger car over Soldier Creek Road or Stateline Road, except during rainstorms

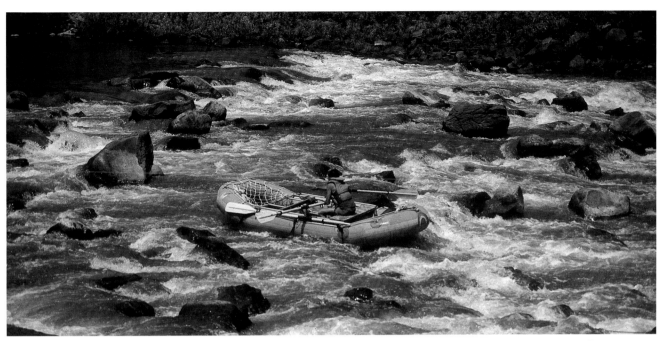

Rock Dam used to be one of the Class IV's that needed to be scouted before the big floods between 1983 and 1994.

(which make many roads here impassable). Here the North Fork, Middle Fork and main stem surge together to begin a plunge into the Three Forks Gorge. Shut off from civilization, this experts-only run is still classic pool-and-drop, allowing breathing room between the hairball whitewater for relaxing, fishing, hot spring soaking and eagle watching.

Even if you never aspire to Class V rapids, a short drive, or a hike/upstream paddle of the main stem leads to Warm Springs Canyon (north), where dozens of warm trickles sprout from canyon rocks, culminating in the Indian Bathtub at the mouth of the canyon. This semi-hot tub (about 80 degrees) lets you sit naked high on the rimrock, water surging like a whirlpool bath, as golden eagles and rare falcons whiz by. Bird hunters often camp

across the river in October; built-up pools and PVC pipe showers attest to the site's popularity. Fishing is excellent for bass and some trout.

The Duck Valley Indian Reservation on the Nevada-Idaho border provides the uppermost access to the Owyhee River at Canyon Mouth Launch Site. From here a float trip of 200 miles might be possible, winding through canyons, portaging waterfalls and impassable sections, finally finishing in the dead waters of the Owyhee Reservoir (actually, Lake Owyhee, but a lake is natural; reservoirs are artificial).

The Owyhee is deep, mysterious, very isolated, and full of surprises. In olden times, many locals truly believed that the river disappeared underground somewhere in the unexplored canyons downstream of Rome.

Rock Dam has morphed into a simple Class II+ rapid since the floods mentioned above.

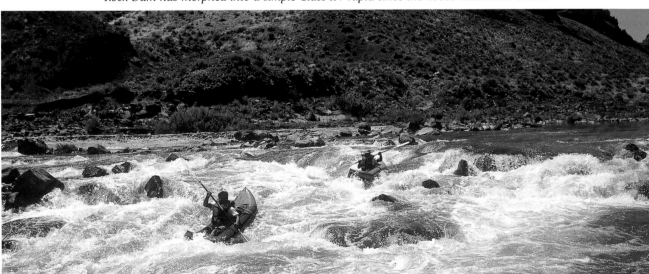

Vertical walls of the upper reaches discouraged exploration and added to the mystery. The river with the quixotic water levels (floods of up to 50,000 cfs in early spring, lows of less than 100 cfs in summer drought) somehow managed to support salmon and steelhead that migrated over 1,000 river miles from the ocean, up the Columbia and Snake in their pre-dam days, then into the shallows of the Owyhee to spawn. The river and side creeks are also home to the enigma that is the redband trout, a rare species adapted to desert life (they can survive in 90-degree water temperatures!).

Things changed with the arrival of enterprising river guides from the Eugene/Springfield area of Oregon. In 1951, Prince Helfrich, a pioneering McKenzie River guide, and Woodie Hindman, a maker of wood driftboats, floated Three Forks to Rome (the "upper Owyhee" to Oregonians, or the "middle Owyhee" to Idahoans). They used the small surplus neoprene rafts that became widely available right after World War II, topped with wooden rowing frames. This first descent is surprising as the upper reaches are considered expert (Class IV-V) whitewater, with one Class V+ (aptly named the Widowmaker).

Their next run was the lower stretch, the same one wilderness lovers and bass fishers adore, another first descent, accomplished in 1954. From this trip, many of the rock formations and rapids were named, the honor of assigning names to things earned by first descenders. Prince's descendant, Dave Helfrich, also a McKenzie River guide (the guides association, formed in 1931, honed the skills of the hardboaters on the rocky, fast McKenzie), joined the guides group in 1960 for a run in McKenzie River driftboats from Duck Valley, Nevada through the Idaho canyons and into Three Forks. One can only imagine the fun of portaging heavy wood boats around

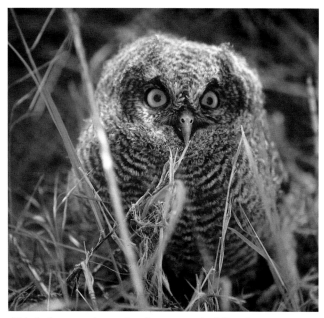

This baby great-horned owl, apparently fallen from a nest on the cliff above, was found on a beach during a lunch break.

Owyhee Falls and lining them through nasty rapids laden with sharp lava rocks.

The Helfriches understood the commercial possibilities offered by the lower run, without those arduous portages and long wilderness reaches endured along the "three state tour" from Duck Valley, and ran five- to six-day excursions for tourists the next three decades. Prince (who had the McKenzie's Thomson Lane boat landing named for him), is no longer with us but his sons and grandsons continue the family guiding tradition.

Personality

The country is strictly high desert, with sparse vegetation. The only trees for most of the trip are a few hackberries, more like bushes than real trees. A few junipers pop up along the lower reaches. In spring, the hills are green

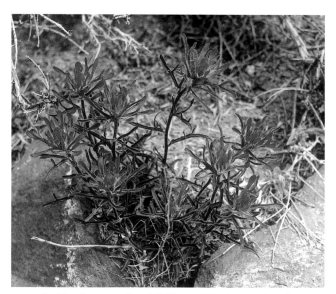

Red Indian paintbrush hides under the sagebrush.

with new growth, often grazed by open-range cattle, so watch out for cowflops in camp, dead cows in the river, and polluted water (everything except the springs is undrinkable unless treated or filtered). Wildflowers are a special treat; there are the usual desert blooms of balsamroot, Indian paintbrush, lupine, wild onion. Then there's the unusual: wild thyme bushes, peppermint, watercress.

The river runs through a series of canyons, none officially named, each one special. The first basalt canyon begins with the confluence of Crooked Creek, and continues to Rustler's Cabin. The next is Chalk Basin, an old lake bed with good hiking/Lambert Rocks, a badlands of jagged a'a (Hawaiian term for sharp lava) volcanic rocks located on river right from Pruitt's Castle. A brief stretch of rhyolite (the volcanic equivalent of granite, often quite colorful) leads to the most awe-inspiring Montgomery Gorge, where cliff walls stretch a thousand feet above the water's edge, and bighorn sheep leap from one precarious perch to the next. Then the gorge opens into Jackson Hole

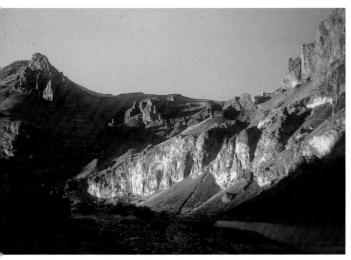

Colorful cliffs near the end of the river's free-flowing water.

and Hole-in-the-Ground. The last wild reach I call Sentinel Canyon, where a huge pinnacle resembles an Easter Island stone face, a sentinel watching over boaters.

The reservoir headwaters boast some colorful formations, as do The Pinnacles (a former private ranch on river right). After a few miles of dull desert, boaters going down the reservoir (usually by motor tow) enter the Owyhee Breaks, a former gorge now partially filled in. A hot springs is located at the head of this last canyon. Leslie Gulch (named for a cattleman killed by lightning around 1880) is a side canyon with boat ramp and the shuttle road, Oregon's most stunning shuttle, with blazing colors, honeycombed slabs, imaginative pillars, such as the Buffalo, and Three-fingers, a giant monolith. A private cabin partway up the road provides fresh, sweet spring water for thirsty boaters.

The fact that delicate McKenzie driftboats make the lower run every spring when optimal levels occur, and that the BLM does not regulate boaters in terms of numbers or experience (with too many floaters at times dulling the wilderness experience) does not mean the Owyhee is the easy family run the BLM and some boaters claim. In contrast to paradise, purgatory may come to mind during the fierce storms that often blow up suddenly, the wrap rocks that seemingly jump in front of boats, or the hatch of two million midges at riverside just as dinner is served (well, they do add high-quality protein to your meal!).

Then there's the arid climate that cracks fingertips open with such cruelty that often only heavy applications of Bag Balm (cow udder ointment) will relieve the pain and disability. Stories of paddling through hurricane-level winds, of stranded or lost craft, of drowned boaters, of snowstorms or giant hail in May, of four-wheel-drive vehicles rigged with chains taking eight hours to drive 12 miles through the muck—all these fail to ward off eager newcomers, and even the jaded veterans push that harshness back out of the mind.

Particularly as you take in the stunning beauty of Montgomery Gorge, and the orange glows of Sentinel Canyon at sundown, so reminiscent of Brice and Zion national parks in Utah (the Owyhee really should be a national park, too). Gaze in wonder at the "Underground River" that gushes pure filtered drinking water into the brown sludge that is the Owyhee at optimum floating flows. Wander through the fairylands of the Chalk Basin, and giggle at the graphic shapes of certain rock pinnacles.

Both brain and soul must accept that this lava-based canyon, so far from the volatile Cascade volcanoes, was possibly created by a meteor strike that caused lava to emerge from deep within the earth, forever changing the landscape. Rivers were trapped inside solid rock, springs

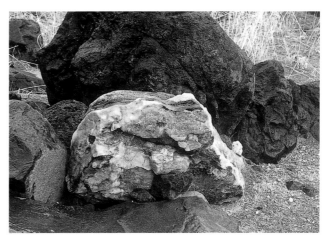

Giant agates are part of the alluvial fan brought down by the creek that squeezed the river to far right.

heated to 68 degrees or better, ash was dumped into ancient lake beds, baking clay into brick.

Changes in the speed of lava flows and cooling rates, as well as composition of minerals, converted what usually would be blah gray-black basalt into bright magenta rhyolite, freezing other flows into columnar basalt, concentrating minerals into geodes (thundereggs, Oregon's state rock), agates, pure quartz hexagonal crystals, even opal and gold.

The Owyhee is a geological time machine, taking you back 100,000 years in time for every mile floated. Some of the rocks and fantastic formations date back 17 million years. The upper run is all sheer basalt pillars and cliff walls down to the river's edge—more intimidating than fascinating to most—but the lower float is a 65-mile parade of ever-changing shapes and colors: volcanic dikes, split fault mountains, cap rocks, green "dinosaur eggs", a boulder the size of a Volkswagen, studded with thousands of calcite crystals.

Add a soak and shower in the delightful 103-degree hot springs, a glimpse of a mighty bighorn sheep, a bald eagle staring down from the pillars of Rome, the surprising battle of a 12-inch channel catfish against your trout lure, 500-pound agates littering the shoreline, the almost

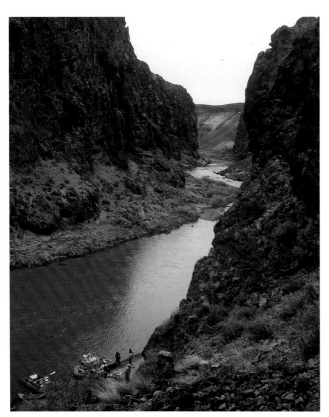

Overview of Hike-out Camp.

total lack of boaters after Memorial Day, and maybe you do have float-fisher's paradise.

The lower Owyhee is one of Oregon's most remote rivers, with no people living along the float except perhaps a caretaker at Hole-in-the-Ground Ranch. Several ranches near the end of the trip are now owned by the BLM and "We the People". Birch Creek Ranch is the closest reliable source of help, as well as a possible takeout to avoid the last 14 miles of flat water and reservoir.

Nearly all Owyhee River fishing is done on the reservoir (downstream of the wild section, a mini-Lake Mead over 50 miles long) and on the road-accessible segment just below the dam, where a tailwater fishery for trout is popular fly and lure fishing. The dam and the drive in are worth a look while you are traveling around this remote region. The drive is scenic and trout fishing often intense in season. There is a wonderful hot spring not far below the dam. At very high water levels, the Glory Hole drain spout above the dam looms like a black hole, sucking in all water and any other matter within reach—bringing a shiver as you recall the universal childhood terror of being sucked down the bathtub drain along with the bathwater.

This long float is infamous among boaters for its fickle snowpack. Recent drought years kept people away, short of the few who gambled on "flashes" that sometimes bring the river back to optimum levels, plus those with the skills, gear and time to pull off the "whitewater limbo" (how low can you go?). The lower river has been

run at levels below 100 cfs, a very tight fit except for the most determined of floaters.

Rome to Leslie Gulch

Location Southeastern Oregon. The Owyhee is about an 8-hour drive from Portland or Eugene, about 3 hours from Boise, Idaho.

From Bend, take Highway 20 to Burns, then follow Highway 78 through the bend around Crane, down to Princeton and ending at Burns Junction, where this isolated desert "road" (sorta paved) joins Highway 95. Turn east towards Jordan Valley. Rome, the put-in site, is located about halfway between Burns Junction and Jordan Valley (46 miles between these outposts of civilization). Both places offer motels, food and gas.

Jordan Valley is a wild cowboy town with taverns, an infamous rodeo, plus the Old Basque Inn (fine home-style food, in super-size quantities), as well as historic Basque sheepherder sites.

Rome now boasts a gas station, a tiny café (even the Tater Tots taste wonderful), an RV camp, rental cabins and fresh water, along with a smattering of boater necessities (paperbacks, flashlights, disposable cameras, plastic bags, batteries, etc.).

Difficulty

Class III+ (Montgomery or Iron Point Rapid is often rated as a Class IV due to the risk of wrapping/flipping and the extreme difficulty of rescue in its narrow gorge setting; Whistling Bird Rapid has killed several boaters and wrapped/flipped many more; it's a IV at lower or very high water levels, at least in my book.)

Gradient

15 fpm

Greeley Bar hot springs. photo by www.alswildwater.com

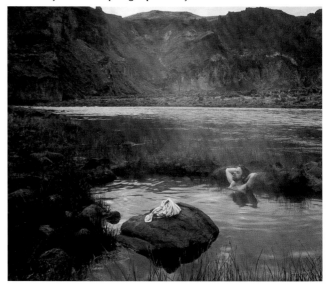

Mileage/Days

Rome to Leslie Gulch, 66.5 miles, 4+ days (at optimum water levels).

This is the most popular run; 5 days is a better minimum as there is lots to see and do. Most floaters bring a motor for the last 12 miles of reservoir water (an exhausting row or paddle) or hire a boat tow from a local. Leslie Gulch alone is worth the bother of crossing the reservoir.

Rome to Birch Creek Ranch, 49 miles, 3+ days (at optimum water levels).

In 1991 the BLM opened Birch Creek Ranch to public boat landing and fishing access. There are usually caretakers present at the ranch. The road out of the canyon to the rim is presently very rough and may become impassable even by four-wheel-drive during wet conditions. You can arrange to have a local shuttle driver meet you here with their all-terrain vehicle if you don't have one.

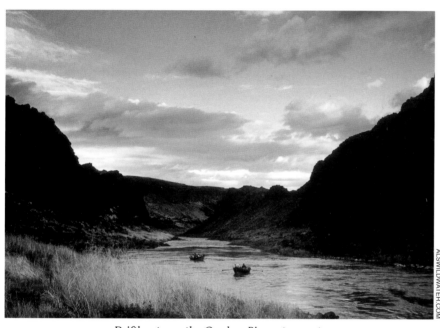

Driftboats on the Owyhee River at sunset.

The BLM may, in the future, open up Hole-in-the-Ground Ranch road as a take-out. I hope not, as the ability to do shorter trips will certainly detract from the wilderness experience of this fantastic float.

Average Float Levels/Seasons

Optimum flows are 1,500 to 4,000 cfs and occur late March through the end of May when the Owyhee snowpack is normal. Driftboats need about 3,000 to 6,000 to cover most troublesome rocks. The gauge is located at Rome.

High-Water Season

Same as optimum season. Flood levels are 8,000 to 14,000 cfs with spurts as high as 50,000 cfs.

Extreme flooding is possible on the Owyhee any time during the spring except during drought seasons. During the last El Niño events, water levels reached 50,000 cfs in March. Even high desert roads were under water, with carp swimming merrily along just above the pavement, stalked by bowfishers.

Hot weather can trigger a big meltoff, as can heavy rainstorms, so boaters need to take precautions. Camp high above the river when floods threaten, keep a watch at night, and avoid being caught in Montgomery Gorge during a high-water event. Use a stick to measure river rise at night; if the river is bigger than expected, proceed slowly and scout any rapid you can't see all of from your boat. If in doubt, lay over and wait; the river may drop after the weather event ends.

High water creates dangerous reversals at innocent-looking rapids as well as increasing the difficulty of Iron Point. Upset Rapid was named during a big-water event when uninformed boaters drifted down a midstream "slick" that lead into a gigantic flip hole. One party flipped all four of their 14-foot, heavily-loaded rafts and decided to hike out, helicoptering their gear from the rim, which is where Hike-out Camp got its name.

A man from Creswell, Oregon, my home of 23 years, died in Upset after the river rose swiftly. He was rowing a driftboat and had his life jacket apparently clipped to the boat. His body was found in an eddy; the boat survived. He would have probably lived if only the "life" jacket had been on his body.

A raft with two beginners blew out a tube while pulled over at river left to scout Iron Point at 12,000 cfs. The rapid had a raging hole in midstream and a monster reversal at the bottom. One raft landed river right and found it impossible to cross the current at the head of the rapid to help the other raft with the "flat tire". They ended up lining the boat rather than risk being trashed in the upper hydraulic. Even the party's strongest member, a professional guide, could not overcome the current to reach the far side to assist the ripped boat.

The beginners finally figured out how to stick a patch on their raft, but stayed overnight at the scout site in Shipwreck Camp. They had a successful run of Iron Point the next morning, avoiding both reversals by staying left past the first, then madly pulling right to miss the second. Moral: Know how to fix your own boat! And keep your party together, closer when conditions are more hazardous.

Another horror story: A party of four boaters in two "rubber duckies" (cheap vinyl rafts) put on at Rome and floated all the way to Whistling Bird on the same day—a distance of 30 miles, definitely not a typical day's float. According to locals, the boaters had been drinking and possibly using drugs the entire day. At Whistling Bird, one raft dumped. Without life jackets on (and even these might not have saved them), the two occupants of the raft were sucked under the slab and drowned. Their bodies were not located until searchers got to the reservoir (another 35 miles). Save your partying for camp; boat sober.

As for fishing, when the water is high, it's cold and quite murky, so only the squawfish and channel cats will strike. Scented baits or worms are necessary.

Low-Water Season

Begins at 1,500 cfs and just gets more difficult as the river drops lower. An intermediate rafter/kayaker can handle 1,000 cfs if bad rapids are scouted. The BLM posts a "Warning! River too low for safe floating!" sign at about 400 cfs. The river never drops below 100 cfs due to all the springs and the underground river, regardless of the level taken at the Rome gauge (except in extreme drought conditions).

A better level for inflatable kayaks and small catarafts is 200 to 300 cfs. Hardshell kayaks can do this level, but must pack light. Rafts need 350-400 cfs or more plus an excellent oarsman/woman.

The rock gardens of the first day take on a Class IV character as the river levels shrink. Tough boats are needed as even the best of us will hit some rocks. These first rapids drop off steeply in low water, making the lead boater responsible for quick river-reading and decision-making. If you find the first ten miles too difficult, getting out of the canyon is easiest at Hike-out Camp (up the cliff wall via a deer trail and 12 miles back to the highway) or further downstream at Rustler Cabin (where it is possible to hike out, hitch a ride back to Rome, and beg the rangers to come in their SUV to get your gear; doing this yourself requires trespassing).

Petroglyphs on the reservoir are seen by few powerboaters.

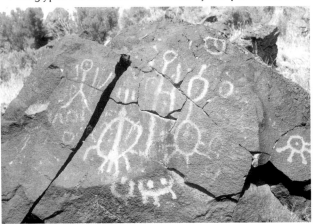

Low flows usually occur June through October most years. In drought years, the river level may never rise, or may just shoot up as a "two day wonder" after a brief storm. Tired of droughts, my husband and I made a run at 190 cfs in inflatable kayaks. Neither of us had ever seen the river lower than 1,500 cfs…indeed, the float was made right after I developed only minimal kayak paddling skills (a few hours in a Tahiti with a non-feathered double-bladed paddle). It's a totally different river at low water, with challenging rock gardens on the first day.

We had fun playing "probe boat" (the person who got stuck with taking lead, scouting an unfamiliar rocky drop with only a glance, then tackling it without much time for second chances. The following boater had the advantage of seeing where to go, or more often, where NOT to go if the probe boat got trashed.) The wind blew so hard that we lost gear and had to hole up for a few hours, as we couldn't make any progress downstream. A sandstorm right out of the Sahara desert drove us into the tent early.

However, the river water warms considerably at this level, improving bass fishing along with removing the need for wearing wetsuits in small craft. Bass struck every trout lure along the rock structure, beginning in the Whistling Bird area.

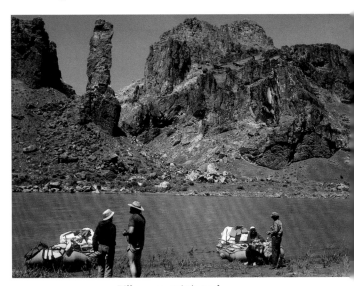

Pillar near trip's end.

As commercial guides, we had run so many rocky, shallow waters, such as the upper McKenzie, at low levels that our river-reading is almost instinctual; we were able to make the swift decisions and mostly take good routes, but as the low-water Owyhee was new to us, and because of the scary warning sign, we scouted the usual rapids—most of which are troublesome only at optimum or high levels.

Below 1,500 cfs the most dangerous rapid is Whistling Bird. This rapid actually gets easier in flood stage, as boats can just sneak over the washboard on river left. Low

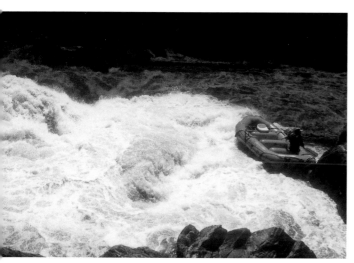

Lining Widowmaker at low water levels—always wear a PFD and beware of loose lines, poor footing.

flows force boats into river right, where a huge slab has fallen into the river. There is an undercut behind this slab that can and has trapped overboard boaters. At least three people have died here (the third a kayaker whose boat became entrapped after flipping, preventing a life-saving Eskimo roll). The slab can also flip or wrap a boat. Consider lining or portaging if the passage is too tight for your skill level. On that memorable low-water trip, a log lodged at the base of Whistling Bird, right where a boater in trouble could flip and then be held under water by the log. Even a life jacket wouldn't help much; it might even hinder by giving the log's branches something extra to snag. I portaged, but the log remained pinned for several seasons, causing much worry among boaters, until at last it was gone. I truly hope that log ended up in someone's firepan!

The next most difficult is Bull's-Eye, which is laden with rocks at low water. Start in the middle and quickly work through slim slots to river left. The current leads right into the "bull's-eye" at the bottom of this rock garden. Scout first from river left. The S-turn of Long Sweetwater is tighter, while the dreaded Upset is a simple boulder dodge with slow current. Read-and-Weep or upper Artillery Rapid is worth a scout from river right (there is a trail leading to a high overlook). Upper Artillery is a washboard of rocks to avoid, with the worst the bottom right. At some flows, a boat can squeeze between this rock and shore; at lower levels, boats must pass left. A wrong decision means a wrapped or overturned boat.

Lower Artillery is more straightforward, the most enjoyable ride when the river is at 1,500 cfs or lower. The main current funnels far left, then drops suddenly into a tight channel with big, fun waves. A splashy reversal awaits at the bottom, and is practically unavoidable, so enjoy it. Below is a long flat section for easy recovery of lost gear or people.

Dog Leg is considered troublesome at lower levels. The river splits around an island into two or three channels. Take the far right channel, dodge rocks, pull off the cliff wall, and beware the merge into the secondary currents, which create strange turbulence.

In Montgomery Gorge, Rock Trap is tight for large boats, but a snap for kayaks. More challenging is Squeeze, known as Cliff-Wall-in-Your-Face, as the best route is far left, with your mug practically kissing a million tons of rhyolite rock. Iron Point actually mellows a bit: there are more sleeper rocks, but the current lessens, so you have more time to maneuver. The Plan B route, far left and dropping between the boulders, becomes difficult at low water (it's best at 2,000 to 4,000 cfs). A large raft

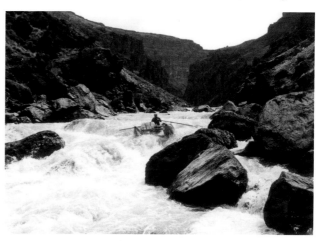

Running Widowmaker on Upper Owyhee.

can have a kayaker scout the drop first before committing to it.

For the Plan A route, pulling away from the big rocks at the bottom is still important, but chances are you can use the "butt-wiggle" technique in an inflatable kayak (get stuck on a small rock on purpose to slow your descent, then slowly wiggle free) to work river right.

Dog Leg Revisited has a big rock to avoid; the eddy at the stop tends to work you around in dizzying circles, sapping strength and nerve. Nuisance, or The Maze, was not an important rapid at all until the collapse of Rock Dam. Now, it's a very difficult rapid at lower flows. You must enter far right behind the boulders, then use the eddies to immediately get left, then swiftly set up to duck more rocks. If the water is a little higher, going down the middle and getting stuck is preferable to wrapping or flipping here.

Rock Dam Rapid has gone from a solid Class IV to a Class II-III. The scout site has changed, too; instead of river right, we now scout on the left. At most levels, it can be scouted from the boat, and involves just a sharp S-turn. Beyond this, the Class IIs that end the rapids contain more rocks, but again, slower current to help you decide and execute maneuvers. Last Chance is very tight but has a slim slot right of center.

The final disadvantage of a low-water Owyhee River float is that the reservoir may not be full, which means motors can't be used until the full pool is reached (at Owyhee Breaks). Boats must also work through miles of mudflats, usually against the wind. One way to avoid this trauma is to arrange for takeout at Birch Creek. Lastly, one note of cheer: the Greeley Bar hot spring is usable only at lower water levels. At 4,000 or more, it's washed out. Also, there are dozens of new hot springs that at optimum levels would be submerged (although few suitable for soaking). Freshwater springs appear more often, too. There is an interesting dripping spring at the back of the Whistling Bird slab "cave" to explore. Even a hot spring may be used as safe drinking water, if you don't mind a hint of sulphur (healthy minerals).

Fishing at low water is fantastic for smallmouth bass and channel catfish. If you explore side creeks entering the river or do a lot of fishing, you may hang into one of the rare redband trout. Please release any redbands without harming them. You can tell a redband from another native trout or hatchery trout by its thick body, bright red streaks, usually pink flesh, and overall brilliant color. Hatchery trout will have their adipose fins clipped.

Craft

Drfitboats at optimum levels, 12-16' rafts at most levels above 1,000 cfs, covered canoes paddled by experts, inflatable kayaks especially at low water (self-bailing preferable), catarafts at nearly all water levels, dories at medium-high levels. Boats must be in good repair and be made of very sturdy materials; leaving a trashed boat behind entails a very rugged hike to get out.

Permits

Self-issuing at the put-in. The rangers maintain a presence in Rome during the spring float season, and usually deliver an environmental lecture, as well as updates on the water level. The permit not only keeps track of boater numbers, but helps rangers to make sure all boaters get off the river safely. Commercial permits are needed for all guides and outfitters.

Hazards

Mostly the area's remoteness and the lack of polished river skills cause problems along this river. Whistling Bird has killed several people, one canoeist died on the first day of his trip (before any major whitewater was reached), Iron Point flips and wraps boats. Perpendicular Montgomery Gorge offers only one way out—downstream.

There are the usual hazards of remote country, of desert lands (scorpions, black widow spiders, rattlesnakes, poison "ivy", water hemlock and death camas). Intense winds and sudden storms are usually short-lived, but may delay float times, blow away or destroy tents, and contribute to hypothermia. Strong afternoon winds that render float craft immobile are common; start early in

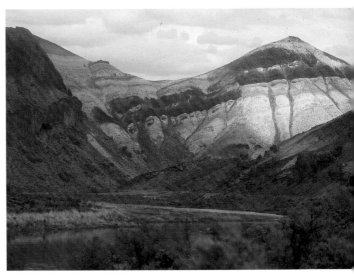

Split-fault Mountain resembles a giant ice cream sundae.

the day. The sun is very intense. Fresh water is limited below Rock Dam.

The river may contain farm chemicals and should be settled (left in a bucket for the silt to separate, as cream rises from whole milk), then filtered only if there is no other water source. Mercury washing down from Nevada mines has been detected in Owyhee Reservoir fish; limit consumption of river fish to one meal per trip or less to be safe. Pregnant women or young children should not eat any Owyhee River/Reservoir fish.

Fishing

Once anglers flocked to the reservoir to catch and preserve a year's supply of catfish, crappie, trout and bass. Since the mercury scare, the fishing is mainly catch and release, so the possibilities of catching very large fish are increasing, as the number of motorboaters declines. The river is best for smallmouth bass at lower levels, with fine catfishing in eddies. These river cats are aggressive enough to strike at trout lures as well as the usual chicken livers or other smelly baits. Channel catfish are often seen at lower water levels swarming in eddies; once I saw hundreds of them circling in an eddy the size of a school bus. They may also be caught right in the current, as a trout would be.

Bass are found around structure, and there is plenty of this along the Owyhee: basalt walls down to the river's edge, boulders and smaller rocks in the river, grassy shallows, the old Rock Dam piers, the occasional downed log. They strike the same lures and flies that the John Day bass do; just bear in mind that the Owyhee water is pure sludge until it drops below 1,000 cfs when it begins to clear as the silt settles. Fish can't see a lure in pea soup, so you may have to resort to scents or live bait (nightcrawlers work well). To chase the elusive redband, try a Rapala and other minnow imitations. Sometimes the saying,"bigger lure, bigger fish" is true.

Because fishing is secondary to this spectacular canyon, I usually carry a telescoping rod in a backpack, with a few boxes of lures and worms for the catfish (eating a few fish is OK). I've seen several of the elusive redbands, but have never landed one. The best places to try are at the mouth of the few creeks entering the main river.

Managing Agency

Vale Bureau of Land Management, P.O. Box 700, Vale, OR 97918; 541/473-3144. For updated river conditions, contact the river rangers in Rome (541/586-2612); they maintain a presence here mid-March through early June, until the river drops and rafters stop coming; then they usually put up the warning sign about low water and go home. Don't call them after 8:00 p.m. or before 7:00 a.m.—they need their beauty sleep. (The time zone here is Mountain and not Pacific as in the rest of Oregon.)

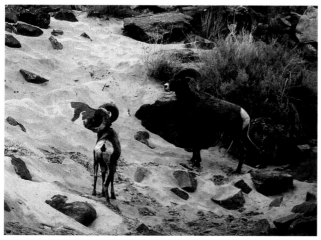

Bighorn sheep are often seen along the Owyhee; many surplus sheep transplanted into other areas came from Leslie Gulch along the Owyhee Reservoir.

Shuttles/Services

Eva Easterday Matteri (541/586-2352) does everything from meeting a group at Birch Creek or taking them upstream to Three Forks in her Suburban, to taking a flat tire out to civilization for a quick patch job. She can also deliver a motor to a group via Birch Creek so this extra weight and smelly can of gasoline doesn't have to be carried. She lives in Arock, near Rome.

Ken Haylett (208/459-1292) of Caldwell, Idaho, runs vehicle shuttles plus boat tows with his powerboat (much faster than hooking all the rafts together and towing them with an 8-horse, as some groups do; you are almost always fighting an upstream wind all the way).

The Rome Café (541/586-2294 or 2295 or 7940 or 7941) can handle shuttle keys and payments (so you don't have to leave these unguarded at your rig), dishes up a great breakfast, rents cabins, sells gas, and can probably find

you a last-minute shuttle if you can't reach Eva or Ken. Jordan Valley and Burns Junction are the nearest options for gas and motels.

Putting in at Pipeline Crossing is possible if you ask around at the café or ask the shuttle drivers. This saves some tough rowing from Rome in low water or when the wind is blowing so hard even the rangers don't launch. The Rome Launch Site is the only public camping in the area.

Mileage/Landmarks

0: Rome Crossing. Put-in site is on river right, east of the Highway 95 bridge crossing. Another site of a small post office, now moved to a larger town, Rome was named for mud sediments from an ancient lake bed, which reminded pioneers of the "pillars of Rome". Rome was the sight of pioneer river crossings, due to the long, calm pool the river has kept to for over a century, as well as the "open bowl" nature of the canyon here. Other crossings of the Owyhee are made impossible by steep cliffs.

Watch for bald eagles that nest among the cliffs here. Cliff swallows and mud swallows swarm over the river, catching bugs and feeding youngsters in nests the swallows construct of mud, carried painstakingly in beaks and patched together to form a beehive-like structure.

0.5: River island. The next 6 miles to Crooked Creek will be a mishmash of natural river islands, meandering side channels, dead-end arms, brush-choked passages, and man-made "wing dams" (bulldozers are used to create a dam of river rocks, which deepens water behind them, allowing irrigation pipes to suck water from the river when it's low). With most wing dams, the current breaks through where the flow is strongest and the dam weakest, generally midstream.

Scout these as you would minor rapids, from the boat. Bumping over them is like jumping a rock ledge on any other river. At high water, you will simply cruise through like a 500-foot yacht. These routes may change from trip to trip, not just from season to season.

Splashing in the shallows near both banks of the river are squawfish (more politically correctly called northern pike minnows), 'cats and carp, busy with spawning duties.

4: Jordan Creek, river right. Named for Michael Jordan (not the 1990s basketball wizard, the 1860s gold prospector) who lead a party that discovered gold on the banks of Jordan Creek in 1863. His group was killed in a terrible Indian fight in 1864. Of the bodies, survivors reported, "They were so cut to pieces that we had to gather them up in a blanket to bury them." Jordan Valley became a town with the arrival of a post office bearing the creek's name. After spring meltoff, Jordan Creek adds little volume to the Owyhee.

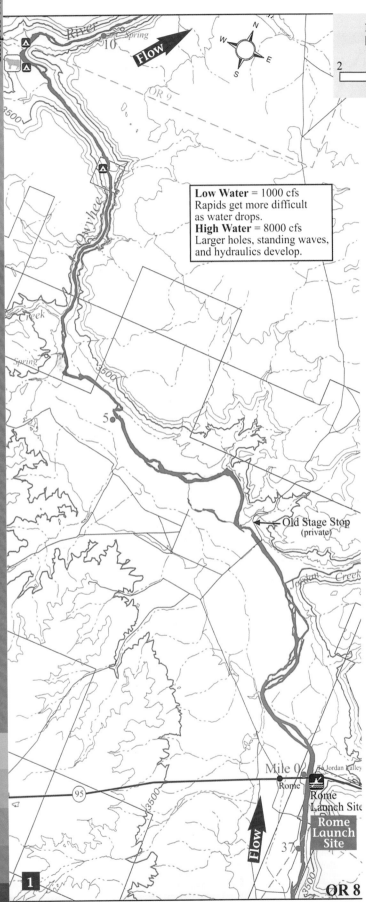

Low Water = 1000 cfs
Rapids get more difficult
as water drops.
High Water = 8000 cfs
Larger holes, standing waves,
and hydraulics develop.

4.6: Pipeline and road/bridge cross the Owyhee. Above the bridge on river right is the Pipeline Launch, a private land put-in that friendly ranchers may let you use (always ask first). The short distance cut by this put-in site is worth the trouble when the infamous Owyhee headwinds (up-canyon, almost always in afternoon) have stalled river traffic at Rome.

Just past the pipeline crossing is the Old Stage Stop, now a private home. Please enjoy this piece of history from the river: Ranchers tend to be reserved around boaters; meet them at the Rome or Jordan Valley cafes to enjoy their wealth of cowboy lore and weird-but-true tales.

8.6: In the two miles from Pipeline to River Mile 5, you float past old-timer ranches along this stretch of the river as it runs broad and slow through flat lands, wing dams, and around islands (where channels change every season). Please respect their privacy and do not land at their ranches.

Enjoy the Rome-like columns and other sediment formations you see along the way. Look high on cliff walls to spot nesting bald and golden eagles. Canada geese and other waterfowl nest this segment heavily; please grant them a wide berth, as the goslings may think a big gray raft is "mommy" and try to follow you. Red-tailed hawks are commonly seen soaring above ranchers' fields, prowling for mice, rabbits, and other crop pests. Additionally, many red-winged blackbirds warble their mating songs from the cattails and reeds along shore, hoping to attract a mate. The Owyhee also has yellow-wing blackbirds (only the males have color), but both are quite vocal. Listen for the Western meadowlark, another colorful songbird found in this area.

7: Crooked Creek enters the Owyhee from a canyon on river left. This junction marks the beginning of the first rhyolite rock gorge, a red rock bordering into pinks and reds. I call this Eagle Nest Gorge as the nests of many eagles may be seen on cliff walls, much closer to boaters than the "rim nesters" of other canyons.

Rhyolite is a volcanic rock that is very stiff and slow-moving in its molten state, and never travels far from its volcanic vent. Fine-grained and rich in silica, it forms much of the colorful portions of the Owyhee. Pinkish-gray rock, layered like sandwich filling, is rhyolite, part of the Jump Creek Formation which extends the length of the Owyhee.

Crooked Creek is a popular body-surf stream (wear your life jacket) and also marks the beginning of the wilderness, where hiking out becomes increasingly difficult.

Several springs dot the canyon walls above and below Crooked Creek; look for the lush vegetation that accompanies them. Water oozing from solid rock is safe to drink without treatment; otherwise, filter or treat chemically, as cattle graze in this area, spreading the water-bourne disease of *giardia*.

In the tight gorge that ends with Sweetwater, many eagles nest on cliff walls. Several small beaches, suitable for lunch breaks, allow for viewing of these majestic birds. They use the same nest of sticks every season until a big storm finally blows them down. You may also see water ouzel (a small gray-blue bird that hops along the shallows and actually walks underwater to stalk insects) and hear the calls of the canyon wren (a bird about 2-inches long with a big, booming voice).

8.25: First good camping area, river left. This is usually a sandy beach with lots of room. The wind blows very strongly here, so anchor your gear immediately. If the winds have been fierce since Rome, this is a good place to camp, gather your strength, and plan to be on the river promptly at first light.

9.0: This is the start of a U-bend that begins to the right at a small camp, river left (cattle graze here) with another camp, also river left, at the bottom of the U-bend, the mouth of another small canyon.

Rapids are beginning to show. At first, picking your way through is easy. The drops will gain in complexity as you continue into Eagle Nest Gorge, ending at Bulls-Eye Rapid.

10.25: Spring, river right. Identify springs in the Owyhee canyons by looking for spots of lush growth. Cattails, peppermint, nettles, watercress, water hemlock, reeds and other greenery explode around springs.

11.75: Long Sweetwater Rapid, Class III (low water). This is an S-curve rapid tight with rocks when run below optimum river levels. The rapid is named for the many springs in this area, not all of which are on the map. These are safe drinking water with no pollutants if collected at the source.

13: Upset Rapid, Class III moderate, Class II low water (Class IV+ in high water). A smooth slick in midstream leads into a gigantic reversal at levels above 8,000 cfs.

Landmark: Watch for red streaks below the rim of the gorge: clay that was baked into red brick by volcanic heat. At the head of the rapid is a large boulder of jagged basalt on river left.

Scout from left at high water. A sneak route exists far left of the big reversal in high water. In low water, this is a simple S-turn. In medium water levels, there is a second, hidden rock on the bottom of the turn with a pourover that may trash boaters. There is also a warm spring at the head of the rapid, but the terrain is slippery and the spring not all that usable for cleaning up.

A sharp right turn warns of upcoming Bulls-eye Rapid, a difficult drop below 1,500 cfs. Watch for the slow eddy on river left for scouting this technical low-water drop.

14: Bulls-eye Rapid, Class III (Class IV+ in low water, washed out in high water except for the big rock dead-center in the channel that morphs into a giant reversal at flood stages!).

Scout river left, small eddy in low water. Rugged ground for scouting. Usual route is to enter middle, work to left to avoid rocks at bottom middle and river right.

Below Bulls-eye Rapid, a debris fan has washed out from river left to form a Class II rapid with large and fun, but very splashy, waves. A strong eddy on river left is the landing for Hike-out Camp. Notice that the canyon scenery is changing from colorful, open rhyolite to the tighter, gray-black basalt rock characterized by high rims, basalt columns, large boulders (some known as "volcanic bombs" as they can be thrown great distances from an eruption site).

14.9: Hike-out Camp was named for a party of rafters that flipped all of their 14-foot rafts at Upset, lost much gear, then decided to call their trip off. They got the remainder of their belongings downstream to this camp and carried them up the hill for helicopter removal. One party member walked the 12 miles back to the highway and the Rome Ranger Station to summon the helicopter.

Another group had a leader who passed around deadly roots from the poisonous water hemlock, common at high water. His party could only watch as he went into shock, writhed in convulsions, and finally died. No one else had eaten enough root to get more than just really sick, but a piece of root the size of a peanut can kill an animal the size of a cow!

Most normal boaters without life-threatening conditions enjoy the climb up a deer path to the rim of the gorge from this camp. The views of the canyon threading its "slot" through the river are incredible. (I have made this hike with a bum knee, so almost anyone can do it, if they move slowly and keep an eye on the terrain ahead). Golden eagles often soar over hikers near the rimrock at the canyon's top. Photography opportunities are excellent.

The eddy next to the camp's beach is known for channel catfish, rather than bass, but remember these are very aggressive 'cats that will strike even trout lures.

Small groups (12 or less) should leave this area free for larger parties (up to the party limit of 20 persons). Large camps are hard to find in the Owyhee Canyon, so everyone needs to do their part in reducing "user conflicts". (Often, if camp site spaces are tight, you may ask another group if you can squeeze into the far side of their camp; ask nicely and you'll make new friends.)

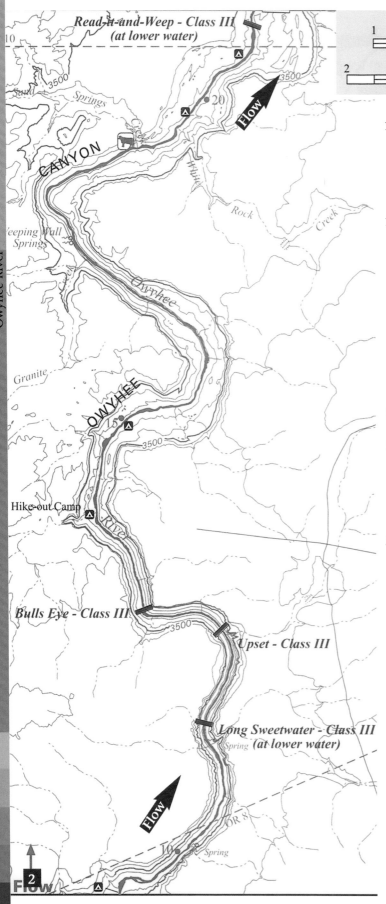

16: Hackberry Camp, river right. A medium-sized camp offers small rugged trees known as "hackberries" due to their thorny coverings; these trees shed wind and provide shelter in extreme conditions. A camp sometimes exists on river left just upstream, suitable for small groups.

18: Weeping Wall Springs, or Underground River, river left. In prehistoric times, this was a side stream entering the Owyhee. Once buried by a lava flow, the waterway converted to an underground river that now "weeps" spring waters in great abundance, technically, the underground water is trickling through the porous basalt. The verdant vegetation alerts you to its presence. Fill all water containers with this sweet-tasting, naturally rock-filtered water, but watch out for a bit of poison oak. Bright yellow monkey flowers, named for the grinning face in their blossoms, grow in abundance here.

18.75: Sand Springs Canyon, river left. A mostly-dry wash, known as a cattle area.

19.25: Campsite, river left. As the BLM map turns to River Mile 20, you are close to the pair of rapids known as troublesome in low water conditions: "Read-and-Weep" (upper Artillery) and lower Artillery. There is another campsite about a mile downstream from this one.

20.50: Read-and-Weep Rapid, Class III, also known as upper Artillery.

A large, roundish boulder on river right identifies the start of this rapid, which begins around a blind corner. There is a trail on river right for scouting. This rapid is most troublesome at low water, when there is a wrap rock at the bottom right of the drop. Scouting from the top of the trail lets you see what you are getting into.

Also, the bowl formation below (river right) is the site of an ancient Native American encampment, and was once farmed by settlers from Rustler Cabin. This site can be seen only from above, another reason to trek the scouting trail.

This area now resembles a meadow. There is a spring, and petroglyphs are visible on river left by scrambling around the boulders.

Upper Artillery is a hodgepodge of boulders and rocks to avoid, with one bad dude at the bottom right. At some flows, a boat can squeeze between this rock and shore; at lower levels, boats must pass left. A wrong decision might mean a wrapped or overturned boat. The ability to scout "on the fly" (from the boat as it moves in current) is vital here.

21: Artillery Rapid. As you finish running the upper section, a calm pool awaits below. Notice that all the rocks (at low water) are on far river right. This means you must ferry left, and quickly. There is one channel of strong current on far left, the only route, so maneuver your boat there and get set up for this channel. Small rocks at the top are troublesome at some levels, but don't let them distract you. The fast-moving left channel drops quickly into big waves, set up to hit these head-on. At the bottom (in low water) a large reversal forms. There's no way to sneak or dodge here: just hit bow-on. Boats may collide with small rocks on the banks, river left. Recovery water below allows for the rescue of any escaping gear.

Relax now, you're entering the slow waters of the Owyhee Badlands, with jagged piles of a'a lava rock on river right known as Lambert Rocks (Mr. Lambert being an early explorer of the region) and sedimentary formations reminiscent of castles and fairy palaces on river left.

21.75: The Lambert Inscription is high on river left, difficult to find. Watch for large rattlesnakes in this rocky area. Many Native petroglyphs, fairly ordinary examples, may also be found on the rocks in this area, river left. This is difficult terrain for walking due to the many boulders.

22.25: Rustler Cabin high on right bank. Hike up using the old roadbed; walking across wet or grassy areas may cause injury in addition to disturbing concealed rattlesnakes. This is a bad area for ticks and cow flops due to private land cattle use.

The decaying shack of quarried rock with wood roof was the site of a 19th-century shootout between a gang of rustlers and lawmen. Like Tombstone's gunfight at the OK Corral, the bad guys lost. The rustlers used a stone corral (still visible) to herd their stolen cattle. A boy who held the horses for the rustlers was an old man telling the tale when the first floaters arrived.

The shack has a cold spring used for refrigeration as well as drinking water; watercress and wild peppermint thrive here. Down by the river is a warm spring, so it could be said the cabin's residents had "hot and cold running water." The cabin is at present in a jumbles due to harsh winters (it was once a two-story building). It is hoped the BLM will acquire the land and rebuild the cabin to its original glory. Stone for the cabin walls was dug from a nearby slope. Up the road past the cabin are wild thyme bushes.

Evidence of later homesteaders remains in the form of rusty farming equipment and artifacts like a remarkably-preserved cast-iron Dutch oven, an essential household tool during the 1800s. This pot could cook stew, bake biscuits, even fry bacon on its inverted lid. (Remember that removing artifacts is illegal. Take only pictures, leave only footprints.)

23.75: Rye Grass Camp, river left, is scornfully known as Cow Flop Camp due to heavy cattle use. Bring your shovel or paddle to clear a kitchen space! The best part of this camp is the hot springs just upstream, which run at an amazing 103 to 106 degrees year-round. (Camping too close to the hot springs is not allowed.) The minerals in the hot springs attract deer as well as cattle.

Build only temporary structures such as PVC pipe showers and tarp bathtubs. Do not use soap in hot springs—the natural sulphur elements serve as an organic cleansing compound. Also, do not "hog" the hot springs; let other groups share. Camping too close or more than one night is not allowed. Passers-by will expect to use the springs even if you are camped there. The general rule of thumb is bathing suits in daylight, birthday suits after dark (carry a flashlight to find your way back to camp).

Sitting in these natural hot springs contemplating the desert night with almost no towns for a hundred miles is one of those perfect river moments to which no hot tub can compare. These springs were caused by the fault line that crosses the river here, which creates a river-wide ledge much like a small low-head dam. The steady hum of this riffle at night sends you off to sleep better than a lullaby. Fishing in the riffles below this dam offers a tailwater-type experience for bass, catfish and some trout.

There are several nice camps on river left and right, but the best is at the base of Pruitt's Castle, just downstream.

24: Pruitt's Castle, river left. A large formation, shaped much like a castle, named for Bobby Pruitt, "probably because it looks like a giant phallus," according to Dave Helfrich (descendant of Prince Helfrich, one of the pioneering boaters on this lonely stretch of river).

About a mile downstream from this formation is an island in the river. This island is a good place to look for agates, as are the many gravel bars and shore lines at low water. You can now see the big, black, rocky loneliness that is Lambert Rocks badlands on river right. About the only creatures walking this rougher side of the river bank are bighorn sheep.

About another mile and the full spectacle of Chalk Basin on river left comes into view, a towering formation made of lake bed sediments, black ashes, clay baked into red brick—all with intricate passages and caves leading inside. Many boaters call this the Wedding Cake as it does resemble a giant wedding cake with all the layers.

A passage through the downstream side of the formation resembles a Fairy Garden of fantastic formations, such as "cap rocks" (sedimentary bases, washing away, topped with a cap of sturdier baked clay, leaving a shape much like a mushroom). Small caves invite exploration, but watch your footing as there is much

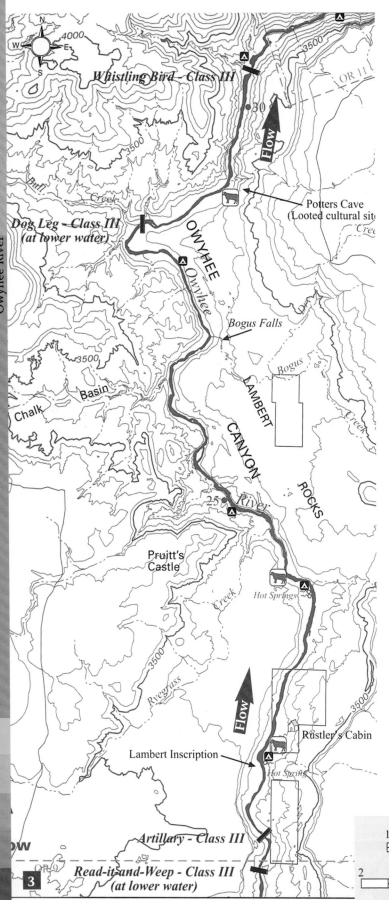

loose soil and scree (small pieces of hard rocks, very slippery) all over the formation.

A large beach once marked the beginning of Chalk Basin, but has been washed away and taken over by weeds such as cockleburr. Several tiny beaches with flat lands above allow for small-group camping. Many people camp near the Rye Grass Hot Springs camp and then spend the next day climbing the over-3,500-foot peak of Chalk Basin, which offers a stunning view of the canyon lands below, and the great, empty openness. Several routes lead to the top, either straight-up for the strong and daring, or switchbacking for the lesser-fit. Crystals and agates litter the top of Chalk Basin.

Don't get too close to the edge at the top, as the loose bits of chalk can give way under your feet, and Presto!—you're the next cap rock!

Many unusual rocks may be found poking around the base of this formation. Opalized chert, as well as true opal, is rare but sometimes found. Fossilized bone, chert and flint (both used by Natives for chipping tools and arrowheads), greenish olivine, petrified wood, rare zeolite minerals, agate, pumice, calcite crystals, and, of course, real "chalk" may all be discovered here. Brick formations leave a red streak when rubbed against another rock.

Along the river shoreline (left), are found the "bubble rocks"—where lava cooled with a "burp", leaving air pockets behind. These are most common by the mouth of the dry stream bed. There is good fishing here, with bass fishing picking up around rocks in the river.

Looking downstream, feel free to chuckle at several obviously phallic rocks that are actually cap rocks but look like the real thing, only many times larger. Guides euphemistically term these the Finger Rocks but they do not look like fingers.

A large island at the base of the Chalk Basin pool can be run on either side at optimum water levels. All islands, gravel bars, and eroded river banks in this area harbor agates and similar collector's delights. Collecting should be limited to several rocks per person, although floods generally wash down thousands of new materials every spring.

Several Class II+s await below the Chalk Basin pool; at optimum levels, these are exciting, splashy drops with a few rocks to dodge. At low water, rocks seem to take over, and locating a floatable channel becomes a challenge. Most channels are in midstream, with some lateral moves required.

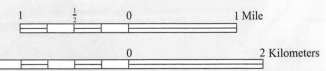

26.25: As you leave the Chalk Basin region, look up to river right to view Bogus Falls, a sometimes-running waterfall formed by Bogus Creek. (A long and rugged trek leads to a road and Bogus Creek Ranch—emergencies only.) This is the beginning of bighorn sheep country. Some boaters hike to the top of Bogus Falls; private land occupies only a tiny rectangle about a mile away.

About a mile downstream is a good campsite on river right.

Landmark: Keep an eye out for a large juniper tree at the top of a tall peak on river left; this is the landmark for Dog Leg Rapid as it is the only juniper visible for miles. Before Dog Leg, the river takes a sharp left bend past the campsite, then bends back northeast (sort of to the right).

27: Dog Leg Rapid, Class II+–III at optimum and low waters. At high water, the river overflows around this otherwise-tight bend, creating a false island and left current. River right is almost always the preferred route, and the only feasible route in low-optimum conditions. Dog Leg sweeps hard to the right, into a cliff wall. In an oar boat, use the "face the danger" technique to stay off the wall. As the river curves around the wall and joins the main current (most of which runs through or under the false island), prepare for strong hydraulics as the two sets of currents converge. In low water, this confluence is quite rocky.

27.8: Potter's Cave, river right. This is a looted cultural site. Don't add more damage to this delicate canyon; leave artifacts as you found them.

The area below Dog Leg signals the beginning of the Whistling Bird Pool, a long stretch of mostly sluggish water that has formed behind this river-damming rapid, much like a reservoir forms behind a man-made dam. Take time to notice overhangs with swallows flitting in and out; in spring, they are usually feeding babies in their mud nests. There are coves to paddle into, but don't stay long to avoid disturbing the wildlife.

This is also the beginning of the Whistling Bird Gorge, a short rhyolite canyon with impressive formations and colorful rock formations. Bighorn sheep are often spotted around the rapid during scouting. Snakes sometimes linger in the deep grasses, too, so clear a path with a handy stick or paddle thrust in front of the scouting crew.

31: Whistling Bird Rapid, Class IV except in high water (above 5-6,000 cfs). Scout river left; scouting highly recommended every time as logs can lodge in the tailout. This rapid was named for the high-pitched call of the tiny (about 2-inches long) canyon wren, "a little bird with a big mouth" as desert anarchist Edward Abbey described it. The group of McKenzie River guides who boated the Owyhee for the first time in 1954 heard a canyon wren whistling at the campsite below the drop, and the name stuck. The canyon wrens belt out notes like opera divas all through this canyon, downstream to Jackson Hole.

Debris has washed down a draw on river left, forcing the water into a narrow slot on river right. (Some of this "debris" is 500-pound agates; leave them for others to enjoy, but feel free to take pictures that show perspective, such as someone in Teva sandals standing on a giant agate face.) On the right, a huge rock slab has dropped into the river, creating an undercut, a dangerous entrapment hazard that not even a PFD can conquer. Plan on staying inside your boat at all costs. Marginal boaters should line or portage their craft.

One group, led by my husband Al Law, a 6'3" boatman, tied up their five rafts to scout this rapid at 650 cfs. A log had jammed at the bottom wrap rock, leaving only a tiny chute between the slab and wrap rock on river left, and the jumble of debris brought down by the creek on river right. The other guides proclaimed they were not running the rapid, then proceeded to line the empty paddle boat by scrambling over the slippery washboard of rocks. Al watched them slip and fall on the rocks, then walked back upstream and took the oars of the lightest cargo boat. He had a very successful run, then walked back upstream to bring the other three boats, each more heavily loaded, down the rapid, one at a time. The last, heaviest 16-foot raft cleared the log by about an inch.

Many guides prefer to walk clients here, when low water conditions cause the channel to shrink. Two guides can "R-2" an empty boat (that is, paddle it like it is a canoe, with a bowman and a stern paddler) without getting into trouble. Rowing is harder as the oarswoman must judge the proper moment to begin pulling. Pull too early, and the stern of the craft will strike rocks behind the stern, unseen by the rower. This leaves about 2-3 strong pull strokes at lower levels (below 1,500 cfs) to "pull or die" but is more of a mental challenge.

To run Whistling Bird at optimum or lower levels, set an oar raft at an angle to the current, facing the danger of the rock slab on river left. Keep the angle, waiting for the right time to pull. (A person on shore or the back of the boat can help by yelling "Now!" once the alluvial fan has been cleared.) Then pull with all your might, using both oars and even but powerful strokes, until you are past the slab and wrap rock on river left. Lining is always an option; you will want to bring long ropes to avoid treacherous footing.

At the bottom of the rapid, there is a nice camp with hackberry trees, good rock-hunting, catfishing, swimming and hiking (up the wash to Hoot Owl Spring). It's also a good place to rest and have lunch after the trauma of running Whistling Bird.

After you safely depart Whistling Bird, keep watch on river left. Just above an island that splits the river,

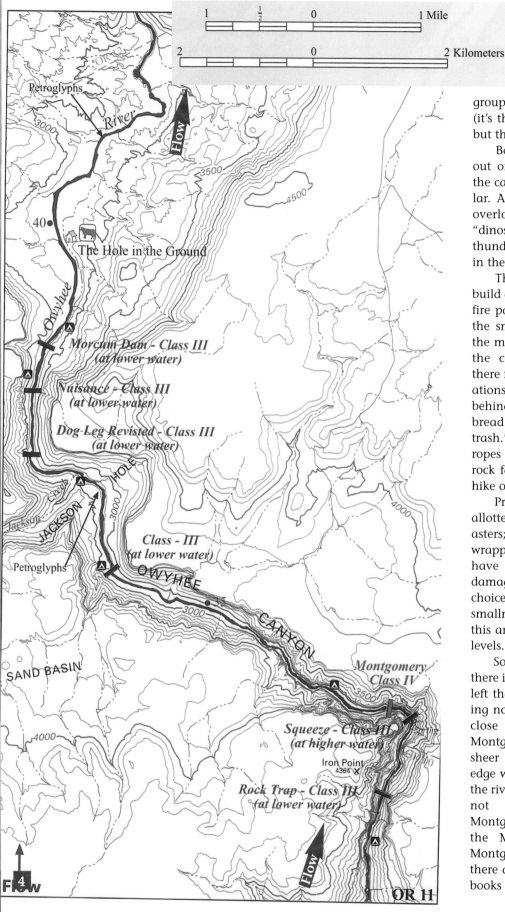

Owyhee River

there is a large cave in the rhyolite formations at river level. This is a good lunch or rest break, but can also be an overnight stay for a group that doesn't mind getting cozy (it's the size of a two-bedroom house, but the rooms are modestly sized).

Both bats and birds whiz in and out of this cave. Photos taken using the cave walls as frames are spectacular. A hike up the wash leads to an overlook of the gorge, as well as "dinosaur eggs"—rocks that resemble thundereggs but are green like oviline in the center.

This cave is a delicate area, so build a fire only at the mouth, using a fire pan, and put your porta-potty in the small side cave just upstream of the main cave (do not poop or pee in the cave sands—both will remain there for a long time, offending generations of boaters). Also, do not leave behind cigarette butts, orange peels, bread twist-ties, and other "microtrash." Tie boats securely, with two ropes per boat, as this is an isolated rock face that is nearly impossible to hike out of should you lose your boat.

Priority for camping in the cave is allotted to the party with the most disasters; any boaters who flipped or wrapped at Whistling Bird, or who have wet sleeping bags and other damaged gear should be given first choice. By the way, catfishing and smallmouth bass angling are great in this area, especially at very low water levels.

Soon after leaving Whistling Bird, there is a large rock formation on river left that resembles a huge, overhanging nose, and the river walls begin to close in. This is the "Gates" of Montgomery Gorge, the closing-in of sheer rock faces down to the river's edge with no escape other than down the river. Montgomery Gorge is named not for Rube and Howard Montgomery, who herded logs down the McKenzie, but for a Doctor Montgomery who tipped his boat over there during a 1950s trip. Some guide books call it Green Dragon Canyon, but it's not green and there are no dragons (just more rattlesnakes).

32: Rock Trap Rapid, Class III (optimum and low water levels), scouting from right may be necessary. A maze of five major boulders presents a river-wide obstacle, with several routes possible, depending on the water level. Use the eddies behind the rocks to move from rock to rock. Watch out for breaking paddles, oars and even oarlocks—be ready to ship oars into the boat. Right is the preferred channel in optimum levels.`

Don't relax here, there are several Class IIs, depending on the water levels. The Little Yellow Tarp Rock is found in this area; I hope it doesn't find you!

"The Little Yellow Tarp"—We were a group 20 strong in a half-dozen boats; rounding a corner, I saw that everyone in our party was pulling for the right bank. As the "sweep," or last boat in line, I followed suit. When we arrived, I saw what looked like a little yellow tarp wrapped around a boulder, beneath the water, with a despondent man sitting on the rock. Three women kayakers had beached their boats and were recovering some lost gear. I quickly realized the "little yellow tarp" was actually a 16-foot-long yellow Maravia raft, worth about $3500 in those days. It looked like someone's lost rain slicker.

Our gang included a Swiftwater Rescue Technician, besides boasting seven men over 6' tall. Our SRT set up a "Z-drag" (a system of pulleys, carabineer, polyethylene rescue rope that floats, and prusik knotted cord that greatly increases the mechanical advantage of people pulling on a single line). About 30 minutes later, their raft was sitting on shore, mostly intact. Plus, we had salvaged most of their gear, including their motor for the reservoir tow. I guess they'd still be there, waiting for help, if our commercial party hadn't come along with the party-limit of 20 people, the right gear, and the knowledge of how to save their boat.

Think about this the next time you hear other private boaters express a negative opinion towards commercial boaters and/or their guests for making/paying money to run rivers. They also help save lives and gear. Truly, the next group was many days behind them, and they might not even have stopped to assist.

33: Tight Squeeze or Cliff Wall in Your Face, Class II+ to III (optimum and low water levels). The best current is on the far left, right with your face pressed close to the 30-ton rock wall. Those who take the wrong route at lower levels, thinking they are safer far from the wall, may end up flipped or wrapped. Don't look at the towering cliffs too long in search of bighorn sheep as the big one is coming right up.

33.5: Iron Point or Montgomery Rapid. The river takes a very sharp bend to the left after the Squeeze, leading into Montgomery. The Iron Point Rapid name is given due to the reddish-orange color of the steep peninsula

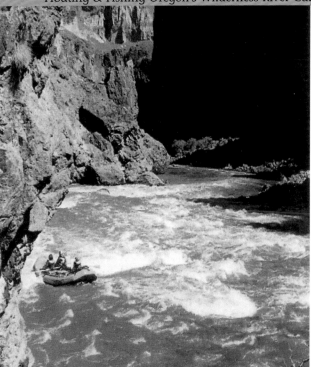

One of our favorite places, Montgomery rapid on the Owyhee. For Plan B stay far left or, Plan A to the right.

of land jutting out from this vertical canyon, its tip 4364 feet in elevation. Scouting on river left is highly recommended. In high waters, scouters can become stranded if they scout river right, and will be forced to line their boats.

The usual run, or Plan A, at optimum or low flows is to locate the large boulders (wrap rocks) at the bottom of the rapid. Boaters must then thread a course through the rocky entrance, and once past these obstacles, face the danger of the wrap rocks and pull for their lives. Face the danger—river left—set up at a strong angle, and pull, pull, pull. A wrapped boat on river left is extremely difficult to recover—far from shore, far from other boaters, no helicopter landings, etc.

This rapid is actually easier at lower levels as the current does not force boats into the deadly left-side boulders. An upstream breeze helps, too. There is enough fallen rock on river right that, at normal to high levels, boaters are forced to start left, then madly pull right once past these outcrops to miss the bottom boulders.

At very low water levels, there is a warm spring at the edge of the scouting outcrop on river left. At any water level, watch out for poison ivy, which thrives here.

At high water, as mentioned earlier, those wrap rocks at the base of the rapid become a humongous reversal, a certain boat-flipper. The rocks in the middle become another dangerous hole. The boater must head left, miss the first hole, then set up sideways to pull hard away from the hole at the bottom. Also in high water, a lost or overturned boat may escape. One

Owyhee River

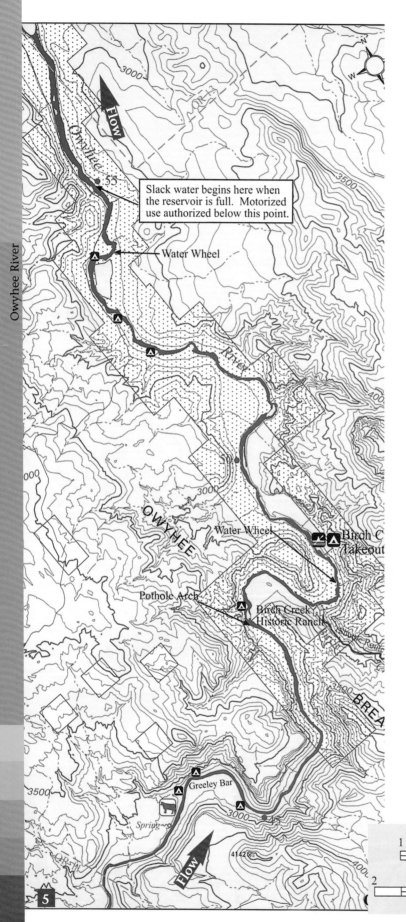

Slack water begins here when the reservoir is full. Motorized use authorized below this point.

Water Wheel

OWYHEE

River

Water Wheel

Birch C Takeout

Pothole Arch

Birch Creek Historic Ranch

Greeley Bar

Spring

4142

BREA

Flow

Flow

1 ½ 0 1 Mile

2 0 2 Kilometers

5

hapless boater who was flipped out swam after his boat in the strong flood currents and finally captured it several miles downstream.

If you miss the pull to the right, or if the river is at optimum levels and you are feeling sure of yourself, there's always Plan B. This requires much more trust in river currents than hard pulls. Set up far left, barely missing sleeper rocks, staying within a few feet of the cliff wall. The current will carry your boat left towards the furthest wrap-rock. Just before you slam sideways into this rock, take a few strokes backward (face the danger and pull), watching for sneaky sleepers in your route. Once your boat is sideways between the two boulders, perform a perfect double-oar turn so you are bow-first (or, in an emergency, stern-first, just never sideways), tuck in or feather your oars, and drop between the boulders.

Don't rest yet, a rock ledge below this drop thrusts out, daring your boat to hit sideways and wrap. Pull away, being ready to highside if necessary. This drop is often too abrupt for small or heavily loaded inflatables and driftboats, and for them is a last-ditch effort only. It can be scouted by a probe boat first.

At the end of Iron Point Rapid, pop a soda or a beer and relax while you wait for the rest of your party. Always keep your group together in this narrow gorge so nobody gets left behind. The gorge walls are over 3,000 feet straight up for the next three miles, and walking out is a joke unless you have cloven hooves.

Fresh potable spring water is available on a beach, river right, at lower water levels. There are several nice camps, including the Bat Cave, river left below Iron Point about 3/4 mile, where a camping beach comes and goes with the vagaries of the river, but nice sandy sites remain at the base of the cliffs, most even providing dry spots during storms due to the overhang. Rattlesnakes are very common on this beach as they thrive on the mouse population in the Bat Cave; don't kill them, just use an oar to push them into the river, where they will swim downstream to the next camp. Larger groups have first pick here.

A number of smaller beaches beckon to smaller groups. Several riffles and pick-your-routes keep interest going as, all too soon you approach the gorge's end, signaled by a large, gray-colored wall on river left. Camping in the gorge should be done at high water only if the river is dropping, as boater camps have been flooded out.

Bass fishing in this gorge is the best on the river. Bighorn sheep can be seen at first light, using binoculars to scan the small green ledges they crop for breakfast. A night in this enclosed gorge provides a special experience to all but the claustrophobic.

The gorge ends with a wonderful camp on river left, with a protective overhang to fend off bad weather and dew. Fishing around the riffle that leads to this camp is good. There are wildflowers to enjoy, but not the closed-in feeling of the main gorge.

37.25: Rapids pick up again once outside the gorge. A Class III drop (lower optimum flow to low water) challenges with hidden boulders. This starts with a powerful eddy on river left, then the current leads into a midstream boulder that must be dodged.

Several more Class IIs (again, depending on water levels, more at lower water) continue, in pool-and-drop fashion, down to Hole-in-the-Ground. You will notice the canyon opens up; this is Jackson Hole.

A beach on river left is now divided into upper and lower sections; at one time, this was one long beach that rivaled the huge beaches of Idaho's Lower Salmon until floods brought pebbles, gravel, riprap and other barefoot obstacles to divide the beach. At the lower end, there are small trees and a good landing spot on the sand. The boulders among the camp sites are adorned with petroglyphs. A long but satisfying hike is possible by following Jackson Creek or the open hillsides, switchbacking your way up, to an overlook of the great gorge (watch for snakes).

37.75: Dog Leg Revisited is a Class III bend of the river with a BFR (Big Freaking Rock) to dodge midstream (at optimum or low flows).

38.25: Nuisance Rapid, or The Maze, at lower water levels, Class III+. This is a river-wide scattering of boulders that, in high water, can be run straight down the middle. In low water, boats must sneak behind the right side boulder, then immediately maneuver to miss the next; much like Rock Trap, only more difficult. Scouting from the right is recommended. Cargo rafts often wrap, flip, or lose gear in this rapid. A paddle of mine was stuck under a rock, dragging me under with it, until I decided to let the river have the paddle. It remained sunken even after an hour-long search—and it was a brand-new, yellow-bladed kayak paddle, easy to spot even under water.

Nuisance did not exist until the next drop, Rock Dam, washed out during heavy flooding. The pool of dammed water kept Nuisance runnable. Now it's far more difficult a run than Rock Dam (inaccurately listed in older manuals as a Class IV).

38.75: Rock Dam Rapid, aka Morcum Dam, formerly rated as a Class III-IV, it's now mostly a Class II+. This was an attempt by the Morcum Ranch settlers to dam the Owyhee for irrigation and flood control, but the river decided it would rather run free and unfettered. One big flood season took out most of the concrete, including the lining channel used by boaters on river right. You can still see rusted machinery scattered around.

To run the modern Rock Dam, scout from river left, if necessary, or from the boat. This rapid is an S-turn at most water levels, with the route left of center. If you scout, watch for rattlesnakes.

39: Possible sandy beach on river right, good camping flat. The land belongs to the BLM (public) now.

39.75: The-Hole-in-the-Ground, or Morcum Ranch. The canyon has opened into a large bowl, with some minor riffles the only rapids to worry about. This ranch has a road leading out to the rim and civilization; sometimes a caretaker is present, making Morcum Ranch a possible source of emergency help. There are rumors that the BLM wants to develop this road and the ranch into a boat landing, which would change the nature of the Owyhee from a long wilderness excursion into a 3-day "splash and giggle". I hope this is not done, as it would ruin the wilderness experience for the few who relish longer sabbaticals from society.

Jeep roads are on both sides of the river. Some cattle are still run on this lonely ranch. We can only trust that the BLM will close these roads to public entry to protect the delicate petroglyphs just ahead. Watch for several small rapids.

41.25: Petroglyphs, river left. This is the best collection of Native carvings in eastern Oregon. You can land at the upper site, marked by two large junipers (the third was burned down). Here are 'glyphs that seem to mark the passage of time with circles. Please do not camp here, touch or try to make rubbings of the 'glyphs, or add your own carvings or markings. These rock carvings photograph very nicely.

A Class II+ rapid is directly ahead; after running it, you can land at its base (look for a small beach that forms at levels below 4,000 cfs or so) and view more petroglyphs (or hike the ridge line from the 3 Trees landing). A "white man petroglyph" is old enough not to detract from the ancient carvings. One of my favorite Native art pieces is the carving of a bighorn sheep, found on the rim trail. Another is a large rock, flat on one vertical side, with carvings of what appear to be "little green men" but are probably meant to represent the tribe's shaman, or priest. Notice that previous attempts at rubbings have left indelible markings on this site. Several small 'glyphs have actually been chipped loose and carried away. Don't do this, or you will be haunted by the ghosts of the ancient Paiute!

Look carefully around the base of petroglyph rocks and you will find many lithic fragments (remnants of arrowhead chipping), as well as actual prehistoric arrowheads. Please leave these for others to enjoy. Also note that obsidian, the chief ingredient in these arrowheads, is not native to the Owyhee Canyon. These Natives traded for obsidian from other tribes much further away, probably from the 6385 foot elevation Glass

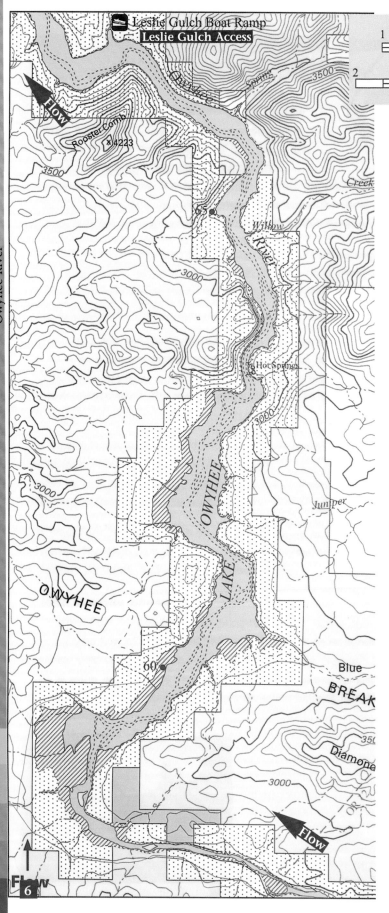

Owyhee River

Butte close to Bend, where a mountain of valuable sharp material was available for the picking. Other arrowheads were made of chert, Oregon jasper and flint. Sometimes agates were chipped into tools or used as-is for "pebble tools" (a pounding instrument, naturally round or oval, held in the hand). The petroglyph sites were probably a sacred area where tools were made under the watchful eyes of the religious carvings, so as to increase their "luck" and to grant the good graces of the spirit world when Natives hunted sheep or deer.

For the next two miles, **rocky rapids** challenge optimum and low water boaters. A large rock formation I call the Devil's Tower dominates the left side of the canyon. (This name reflects this columnar basalt mountain's eerie resemblance to the Wyoming tower in the movie, Close Encounters of the Third Kind.) Once more, the canyon changes into great formations that are mostly orange from iron oxides. I call this last canyon of the free-flowing Owyhee Sentinel Gorge after a large rock face downstream of several camps.

42.5: Greeley Hot Springs, river left, marks the end of major rapids. The last drop before Greeley Bar, Last Chance, is tricky at low water. Mid-channel or just to the right of it is the best route to dodge most of the rocks. Greeley Bar is the name for the big sandy beach with real trees located about 1/4 downstream on river left. There is a large boulder loaded with calcite crystals near this camp (don't chip away at it, many are laying on the ground if you want a souvenir), in addition to petrified wood, Owyhee River Picture Rock (named for the streaks on this rock's slab faces, which often resemble paintings), and other goodies.

Greeley Hot Springs are submerged at river levels over 4,000 cfs or so. They are a good walk upstream from the main camp, so take your flashlight if you go there at night. One brisk night I just couldn't get warm in my sleeping bag, so I walked upstream to the hot springs and soaked for about 20 minutes. Afterwards, I dried off, dressed, and returned to my tent, where I fell asleep in moments. I also spent an enjoyable night here watching Hale-Bopp comet sweep across the dark desert skies.

43.5: Greeley Bar Camp, river left. The shelter at the downstream end of the camp has been trashed by cow flops. The cabin on river right is where Greeley lived as a sheepherder. A tiny rock shelter protected him from the chill winds of winter. Locals say

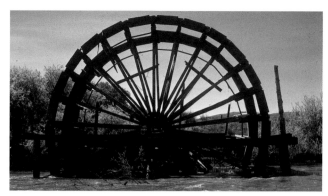

Old water wheel helped irrigate fields at the head of the reservoir.

that when the weather was particularly nasty, Greeley would take in several ewes to sleep with, as the Eskimos sleep with dogs. Thus the term, "a three-ewe-night".

If the river-left camp is occupied (large groups only in the busy season), there are many good sites on the huge bar, river right, which offers good rock collecting and a wild explosion of yellow balsamroot flowers in spring.

This is the last of the free river; soon enough the stagnant pool of the lake will be encountered, so enjoy your camps here. All of Greeley Bar, both river left and right, has many channel catfish waiting to be caught. Using meat scraps or nightcrawlers on a set line is effective.

At a camp downstream, a large pillar resembles an Easter Island statue, a stern rock face, especially when viewed from downriver of its location. (While floating, don't forget to look back upstream once in a while.) What appears to be a cave high on this formation is actually a huge eagle's nest (use your binoculars to check more closely). This is the formation that gave this orange-tinted canyon the unofficial name Sentinel Canyon.

If you have a good imagination, you can spot the Statue of Liberty pillar, which also resembles a cigar-store Indian at some angles. This formation is located on river left. Signs of scum and reeds at low water levels usually indicate the presence of more warm springs that are under water at optimum levels.

46.75: Water wheel, river right. There were once three water wheels along this segment, where downstream ranches tried to use the power of the river to irrigate crops and grow grass for cattle. But the river keeps destroying them. This one has a rocky drop next to it, probably the result of a wing-dam flooded out. Another water wheel, further downstream, was left high and dry when the river changed to the left channel.

47.25: Birch Creek Ranch, newly developed BLM takeout and recreation site. The road is, so far, very much a 4-wheel-drive affair, and undriveable after a storm. Many camps, wildly colored formations, and small

rapids are found between Greeley and Birch Creek. On river left is the Pothole Arch. One boulder, if you paddle past it during very low water, exudes boiling water from a hidden hot spring. Don't test it with your hands!

The large mountain downstream, which looks like a tilted ice cream sundae, is sometimes called the Split Fault Mountain. Most of the river follows a fault line during its course; here, the fault line has shifted, creating the "tilt" effect of this black, gray and white layered hill.

50.50: Island splits river. Right channel is more interesting.

Several good camps on river left. This country is the Owyhee Breaks. Cameras at sunset click away at the fantastic rock formations bathed in glow. Remnants of old shack, river left, are all that are left of a community of long-ago.

53.50: Water wheel #2, around a sharp bend to river right.

55: Slack water generally begins here, unless the reservoir has not filled. There are long gravel bars suitable for stopping to hook boats together with rope and carabiner in this region. If the reservoir is low, do not use a motor with prop; wait for deeper water.

60.25: Blue Canyon enters, reservoir right. Cormorants, egrets, bald eagles and the rare wild swan are sometimes seen on the reservoir. Fishing for crappie and bass is usually good. If you are under tow, try trolling.

63.75: Hot Springs, reservoir right. The PVC pipe shower is visible for a distance. About seven pools of varying temperatures tempt tired floaters. Rough land for camping is available on reservoir left. Remember this is an area frequented by motorboaters, so you may not want to skinny-dip.

The springs also begins a colorful, tighter canyon as you are half way to the take-out. Watch for eagles here.

66.5: Leslie Gulch, reservoir right, appears as a large side channel. A concrete boat ramp accommodates both powerboaters and float boaters. Keep one side of the ramp open for trailered boats. Three Fingers Formation is located just up the gravel road from the boat ramp. One night after leaving our motor mount behind on the beach at Greeley Bar, we cobbled a new one at Pinnacles, the ranch downstream of Birch Creek. Due to lost time, our group of river guide trainees found themselves putting along in the dark. We were able to locate Three Fingers by starlight, and soon were at the ramp. With the Coleman lantern lit, we didn't leave any gear behind in the dark. There was a beautiful agate laying on the ramp that everyone kept tripping over, so I brought it home.

Don't be afraid to ask for a tow if your motor conks out, most folks are friendly (plus, your gas, beer, and film all make good trading commodities).

Owyhee River

Chapter 8

Rogue River Wilderness

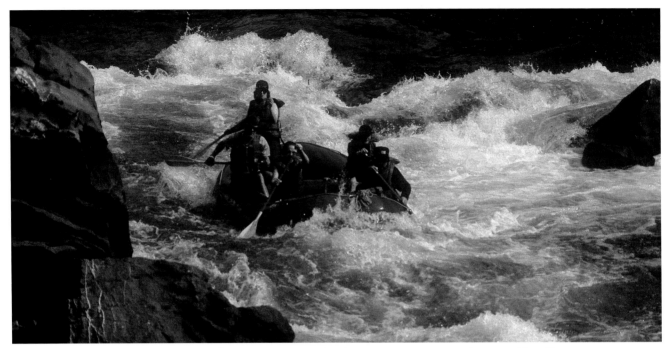

Running Upper Black Bar Rapid on river right, the proper position at optimum and low flows
(looking upstream, it appears to be left).

THE WILD & SCENIC ROGUE WAS AMONG THE FIRST eight rivers designated as a federally-protected waterway. It is world-famous for both wilderness and civilized fishing. Recent runs of salmon in the years after 2000 have featured huge fish, and a world-record salmon was caught near the mouth of the Rogue.

The name "Rogue" has several possible origins (it's pronounced "rogue" as in "scoundrel" and not "rouge" which means red in French). "Rouge" was employed by early French trappers for the reddish color of the Rogue in flood; the "Colorado" or "Red" river, named by Spanish explorers, is definitely more red. The Rogue is more like mocha coffee in spring flood. Red may also have derived from the many bloody battles between Rogue Indians and Cavalry. More likely, because of the trouble caused by Rogue tribes when invaders tried to take their lands, the English version of the French name for these Natives; Les Coquins (the Rogues), stuck.

The river has a long and colorful history. Inhabited for many thousands of years by Native Americans, tribes from the Umpquas to the north as far as the Klamath to the south passed from generation to generation tales of the great mountain god Mazama, who vented his anger on the Earth by raining down ash, fire and mudslides. We now know that Crater Lake, one of the deepest in the world (deeper than 2,000 feet), was formed in the caldera of this mysterious missing mountain. The eruption is estimated to have happened about 8 to 12,000 years ago, and would have been large enough to put Mt. St. Helens to shame. The Rogue headwaters near this national park.

Lesser battles were fought among mortals for control of the Rogue region, between Natives and cavalry, neighboring hermits, and commercial fish-netters. Some of the most intense battles for control of Native lands were fought in the Rogue River and southwestern Oregon area, at Battle Bar, Big Bend and other sites. The area was rich with wildlife, so beaver trapping was profitable; then came the Gold Rush, and pioneers who found the Valley of the Rogue's mild weather perfect for growing crops. Mail-order gift magnate Harry & David's famous "Royal Rivera" pears have been grown around this area since the early 1900s.

Enormous amounts of gold were removed from the Rogue; $28 million in 1800-era dollars was mined from the Almeda site alone. There are still private mining claims that reap enough gold to make the hard work worthwhile, while the wilderness can be panned by anybody for fun (not commercially). Floods bring down more gold every season, while increases in mining technology allow hidden gold to be extracted more profitably (outside the wild zone).

Almeda Campground or Grave Creek to Foster Bar

Location

Southwest Oregon, near the border with California. This is the easiest wilderness river to access by car, as the launch sites are only about 30 minutes from the freeway. From Interstate 5, take the Merlin exit (located just north of Grants Pass). At the stoplight, turn left. Here a sign indicates Indian Mary Park—a very luxurious public camp—in case you forget which way to turn. Stay on this road through Merlin (named for the small bird of prey, "pigeon hawk" and not the medieval magician). Here you can get groceries or rent boats.

The Rogue headwaters at Boundary Springs near Crater Lake National Park, flowing though a spectacular, tight gorge, before settling down into a warmer, lazier stream near Shady Cove. The section known as the Gold Hill or "Nugget" run drops over two steep ledges into large reversals (one is actually a jump over the old dam site). Below this spot, the Rogue wanders again as it comes into Grants Pass, looking much like a tame city river until the Galice area, where the classic pool-and-drop rapids begin.

The road from the Merlin exit continues through spectacular Hellgate Canyon (an easier day trip) to Galice, the last-chance and a must-stop for boaters, with shuttle service, T-shirts, glasses straps, sandals and other river necessities. There are over a dozen public boat ramps in this area. Most boaters prefer to launch at the beginning of the wilderness section, Grave Creek, creating a crowded situation at times. Launching at the paved ramp of Almeda is often easier, and you can camp there the night before (no overnight parking at Grave Creek is allowed, and in flood season, your cars may be washed downstream—"no overnight parking" enforced by Mother Nature). Argo is a primitive site with camping and boat ramp, but the ramp is sandy, so take care not to get stuck.

Zane Gray's cabin. It's easy to imagine living here alone, as Zane Grey did, writing about feuds over gillnetters after salmon.

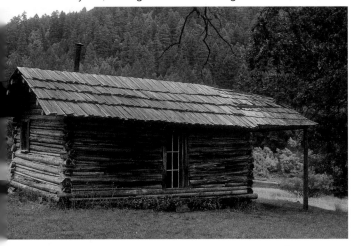

Ennis Riffle is another popular site (free camping), but with the same type of sticky sand.

Personality

The Rogue has several wilderness lodges (wonderful but sometimes hard to book without an outfitter), old miner's cabins and equipment, a caretaker's cabin at Brushy Bar, and lots of people despite a permit system (120 a day are allowed in the wilderness in season), outhouses, a hiking trail along its entire length, shelters at two camps, rapids made runnable by dynamited boulders, giant jetboats loaded with tourists outside the no-motors stretch, rich private-land owners, and sometimes movie stars ("The River Wild" and "A Killing at Hellgate" were filmed here, as are some other movies).

Yet, all of these combine to make the Rogue a special experience. Wilderness can still be found during the off-

Bushwacking up to Dulog Falls.

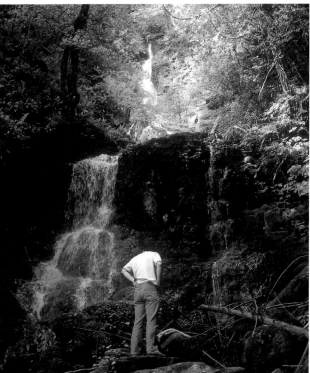

season (in March and April, traffic is so sporadic that the ranger station is closed).

Tame wildlife is another Rogue distinction. Although it's now illegal to feed black bears and the blacktail deer, they still wander into camp looking for handouts. Hunting is not allowed, so the wildlife has no fear of humans. I once lured a fawn to "kiss" me for a photo by holding a Ritz Cracker in my mouth. Mink, river otter, muskrat, raccoons and squirrels are often seen on shore. Bald eagles favor the segment from Almeda to Russian Rapid, but can be seen anywhere. Osprey are common, as are waterfowl, heron, killdeer, kingfisher, cormorant, and wild turkeys. This river is one of the last refuges for the endangered western pond turtle, many almost the size of dinner plates, which can be seen in slower waters such as just above Tyee Rapid. (The predominance of large turtles, however, means that many of the younger ones have been eaten by predators.) There are 11 different types of bats, animals that should not be feared (they won't fly into your hair, not only because of their radar, but because they know what your hair looks like after a week on the river). For the discriminating birder, four species of woodpeckers and 11 types of warblers have been seen in the canyon.

Unique to the Rogue are some man-made rapids. Early boaters faced a very rocky river, and used dynamite to clear channels of pesky boulders (a practice now banned). Glen "Boom-Boom" Wooldridge, the Rogue's first and most famous guide, accomplished most of the bombing by rowing up to the offending boulder, lighting the dynamite, placing it in a paper bag weighted with sand, tossing it off the boat, and then rowing like hell. Before such improvements, Blossom Bar was so choked with boulders that it was not runnable and required a day-long portage of the heavy, wood boats and gear used before World War II brought neoprene rafts into surplus stores. Glen made his first float trip in 1915 and was also the first person to motor up the river from Gold Beach to Grants Pass.

Also in the good old days, a boater had to launch at Grants Pass and float to the ocean. Today, only the occasional adventurer who has several weeks to play with makes this journey (no dams or impassable rapids to portage, only one spot, Rainie Falls, that can be lined). Now the Rogue has easy road access (although the shuttle roads are long and winding), and the stretch from Hog Creek to Grave Creek attracts many beginning boaters, who frolic in rented boats or on guided trips.

A perfect climate attracts boaters and anglers, as well—the water is 70 degrees or higher in summer, great for swimming. The canyon breezes cool off hot days. The river meanders through a beautiful canyon carpeted with Douglas fir, oak, Pacific madrone (an unusual tree that naturally peels off bright red bark, leaving an ivory trunk), chinkapin, dogwood and Oregon myrtle, with leaves that flavor spaghetti or soup like bay leaves. The diversity of the Rogue Canyon can be seen as you float, the canyon itself broadening from a tight rocky gorge formed by hard volcanic rock into open meadows where conglomerate rock has been eroded into pot-holes, caves and other strange formations.

Watch for the Tree Rock, where a sturdy scrub oak grows directly out of a boulder, and for Dinosaur Tree, a bent pine that really does look like Dino. Wild rhododendrons and azaleas provide a burst of colorful blossoms in spring. Huckleberries, salal, salmonberry and the introduced nuisance, Himalayan blackberry (which makes a great cobbler!) are enjoyed by both humans and bears.

Difficulty
Class IV. Most of the river is Class II & III, but Mule Creek Canyon and Blossom Bar do require advanced skills. Rainie Falls is a Class V+ that has drowned a guide, and should be lined.(This is the falls where the log raft goes over in the classic movie "How the West was Won".) Rocks in the middle of the river, as well as weird boiling currents, make the run for expert driftboaters only.

Gradient
13-14 fpm. Classic pool-and-drop river.

Mileage/Days
Grave Creek to Foster Bar, 34 miles, 2+ days, is the most common trip. Allow at least 4 days for fishing. Bear in mind that this launch starts with a bang! with the Class III Grave Creek Rapid, followed closely by Grave Creek Falls, which allows no warmup time.

Almeda boat launch to Foster bar, 37.8 miles, 3+ days. This launch is less crowded, has water and camping, and adds only about an hour or two to your trip. Bald eagles favor this section, and you have some warmup on Class IIs before hitting the IIIs. Argo Rapid at higher levels has a large hydraulic that's entertaining for rafts; Almeda Riffle has a playspot for novice kayakers.

Hog Creek to Grave Creek, 14.4 miles, 1-2 days. This easier (Class II) stretch of the Rogue runs parallel to a road, but the scenery is grand, the rapids are easy, the fishing is good, and floating it first gives you a better idea of what the wilderness section looks like. Argo Rapid develops a rock or reversal at the bottom, depending on water levels, so you may want to sneak far left or right.

Rogue River steelhead caught by covering waters around camp in a small inflatable kayak.

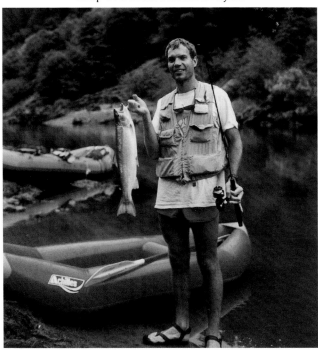

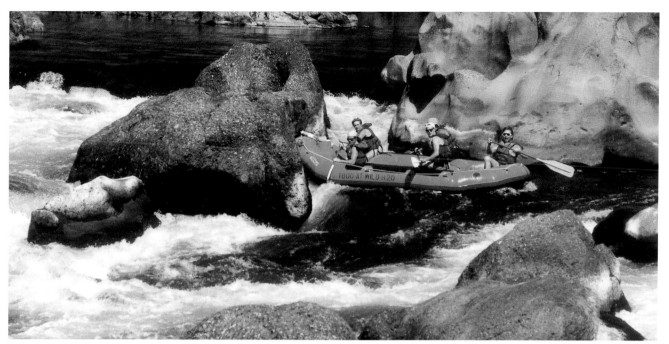

Pinball! Raft doesn't quite make the slot, but bouncing off entry rocks is easier than striking Picket Fence in Blossom Bar (note that raft hit head-on not sideways).

Average Float Levels/Seasons

Runnable all year. Optimum flow is 2,500-6,000 cfs. Gauge is at Agness.

High-Water Season

Before dam controls, the Rogue reached an incredible flow of 500,000 cfs—a flow that puts the Columbia to shame—back in December 1964. The water reached the Grave Creek Bridge (which is high enough for bungee jumping) and lapped at the edges of Paradise Lodge, located high on a cliff at the end of the Wild Section.

Most high water happens during the rainy season from November to March, with snowmelt adding more punch in April and May. Levels of 8,000 to 12,000 are not overly difficult, with most problem rocks covered. However, some of the rocks become dangerous flip holes in high water. Rainie Falls' main chute, Upper Black Bar, China and Blossom Bar have strong reversals in high water. The reversal caused by water covering Telfer's Rock in Mule Creek Canyon (named for three people who died there—no life jackets) can flip or trash a boat, and Mule Creek can be a difficult swim.

Many rafters equipped with the latest techno-gear float during the winter, doing the trip at faster flows in two days and staying at Paradise. Moderately high waters (6,000-9,000 cfs) cover many troublesome rocks and make some rapids easier (Mule Creek in particular "fills in" at higher levels). High water is good for salmon or sturgeon fishing, but most anglers prefer late-summer to autumn levels for trout and steelhead (particularly for fly-fishing).

Low-Water Season

River levels seldom drop below 1,500 cfs but during drought years can get lower. One April of such a year, I ran at an estimated 800 cfs and had my rafting trainee get the 16-foot-raft stuck sideways between the walls of the Coffee Pot (which are supposed to be more like 17 feet wide). This was very dangerous as the swirling action of the Coffee Pot is a cross between a reversal and an eddy, and can pull boaters under water, as well as "surfing" boats for a long time. If you're overboard with the raft above you, you will have to grab the lifeline or get downstream. (If someone is stuck under a raft while the boat is stuck or surfing in Coffee Pot, the last resort may be to cut the floor out.)

In lower flows, Fish Ladder (the lining chute at Rainie Falls) is difficult, and may cause traffic jams when boats get stuck. The Middle Chute, also at Rainie, may be too narrow for many rafts (and is always an abrupt and bumpy drop). Mule Creek Canyon and Coffee Pot are definitely a Class IV, with tight passages and the need to ship or feather oars and paddles quickly, a skill challenging for beginners. Boaters also need to keep arms and legs inside the boat, as the quirky currents here slam boats willy-nilly into cliff walls. The only way out is downstream, vertical rescue is almost impossible.

Craft

All craft run the Rogue at optimum levels in summer, from driftboats to rubber duckies and vinyl inflatable kayaks. Many outfitters use 18-foot rafts, but these must be carefully controlled in Mule Creek Canyon.

Permits

Advance lottery permits required May 15 to October 15 from Grave Creek downstream. Applications are accepted during the winter. Last-minute spaces may be drawn from the common pool by calling the Rand Information Center nine days in advance of the date, or by showing up with a small group and waiting for no-shows. The permit season was extended to control the number of boaters during the peak fishing seasons of late May-early June for salmon and fall for trout, steelhead and half-pounders.

Hazards

Rainie Falls is a 12-foot drop with strong hydraulics at the bottom that can surf boats and trap people underwater. Most boaters line their craft on river right. Rafts and catarafts can be manipulated by oars or paddles through the Fish Ladder lining chute, easier than using rope for skilled boaters. Have others stand by on shore to assist by pushing the boat off rocks. Small boats like kayaks just paddle through. The Middle Chute has a difficult entrance (tight and rocky) and takes you perilously close to the main drop. The Middle Chute drop is very abrupt and can cause serious injury. Even the Fish Ladder can break bones or trap people, due to wading in slippery conditions, and using rope in fast current. Wear life jackets and knives while lining. Weaker passengers should be dropped off on the left bank to walk the easy trail around the falls.

Boating the "easy" run listed above, Almeda to Grave Creek, is worthwhile to get a feel of the river. In higher water, there are waves and small hydraulics; at lower levels, more rocks and many tons of boulders. Boaters quickly learn that the Rogue has many rocks right in the middle of the river (just after you learned to stay in the middle current, to avoid rocks and gravel bars near shore).

Looking upstream at Mule Creek in higher waters.

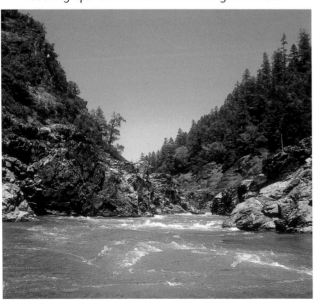

Isolation is not a problem here; in case of accident or illness, row downstream to a lodge (although Marial and Black Bar are seasonal, and Black Bar has limited road access, requiring helicopters for emergencies). Paradise Lodge is very accommodating and will even convey important messages for you. There is a caretaker in summer at the Rogue River Ranch who can drive an injured person out to Grants Pass. Jetboats can also assist in an emergency, once you are out of the no-motor zone.

The usual problem animals exist, with black bears a special Rogue hazard. Accustomed to years of free handouts from campers, the bears have no fear of humans and regularly attack food supplies, whether in the camp kitchen or on the boat. In problem bear areas, there are slings for hoisting food into trees, and electric fenced areas to store your food overnight. Most bears will back down from a person banging pots together. Bears have ripped open coolers, torn holes in rafts, chewed up Ethafoam and otherwise committed kitchen mayhem, but have not clawed campers. Dogs in camp may be a deterrent, or may tempt a bear to play King of the Hill, with the dog usually losing. Ammonia in small contain-

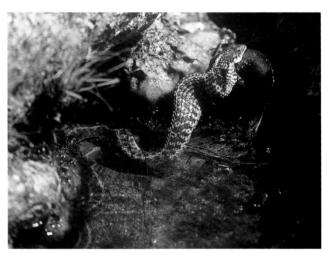

This water snake has a big appetite, swallowing a frog whole.

ers is said to repel bears. A small air horn might help, too. Check with Rand for current bad-boy bear locations.

Cougars are making a comeback on the Rogue, as elsewhere in the state, since the banning of hunting cougars with dogs. Since Rogue black bears grew bold with no-hunting rules in the river corridor, it's likely cougar will also lose their fear of humans. They probably won't raid your camp, as they prefer food that is still moving (bears like steak, cookies, bread and have been known to carry beer off), but keep their presence in mind when trekking along the shore.

A few years back, I observed a cougar chasing an otter through the Rogue's shallows near the mouth of Watson Creek, just above the Foster Bar take-out. To my surprise, the cougar jumped right into the river after the otter.

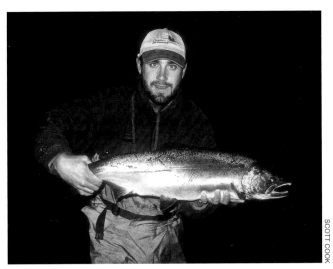

Fly-caught silver salmon on the Rogue River.

SCOTT COOK

However, the otter swam like, well, like an otter so the cougar gave up after a few splashy attempts, then swam back to shore. With its body immersed, the cougar resembled an otter at play. Once on shore, it resumed its feline appearance, shaking off the water in obvious disgust, as would any domestic kitty after an unexpected dunking.

Poison oak is everywhere, especially along the Rogue River Trail, so stay alert. Boating with dogs is popular here, but remember that dogs can carry the poison oak oil on their fur with no symptoms, then pass it along to you. Carry poison oak prevention lotions (available over the counter) and remedies, especially if you have a strong sensitivity. Ants inhabit some camps, particularly those not kept clean. Try to eat by the river so you don't leave crumbs behind to encourage these pests. Beginning in late summer, yellowjackets buzz camps looking for your meat scraps, or even flying into an open can of soda. Bring a yellowjacket trap, bait it and place it near your kitchen area. Anyone allergic to stings should carry an ana-kit.

Most accidents happen when people stumble over rocky bars while on shore, or while entering or exiting the boat. Learn to rock-jump when scouting.

Ticks are most common in spring. In marshy areas such as Brushy Bar, mosquitoes can be a problem. Stay near the river to avoid them, and don't curse the bats that can eat a thousand mosquitoes a night.

Fishing

Renowned for fishing since the days of Western writer Zane Grey (Rogue River Feud was written at his cabin on Winkle Bar). Many famous people have floated the Rogue with fishing guides, usually in comfortable, fairly dry driftboats. The Rogue has steelhead, salmon, sturgeon, half-pounders, trout, shad, even lamprey (resembles an eel, but is uglier and has a sucker mouth instead of jaw structure).

Salmon fishing has recently eclipsed steelhead fishing in popularity on the Rogue, due to recent runs of very large chinook, but both ocean-goers put up grand fights. The silver salmon, smaller than the chinook, averaging eight to 12 pounds, also migrates up the Rogue. (The inside of a chinook's mouth is black, while the silver's has some white.) Salmon runs occur in spring and fall, but a few salmon are in the river at any time. Early gill-netters took a heavy toll on all three fish, but the fishery is recovering and interest in Rogue fishing is booming.

Gold Ray Dam to the mouth of the Illinois River is considered the Middle Rogue. Two strong fisheries of chinook salmon and steelhead dominate most anglers' attention; with the chinook boasting both spring and fall runs, in addition to summer and fall steelhead. These distinct populations each spawn in a different tributary, some head for the Applegate, some continue on the main river.

The famous half-pounders are immature summer steelhead that have arrived early from the sea and are usually around 12 to 16 inches. Don't let their size fool you, however, these mini-steelhead fight like the big ones. The best time to fish for them is late summer into autumn. They travel upstream in schools, then begin to act like trout, staking out a territory to winter over. Tens of thousands of these tenacious fighters are in the Rogue in season. Fish for them as you would trout (they are considered trout by the ODFW, and only fin-clipped fish may be kept). They readily strike flies when a hatch is on, or try nymphs. Large trout flies such as Hare's Ears, Prince Nymphs, and large beaded soft hackles will draw strikes. Sinktips are used for fly-fishing in deeper waters, with nymphs used with a strike indicator.

The "halfsies" like riffly water, with its increased oxygen levels, when the water is lower in fall. Some guides like "twitching" or holding the fly in front of the boat on the water directly ahead, then bouncing it to have it move on the surface like a real bug. Use size 8 Red Ants, Gold Demons, Nymphs, Ugly Bugs silver sedge, Juicy Bug, Pheasant Tail Nymph, plus the good old standbys like the Woolly Buggers and other imitations. "The standard stuff all seems to work," reports Rusty Randall. Flies can be bead-head or standard. Serious fly-fishing from the boat makes the best use of float-in advantages (carrying a fly rod and a spin casting rod, or a fly-tying kit - all the extras you would leave behind while backpacking or fighting through brush to get to the river).

Guides at Morrison's Lodge, located just upstream from the Galice Resort and the put-in sites, suggests anglers bring lots of flies. Light caddis can be a light tan or white. The Green Butt Skunk works on the Rogue. As do Tiger Paws (yellow, black and gold), red caddis, Western Coachmans, Golden Demons, Juicy Bugs, flies with red on the tail end, the Chevney (silvery-gray with orange and white), and lastly, the Rogue River Special.

Most serious trout and steelhead anglers work the Rogue in fall, when the river cools. Randall recommends

Rogue River Wilderness

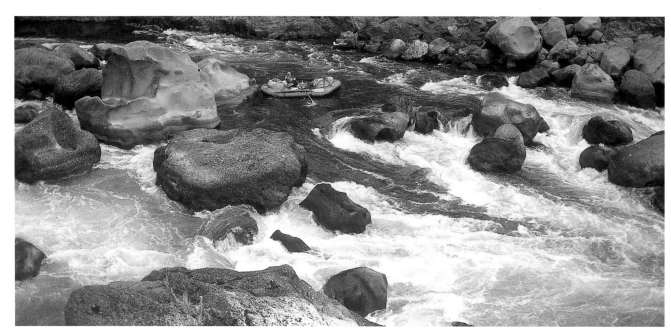

Making the pull into the eddy at the entrance to Blossom Bar.

September to December as a good time. Bad weather is not a concern for anglers riding in driftboats and staying in lodges. Size matters: summer's early-bird steelhead average 4-6 pounds, while fall brings the 9-plus-pounders. Use trout flies, super sized for steelhead. Randall likes a Tiger Paw for "right now or year-round."

The aggressive half-pounders will hit almost anything: flies, bait, spinners, and other small lures. This makes up for the more sluggish large fish during the half-pounder feeding frenzy September through early November. (Consult an ODFW catalog regarding current bait regulations on this run.) While steelhead can be in the river any time, most are caught September through February.

The Rogue's many riffles and gravel bars provide ideal habitat for trout and half-pounders, while the tailouts shelter salmon and steelhead. Toss in 100-foot-deep eddies, and you have sturgeon heaven. Fish the heads of rapids, either by holding in the current with oars, or using an anchor. You can also "plane" with lures while the boat sits still with the current moving ahead. Work a lure back and forth to tease the trout.

On southwestern Oregon waters, John Hazlett of the Ashland Outdoor Store recommends small red nymphs, large stoneflies, and Red Coppers with a 7- or 8-pound weight line and an 8-pound tippet. Most sporting goods department personnel know what lures work in their area.

Steelhead will respond like a half-pounder (they are the same fish, after all, half-pounders are just sexually immature steelhead). Use larger steelhead flies for bigger fish, and fish a little deeper. Look for pocket water, riffles and current lines rather than deep and slow water. In summer to fall, use big nymphs like the stonefly or caddis fly, with weight. Egg patterns are used in winter and early spring. For the lure-fisher, the old reliables for

trout—the Roostertail, and the Rapala Minnow, also spinners—sometimes get action that new-fangled lures don't. For steelhead, the Hot Shot and other plugs work. Even baits will snare the hungry half-pounders. Plugging from a drifting craft, usually held in current by the rower, is popular and productive.

Salmon fishing is good April through October in the wild section and above to the Savage Rapids Dam, with chinook in spring to fall and coho found from mid-September into winter. The non-wild section gets a lot of angling pressure, with hike-in fishermen at Rainie Falls on the river left trail, while the limit of 120 boaters per day (not all of them serious anglers) below Grave Creek ensures a quality fishing experience. Hatchery fish may be kept; wild coho released. Plunkers use salmon roe, shrimp or herring (sometimes combined with spinner blades), side-planers, or Corkies and Spin'n'Glos. Kwikfish and Flatfish plugs are sometimes used for spring salmon. Think of salmon as a commuter interested only in getting to its destination. The river is its freeway, it makes only short rest stops and seldom feeds. But plunk something in its way, and you have a fish on. Many anglers fish the Rogue for salmon at high flows, or a day and a half after the river drops.

In July through August, the wild section is the place to be for steelhead, coho, fall chinook and the occasional half-pounder, as well as trout.

On one special Rogue trip in May, the river water was low and too warm for the spawning salmon; when I pulled into Staircase Falls for the tourist photos, the pool where the cold creek entered was swarming with giant fish. I also saw huge numbers of spawned-out fish dead in some eddies, with scavengers ranging from ravens to bald eagles and black bears feasting. Some gravel bars stunk of rotten fish, limiting our camp choices. One very large male bear, the largest black I'd ever seen, was gorging on salmon right across the river from our camp at Brushy Bar. He chased off a younger bear, then ambled downstream, swam across the river, and wandered behind our tents. I was very glad he was full of about 100 pounds of fish!

Steelhead are large rainbow trout that travel to the ocean, then back up rivers to spawn. Unlike salmon, steelhead don't die after spawning; they can spawn more than once, returning to the ocean to feed. The first steelhead, traveling up to 150 miles to spawn, begin arriving in late July. The Rogue is unique in that it hosts half-pounders, they're fun fishing, giving a lot of play on the line. The larger steelhead arrive in fall, peaking in size in winter. Salmon favor deeper waters, while steelhead, like the trout they are, will hold up in shallows if conditions are right.

If you spend time at Rainie Falls, especially in May or autumn, you will see both salmon and steelhead trying to jump the falls, before they finally locate the Fish Ladder channel. Steelhead were undoubtedly named for their Rottweiler-like hard heads, which they pound repeatedly against rocks while migrating up rapids. Shad roam up the Rogue as far as this big drop before they are stymied by the climb.

Sturgeon are found in very deep waters (usually Sturgeon Rock, Sturgeon Hole near Marial, Mule Creek Canyon, Huggins Canyon). The limit is usually one sturgeon between 42 and 60 inches per day. Since they are usually caught with bait, check ODFW regs for bait restrictions on the Rogue before fishing for them, as baits are restricted at times. They are bottom feeders, seldom seen, but occasionally surprise a boater by surfacing.

Managing Agency

River Permits Office, Rand Information Center, 14335 Galice Road, Merlin, OR 97532. (541) 479-3735. Bureau of Land Management, Medford Resource Area, 3040 Middle Road, Medford, OR 97504. (541) 618-2275.

Boaters in the Wild Section (Grave Creek to Foster Bar) must check in at Rand on the morning of their trip to receive a permit; any dropouts will be added to the common pool for other boaters to share.

Contact these offices for a list of Rogue wilderness lodges, licensed outfitters, permit application information, and river conditions.

Shuttles/Services

Many shuttle services.

The Galice Resort, 11744 Galice Road, Merlin, OR 97532. (541-476-3818) website www.galice.com. Shuttle service, van/bus transport for groups, raft and gear rentals, store and restaurant (with live music on summer Saturday nights), lodging (cabins, some with hot tubs), boat ramp, gas pumps, fishing supplies, source for fishing guides, day trips, etc.

Morrison's Rogue River Lodge, 8500 Galice Road, Merlin, OR 97532 (541-476-3825); guided fishing trips, lodging for nights before and after doing a long trip, plus advice (ask for Ronnie).

Mileage/Highlights

Upstream of the first launch is Jump-off Joe Creek, river right, named for the son of Dr. John McLaughlin, who, around 1828, was with a fur-trapping party when he fell to his death off a high bluff.

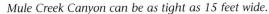

Mule Creek Canyon can be as tight as 15 feet wide.

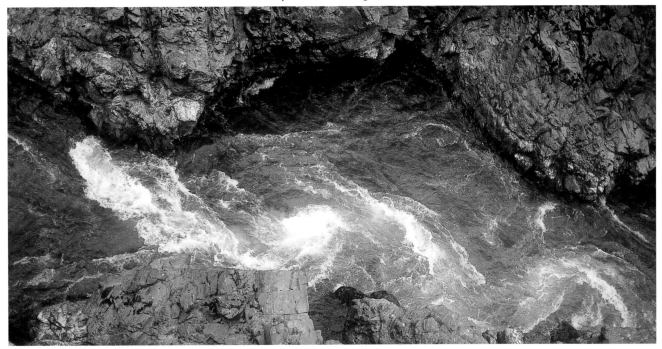

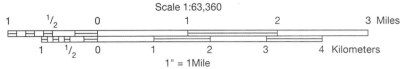

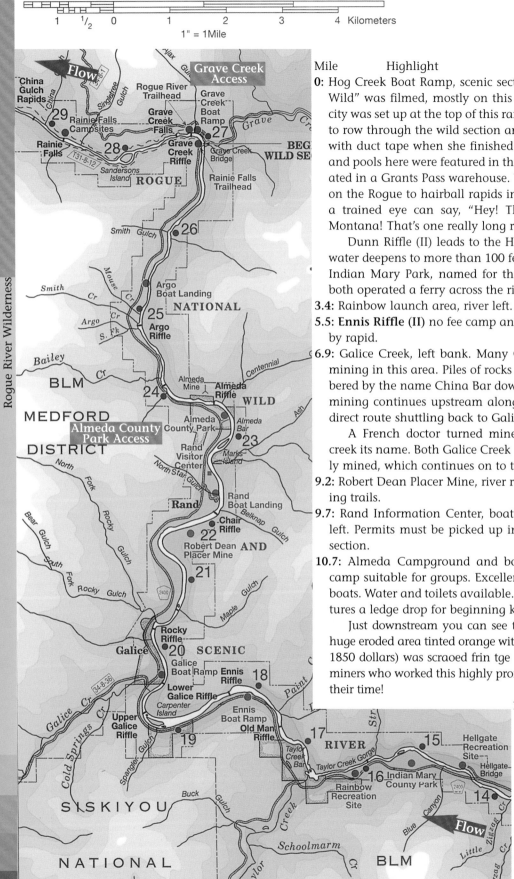

Rogue River Wilderness

Mile	Highlight

0: Hog Creek Boat Ramp, scenic section. When the movie "The River Wild" was filmed, mostly on this easy stretch of the Rogue, a tent city was set up at the top of this ramp. Meryl Streep actually learned to row through the wild section and reportedly had blisters covered with duct tape when she finished. Many of the cliff walls, beaches and pools here were featured in the movie...some scenes were re-created in a Grants Pass warehouse. The movie shifts from whitewater on the Rogue to hairball rapids in Montana so smoothly that only a trained eye can say, "Hey! That's Blossom Bar! No, now it's Montana! That's one really long rapid!"

Dunn Riffle (II) leads to the Hellgate bridge. Hellgate Canyon's water deepens to more than 100 feet in places. Calm water down to Indian Mary Park, named for the daughter of Umpqua Joe, who both operated a ferry across the river.

3.4: Rainbow launch area, river left.

5.5: Ennis Riffle (II) no fee camp and boat landing, river left followed by rapid.

6.9: Galice Creek, left bank. Many Chinese laborers worked on gold mining in this area. Piles of rocks attest to their hard work, remembered by the name China Bar downstream in the wild section. Gold mining continues upstream along the Bear Camp Road, the most direct route shuttling back to Galice.

A French doctor turned miner, Louis Galice, gave this small creek its name. Both Galice Creek and its forks have been extensively mined, which continues on to the present day.

9.2: Robert Dean Placer Mine, river right. BLM campsite with old mining trails.

9.7: Rand Information Center, boat landing and river permits, river left. Permits must be picked up in person before entering the wild section.

10.7: Almeda Campground and boat landing, river left. Large fee camp suitable for groups. Excellent wide, paved ramp for trailered boats. Water and toilets available. Almeda Riffle (II), just below, features a ledge drop for beginning kayakers to play with.

Just downstream you can see the mine tailings on river right, a huge eroded area tinted orange with iron oxides. Over $10 million (in 1850 dollars) was scraoed frin tge /rigye area in just nine years. The miners who worked this highly profitable claim were the Bill Gates' of their time!

12.3: Argo Riffle (II) becomes a Class II+ in higher water, with big waves, a reversal at the bottom, and hidden rocks (which are more hazardous in lower water).

Just past on river left is Argo, a boat landing and campsite similar to Ennis Riffle—a gravel/sand ramp where rigs sometimes get stuck launching, and a no-fee campsite handy for those who arrive

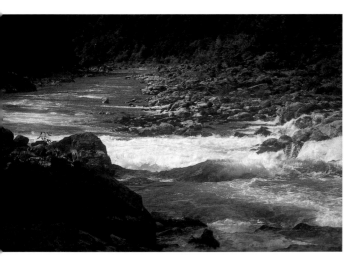

Contemplating Rainie Falls at high water. Scouting of all three passages is possible only on the left side, downstream of the falls looking back.

the night before and want to camp at a no-hassle launch site.

13.9: Class II moderate "S-turn" can be tricky. Start river left and work right at bottom to avoid hidden boulders. Watch for jetboats coming upstream before you commit to the rapid. You have the right- of-way as a downstream and non-powered craft, but it's like a bicycle taking on a Mack truck.

14.4: Grave Creek enters, river right. Named for the daughter of settlers, Martha Leland Crowley, buried under an old oak tree near this creek in 1846.

Grave Creek Bridge towers over you. Signs warn of the upcoming restricted section. Bungee jumpers are sometimes seen here. Watch for bank anglers as you maneuver. A trail on river left leads to Rainie Falls (2 miles).

The Grave Creek boat ramp is often a busy place in summer. The ramp is for unloading only; no raft inflating or rigging allowed. Trailered boats are best for launching here. Remember there is no overnight parking, your vehicle must be shuttled. The Rogue River Trail head begins at the downstream end of the parking area. Restrooms are available.

A quickie cheat sheet for the first leg of big water: Be right. River right is the usual safe run for Rainie Falls, Tyee, Wildcat and Upper Black Bar.

Wild Section

0: Grave Creek boat ramp.

0.2: Begins with a punch as Grave Creek Riffle (Class III) introduces you to waves in the face. An island divides the river channel, stay left. Enter right of center, where an obvious tongue leads into bouncy, splashy haystacks. At the bottom is a cliff wall and at optimum or low levels, a nasty sleeper rock where the river bends to the right. A strong eddy against the low cliff wall can thrash your boat around, so you need to set up to

pull away as soon as you have ridden out the wave trains, a quick decision. Zane Grey punctured his driftboat here during his maiden voyage.

0.3: Grave Creek Falls, Class III. Not a true waterfall, but drops from three to five feet over a rock ledge. The best route is river left, as the middle and right have a hard drop over the rock (a big reversal in high water). Sight in the obvious V-slick on river left, standing in your boat if possible, careful not to get too far left as rocks jut out. In an oar boat, approach slightly sideways, which improves your view, push and pull gently into position, then make a quick double-oar turn (pull on one oar, push on the other) to drop straight through the slot. Sideways will trash you. If you can't turn with both oars yet, use one, but learn the turn, you will need it later on in the trip.

1.0: Sandersons Island. The foundation from the Sandersons' cabin, constructed in 1940, is high on the right bank. They arrived around 1903 from Ohio, worked the Whiskey Creek mine, then the cabin was taken down by the BLM in 1971.

Take the riffle (Class II) to the left side of the island; at some levels, there is a false channel on the right that dead-ends. Old concrete structures mark a bridge for miners with mule trains to cross the river until it was wiped out by a 1927 flood.

1.7: Rainie Falls campsites. Small sites on river right and left are suitable for latecomers to the river who don't want to risk Rainie in the dark (as you must float below Grave Creek on the day your permit specifies). These also serve as lunch sites if you have floated from Almeda.

1.8: Rainie Falls (Class V+) is a true waterfall, dropping 12 feet into a boat-eating hydraulic. The main drop takes up most of the left side of the river, while the best scouting is from the left, requiring you to ferry your boat across the pool just above the falls. The trail on river left allows for easy hiking and scouting without the dangerous scramble on river right, where the Middle Chute is not visible. Take your camera for pictures as you scout left. Weaker passengers can walk around and be picked up below the drop. Watch for poison oak, which thrives on the edges of this trail.

From far enough downstream, look back to view the main falls (now on your right), the Middle Chute (the tricky, rocky, trashy drop in midstream) and the Fish Ladder (now on your left). At higher levels, the Middle Chute can be run by experienced rafters, but the risk of injury is always present as it's an abrupt double drop. The chute may be too tight for your boat at lower levels, and this is not a good place to be stuck. Driftboats and most rafts choose the Fish Ladder, on far right, where an experienced inflatable boater at optimum levels can row or paddle through without getting stuck (be careful of outstretched oars, which can knock you to the floor). Driftboats always line.

In low water, rafts get stuck in Fish Ladder, and must be lined and yanked. Always wear life jackets while lining or scouting. First, tie one rope to the bow, the other to the stern, then have one upstream person lead the boat like a dog on a leash, slowly releasing line, while the downstream person keeps the bow straight (sideways will get it stuck harder). Driftboats have it easier, as their hard bottoms slide over the rocks while the "rubber" raft floors seem to stick like Super Glue (PVC rafts such as Maravias slide easier than Hypalon or neoprene-type rafts). In season, there are other boaters to assist you since they are stuck behind you. This usually involves an exchange of river curren-cy, such as fine chocolate or liquor.

Before committing to Fish Ladder, check the chute to make sure no boats are stuck, or you may end up in a neoprene sandwich.

The falls is not named for the infamous spring rains on the Rogue, which shares part of the Oregon coastal climate's wet reputation, but for Old Man Rainie who lived at this site for the fishing. Instead of a fly rod, he used a gaff to harvest salmon for market. Anglers should remember it is illegal to fish too close to the falls (usually 400 feet), as the fish are stressed from their attempts to migrate this obstacle. Look for the signs posted below the falls.

Bank angler and boater conflicts happen here, as they do on other rivers. Once I observed a bright orange bobber in the river, an obvious fisherman on river left, and I maneuvered well out of his fishing zone. The rafter behind me was oblivious, floated over the line, which then hung up on his raft. Still without a clue, the rafter kept going, with such force that the rod was yanked from the irate fisherman's hands! He then chased the rafter downstream while yelling loud curses. The moral: Pay attention to your surroundings, and exercise common courtesy. Former bank anglers who now boat should understand that walking limits the amount of river you can cover, while floating increases it. Yield to the shore anglers. A friendly wave, as well as moving to miss their lines, goes a long way in lessening what the Forest Service terms "user con-flicts."

2.2: China Gulch Rapids (Class II). The gulch, named for 1800s-era mine workers, enters river right.

3.1: Rum Creek, left, is a nice place for lunch or a swim break. Salmon pool up here due to the cool water. Early gold prospectors were responsible for the naming of this water as well as Whiskey Creek (river right). Wishful thinking, as there are many "bars" on the Rogue, but they serve only sand, gravel and rocks.

Two big campsites are separated by the creek and share an outhouse. A good trail along the east side of the creek leads to the Rogue River Trail and then a cut-off heads uphill to the Whiskey Creek Cabin, about 1/8 of a mile past the trail bridge. This well-preserved

prospector's shack was built around 1880, and is listed on the National Register of Historic Places. A succes-sion of placer miners occupied the cabin, one who had a beloved pet, Kitty Mac, buried at a grave with a tombstone in the front yard.

Many interesting artifacts have been left here for visitors to enjoy; it's both illegal and immoral to remove them. Take plenty of pictures, including the bare-springs bed, the old tin cans, and the first solar shower in Oregon, in the backyard.

3.4: Big Slide Riffle, Class II. There really is a big slide, a giant landslide that occurred in the late 1800s. The entire river was blocked upstream to Hellgate Canyon. There is a hiker's camp, river right, up high, but boaters should not attempt the hazardous climb.

3.6: Doe and lower Doe campsites, river left, with lower Doe offering a big flat beach suitable for groups. Doe Creek enters river left.

4.3: Tyee Bar, river left. Tyee is Chinook jargon (a Native trading language) for "Chief". This was a busy site in th 1800s with over 300 Chinese miners laboring for about $5 million in gold dust; there was also a store and boat crossing.

Now the quiet reaches are home for endangered Western pond turtles: look for them sunning on top of small rocks, usually river right in the shallows. To grab a glimpse of these shy critters, ship those oars in and float quietly by. To show others where the turtles are, use a hand sign and point (make the "turtle on a rock" sign by holding one palm open over a closed fist).

4.4: Tyee Rapids, Class III+. This is a Class IV for drift-boats and other hard boats due to submerged rocks. Scouting from river right is recommended if you are uncertain at all.

A house rock (boulder the size of a small house) guards the center of the rapid, and there is an outcrop-ping of serpentine mineral rock (which often appears as an oily green color and is common in the Rogue area) pushing the river into a right bend, with current that forces boats into this ledge. Rafts usually bounce off, but driftboats don't. Check the entrance carefully, as a series of ledges can bump boats, especially at lower water. Set up for river right, picking your way through rocks and ledges.

I like to run at optimum levels by going right of the first rock, right of the second big pourover rock, then work back right again, maybe about ten feet right, to miss the most dangerous part, a big submerged boul-der with a strong reversal (hazardous at most levels, but often run by rafters when the rock is sufficiently covered, for thrills and spills). Nudging the right of this powerful current puts you close to the rocky right shore. Once past this boulder, work back to center to avoid being jammed into the rock ledge on river right. Don't relax, as the current usually carries you to a sleeper rock hiding at the end of the tailout. (In high water levels, there is a runnable channel left of the house rock.)

The deep water on river right below the ledge is good fishing. There is a camp river right with an outhouse located mid-bar in an oak grove, up the hill. You will soon master the art of locating these hidden potties by following foot trails from flat campgrounds usually to the upper tiers, but remember you have to carry your own facility, and it may be easier to set it up conveniently nearby (and eventually, the left bank outhouses will probably close as they fill up and are hard to clean out).

4.8: Wildcat Rapid, Class III. Following right on the heels of Tyee, Wildcat looks to take another bite from your boat. Most current goes into the right side of the island that splits the river; most boaters follow the big fun wave train, almost with heads under the river right overhanging bushes, until the end of the island is reached. The river drops over Alligator ledge rocks on mid-right, which can be avoided by going left (far right usually brings a raft through). You need to be aware and maneuver, as the free ride from the friendly waves and current is over.

After you have avoided crunching this ledge, you will notice another house rock where the side channel rejoins the main current, to your left. This boulder seems to have a Hoover effect, sucking in unwary boaters with its strong hydraulics. Boats that venture too close and get sideways usually wrap; this is ugly and takes much work to undo. You need to be able to turn quickly, face the danger of the house rock, and pull away again.

On all rated rapids, but especially Class III and above, be sure to wait for all of your boats to get through safely before you proceed downriver. This is important on all rivers, but sometimes overlooked on the Rogue as it is not as remote, and has a trail to hike back. However, the trail on river right is sometimes high above in rocks, meaning if a boat behind has trouble, lots of scrambling is necessary to backtrack. In places like Mule Creek Canyon, even a bighorn sheep would need a climbing harness to get up to the trail. If you lose your group, you will have to go downstream to a place where you can access the trail and hike more miles upstream. Communication between boats will solve problems.

5.1: Wildcat Campsite—aka Russian Bar—river left, large camp. This is a large gravel bar with lots of room overlooking Russian Rapid. Russian was named for the nationality of an emigrant gold prospector who lived here. So many settlers, but so little evidence of their struggles is left.

5.2: Russian Rapid, Class II+. This ride is one of the best at low-water levels for rafts and small craft, as a good backcurler wave develops here. Russian funnels through a chute (get used to tight chutes, they just keep getting tighter as you float the Rogue). There is a broad tongue leading into a clean wave train at optimum levels. The tailout current heads into the left bank, so be prepared to pull away.

5.5: Montgomery Rapids, Class II+. Upper and lower Montgomery drop over submerged ledges and boulders, forcing hard boats to choose carefully. In very low water, I call these the Velcro Rapids as you can get a raft stuck on the sneaky sleeper rocks. Montgomery Creek is on river left. The river looks fairly natural, making it easy to forget that once there were over 25

Getting around Rainie Falls using the Fish Ladder chute means lining for driftboats, which slide over rocks. At optimum or higher levels, an inflatable can be rowed or paddled through, with assistants following on shore to push when necessary. Keep boats straight-on and not sideways (backwards is OK).

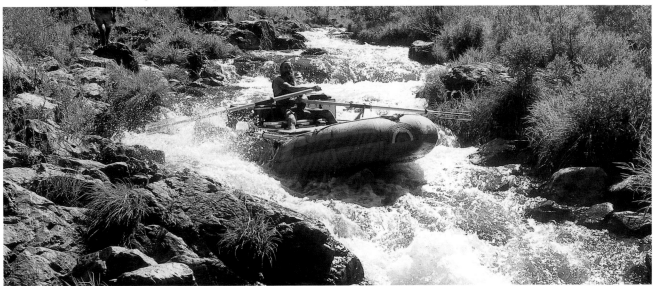

buildings here, put up during the desperate Depression years. A flood in 1955 wiped them out.

6.1: Howard Creek Chutes, Class II+. This begins a series of three chutes, drops down ledges. The first is run down the middle, with an enjoyable wave train (remember to keep your boat straight-on, never sideways, in big waves).

The second chute is down the center, but the current from the third set of waves leads into rock on river left, so be ready to pull back.

Just below the last chute, the water slows. Keep left to see Howard Creek, a beautiful clear stream that offers a shocking dunk in cool water on a hot day. The pool is deep enough to jump into from a Lemming Rock above. (Jump only, on any stream or river, never dive head first.) The landing here is rough and rocky, but the lack of current allows time to scramble ashore and secure boats. This is a nice place to eat, swim, soak sore muscles or just take a nap on a warm afternoon.

6.9: Slim Pickens Rapid, Class III. The landmark for this classic Rogue rapid is an old metal barge on river left (left by the 1955 flood). A house rock can be seen right of center in the drop. This rapid was one blasted by Wooldridge to make passage easier, but you can still find plenty of trouble. The choice is, do you take the obvious channel on river left, or the Slim Pickens tight channel on river right?

I once chose the slim route in a 16-foot raft to show off and wound up with a broken oar. This right route is suggested as a driftboat route, but the skill involved in setting up and shipping oars fast is not for the slow of reflex. The left channel is more enjoyable if run correctly at most water levels; in low water, the right channel may seem safer. If you aren't sure, scout river right. Remember, as at Rainie Falls, lining the boat is always an option.

For the left run, ferry left of center, setting up on the V-slick to dodge left-side rocks, then face the danger, the house rock, angle your boat, and pull, pull, pull. (Sometimes it seems you won't make the pull, but keep pulling; don't give up. That last stroke will help!)

7.2: Washboard Rapid, Class II, two chutes. A ripple of waves creates the appearance of a washboard, the manual washing machine of pioneer days. ("Washboard" is also a common river term for a rapid where currents are studded with moderate-sized or small rocks, so when you cross, your boat gets worked over like dirty laundry. "Speed bumps" might be a more appropriate term.)

7.7: Plowshare Rapid, Class II. Long ledge above surface on river right has sharp edges thought to resemble a plowshare. Stay middle to avoid being plowed under the field.

8.0: Big Windy and Windy Creek Chutes, Class II. Run these two narrow drops in mid-channel (center of river).

Why Big Windy? Well, there is often a strong afternoon breeze here, slowing progress as boaters hunt for camps. You will want to get at least this far on this first day of a 3-day trip. There is a nice campsite high on river left, but gear must be brought up over rocks. Very suitable for go-light trips.

8.2: Windy Creek, left bank, is a pretty spot for lunch, with swimming in clear, cold pool.

8.5: Upper Black Bar Falls, Class III+ (Class IV for driftboats). Scouting on river right is recommended. The river drops over a ledge with rocks and boulders scattered across the channel. At lower levels, below about 4,000 cfs, the only practical route is the far right channel. Most boaters tuck into the eddy behind the rock on far right at the entry to slow the boat. Watch for the small sleeper rock that sticks up at the edge of the tongue when the river is lower. Hug the right side, avoiding a rock about 1/4 width of river off the right side, not a problem if you don't start pulling away from the sheer rock face staring at you too soon. Then set up to pull away as the rapid ends, since the current pushes hard into the rocky right side. Watch oars and paddles sticking out on river right; they can smash into the rock wall.

In higher water, mid-channel routes are possible, especially for inflatables. Large holes develop over the midstream boulders, too; these drop off so quickly that they are hard to see and identify from water level as you approach.

8.6: Lower Black Bar Falls, Class II+. A short pool allows recovery and setup for the next drop. This one is a straight V-slick into big rollicking waves. Sometimes used to practice swimming in big water (wear life jacket and shoes).

8.8: Black Bar Lodge, river left. The long bar is home to this small wilderness lodge, so well-hidden you might not know it was there. Look for the stairs and boat tie-up on the left bank. Not open for casual visitors; guests and emergencies only.

Black Bar was named after Mr. Black who was murdered, then put into a boat that was pushed off into the river. The body was found downstream. In 1932, the lodge was constructed; most of the overnighters today are on spring to fall fishing trips. closed in winter.

9.3: Little Windy Campsite, river left. A small sandy beach featuring a terrace with flat tent sites up the hill. Trails lead to private sites, blackberry bushes, and the outhouse up the hill. Bears sometimes enter this camp, so keep it clean and secure. Little Windy Creek enters at the end of the beach on river left. I have spent a few nights here in May listening to the sound of big salmon jumping; they sound remarkably like a bear splashing around if you have an overactive imagination.

Little Windy Riffle is a Class II with small rocks. There are several good camps around Jenny Creek on river left, with a common outhouse in the trees. In 1855, a battle raged between Rogue Natives and over 400 personnel with the Army (plus volunteers) for six hours before the Army gave up. Many fierce, but brief battles were fought for control of Rogue territory, with its rich gold deposits provoking confrontation.

10.4: Horseshoe Bend begins, river right. This huge, high bar hosts dozens of good tent sites. At optimum levels, heavy kitchen gear can be set up on flat spots near the river's edge, so it doesn't have to be lugged uphill.

Horseshoe Bend Rapids is a series of three drops (Class III) where the river has been diverted by harder rocks from mostly straight into a sharp right turn, a classic U-bend or Horseshoe shape.

The first rapids involve dodging rocks, with the best current on river left. This stronger current then leads directly into a submerged undercut rock and rock wall on river left, a nasty swim. Small craft should "cheat" well to the inside of the current. Oar boats can stay middle, or if swept left, must promptly set up an angle for pulling away from the left side, as the current piles into the rock wall harder than it appears.

At the end of Horseshoe Bend Rapid, river right, is a favored campsite suitable for large groups. Catch the eddy (a good landing spot for boats at optimum or lower levels). A lower flat spot provides a riverside kitchen area, with a flat upper terrace that boasts a panoramic vista. A bit further up the hill is an outhouse and access to the Rogue River Trail.

Lower Horseshoe Campsite is on river right, downstream, separated from the upper camp by a riverside rock ledge. Deep waters here conceal sturgeon.

10.7: **Telephone Hole Riffle** is just one name (also, Mary's Hole) for the next rapid. Be alert for rocks that can create a surprise reversal at some water levels. A gravel bar, left, and a house rock in the river identify this Class II S-turn. A Forest Service phone line once crossed the river here.

In whitewater tradition, a "riffle" or "ripple" is usually considered a minor rapid, while "rapid" denotes a more serious drop. Other than the Rogue, few Oregon rivers have official names for riffles or Class I+ currents. Due to the Gold Rush, the Rogue's

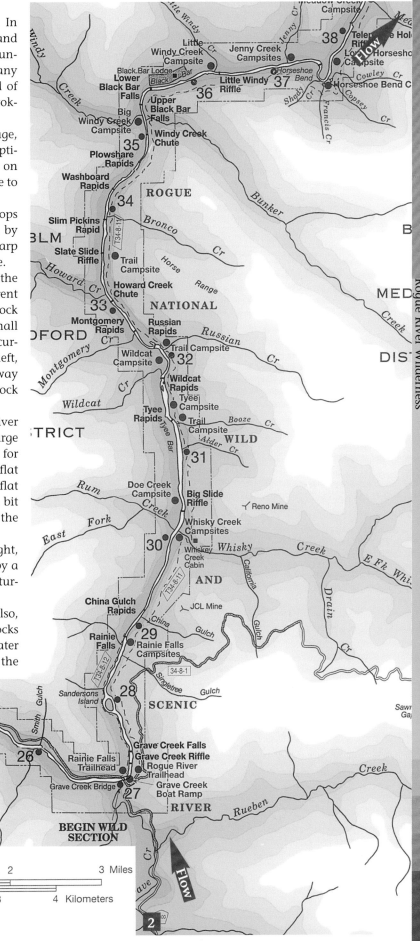

Scale 1:63,360

1   ½   0   1   2   3 Miles

1   ½   0   1   2   3   4   Kilometers

1" = 1Mile

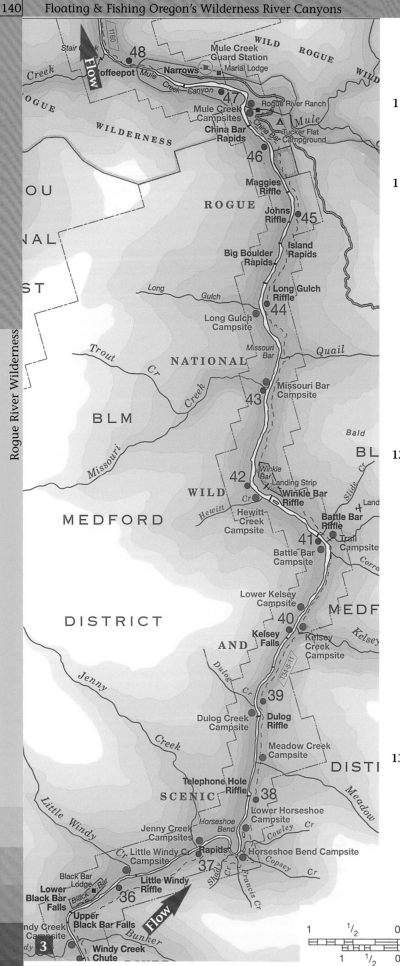

early boaters had a lot of history to provide names for canyons, bars, rapids and falls.

11.5: Meadow Creek, right bank, marks a good campsite used by hikers.

Bear in mind that on the Rogue, the left bank is accessible only to boaters; some sites on river right are shared with hikers, others can be reached only by trail.

11.8: Dulog Riffles, Class II+. Of the smaller rapids in this stretch, these two require the most maneuvering. The upper run is identified by large boulders in the river, and the obvious trail cut into the cliff wall ahead. The river bends left around a corner. Follow the inside current around the bend, working away from the big boulder, and around smaller, partially submerged boulders at the end.

Dulog Campsite, river left, is at the tailout of this rapid; a pretty site for large groups. A short scramble up Dialog Creek (end of camp on river left) reveals Dulog Falls.

The second drop, past this creek, is known by some guides as "Let's Make a Deal" because you have three "doors"—three routes through a tight boulder garden. The channel on river left is the correct choice. Tight drop may require tucking in oars.

12.2: Entering Kelsey Canyon, a milder preview of the tight confines and strange turbulence that lurks ahead in Mule Creek Canyon.

Three Class II-II+ drops introduce you to claustrophobia with vertical rock walls, boiling eddies and sometimes the need to pull in or "feather" oars (laying shafts flat along sides). Oars that stick out in tight confines can bend, break or be jammed back at the rower, causing injury or ejection from the boat. Oars should also not be buried deeper than blade-level, as this lessens mechanical advantage and increases the risk of losing the oar or control of the oar, especially when oars are positioned too far in swirly, bubbling eddy waters.

These rapids are known as **"Oodle" (the S-turn), No Name, and Kelsey Falls,** the last one of many rapids dynamited by Wooldridge to open a passage. There are still submerged boulders at lower water levels.

13: Kelsey Creek, river right, is the landmark for an interesting camp. This is one used by hiker groups, especially those with raft support ferrying their gear from camp to camp. Over the boulders is a nice flat spot and pools along the creek to splash or swim in. In warm weather, salmon school up at the creek's mouth. Also, you can hike up the Rogue River Trail to a bridge crossing with a grand view.

Scale 1:63,360

1   ½   0   1   2   3 Miles

1   ½   0   1   2   3   4 Kilometers

1" = 1Mile

Colonel John Kelsey, who led volunteer forces against the notorious Chief John of the Rogue Indians in 1856, provided the inspiration to Glen Wooldridge to name this area.

13.4: Lower Kelsey, river left, is two camps (depending on water levels and how much sand and gravel washed in during the previous winter) split by a boulder.

13.5: Sturgeon Rock, left side. A large rock that marks the beginning of good steelheading, as well as a 50-foot-deep sturgeon hole. Sometimes boaters leap (feet first only) from the tip of the rock into the deep pool.

14: Battle Bar, river left, remembers two long-ago struggles: one large and one small. In 1856, Kelsey attacked Rogue Indians with his cavalry of 536 men; it was mostly a standoff due to the distance between the two riverbanks (and the refusal of his men to cross the river in flimsy boats).

A bizarre feud began between two neighbors 17 years after Robert Fox built a cabin on river left, on the high terrace above the river. Neighbor Jack Mahoney lived a short distance downstream. In 1947, supposedly Fox shot Mahoney's pet deer. Mahoney lay in wait for Fox, ambushing and shooting him. Fox lay seriously wounded for days. Unable to go for help, Fox fired off his rifle repeatedly, but others in the area thought the feud was still on, and avoided the area. Fox died in his cabin.

Mysteriously, Mahoney was also found shot dead, his body far downstream at Half Moon Bar, leaving others to wonder if one of Fox's wild shots had scored a hit, or if Mahoney shot himself in remorse.

Fox's cabin was mostly washed away by the 1964 flood. Recently, the Forest Service rebuilt a shelter over the old rock fireplace. Boaters landing into a small eddy on river left can have lunch, hike up the steep switchbacks to the shelter and a lovely meadow. Another open grassy area on river right is often visited by deer. It's difficult to imagine such fierce battles taking place while viewing the peaceful setting.

From here into the Battle Bar and Winkle Bar riffles, there is good steelhead fishing. There are many shallow spots and gravel bars at lower water levels.

14.8: Winkle Bar Riffle leads into Hewitt Creek Campsite on river left, a former large site reduced to a small flat by winter floods, and the cabin of Western writer Zane Grey (*Rogue River Feud*) on river right.

15.2: Winkle Bar is privately owned, with a large house, a smaller caretaker place, a caretaker much of the time, and, of course, the dime-novel author's shack. Grey bought the site from a gold miner in 1926. Some of his old boats are preserved here under shelters. Visitors are welcome, but should avoid eating lunch (bears are known to attack ice chests while everyone is gone to look at the cabin) or disturbing anything (except the free produce sometimes offered by the caretaker). The field is used as a private airstrip, sometimes

requiring pilots to "buzz" over first to chase deer out of the way.

In lower waters, Zane Grey's Riffle bumps over a gravel bar and the left current runs into rocks.

16: Missouri Creek/Campsite, river left. The former caretaker of Winkle Bar, Gerald Frye, lived here for many years. There is an outhouse up the hill and a small shelter.

16.4: Quail Creek, river right, marks the site of a large 1970 wildfire which burned 2,700 acres and killed two firefighters. Dead trees are visible on both sides of the river. Fresh landslides may be encountered along these fragile riverbanks.

This begins a section of pools and riffles with excellent fishing.

17: Long Gulch Campsite, river left (very small site) still has footings of a Glen Wooldridge cabin. Followed by Long Gulch Riffle (Class II) just beyond where the creek enters on river left, which requires some rock dodging.

17.6: Big Boulder Rapids (Class II) features large boulders in the river, brought down by landslides. One large monolith guards the left side. This is usually navigated right of mid-channel past this monolith, then back to center to avoid outcroppings on river right.

17.8: Island Rapid, Class II. Again the river runs around a monolith with a gravel island at the tail. In this stretch, many "fluted" rocks—carved by pounding surf—can be found, including one with the "flutes" visible only when looking back upstream, which I call the Doug Rock (for football player Doug Flutie).

18: John's Rapid, Class II+. I also call this "Where's the Channel?" as the river appears to disappear into rocks when viewed at a distance. Up close, there is an obvious channel in the center, between boulders and rock outcroppings. At lower water levels, approach from left of center, then tuck into the eddy behind right side rocks, aiming for the center chute between two larger rocks. Named for the Chief John, who lead the Rogue tribe's uprisings against invading gold miners backed by Cavalry might, during 1855-56.

18.4: Maggie's Riffle (Class II) was named for one of Glen Wooldridge's fishing guests, Maggie Stoddard, the place where she caught her first steelhead. This area remains excellent for steelhead and half-pounder fishing.

19: China Bar, river right and **China Riffle (Class II)**, reflect the history of Chinese gold mine workers brought to work on the Rogue.

19.3: China Rapid, Class II+. Big boulders in this stretch command attention,, but boaters also need to watch out for a sneaky, sharp-edged rock, the Can Opener, in midstream. A reversal can develop here at certain water levels.

19.5: Mule Creek campsites and trail to Rogue River Ranch, river right. Homesteaded in 1887 by George Billings, the ranch and outbuildings were purchased by the BLM under the Wild & Scenic Rivers Act in 1970 and are maintained in a preserved state for the public. Even today, the buildings look more like a country ranch, including a white picket fence, than a rough and rowdy town in the wilderness that had a post office, a barn known as The Tabernacle (that had been a dance hall), trading post and general mercantile store serving gold miners, cowboys and soldiers.

Visitors are welcome, although they may have to run through sprinklers watering pastures. The ranch complex has a caretaker in season (emergency evacuations are possible here, by car or helicopter). The buildings feature displays of frontier furniture, a tack-house, blacksmith shop, a coffin where drunken cowboys were placed to "sleep it off" (talk about a rude awakening!) and Native artifacts. You can easily spend an hour or two exploring the ranch.

You can also hook up with the Rogue River Trail and walk downstream to Mule Creek Canyon and Blossom Bar. Inspiration Point, where hikers overlook the cascading Stair Creek Falls, is aptly named.

There are three or four good landing spots at Mule Creek for camping (depending on how winter floods treat the beaches), two upper and two lower. All areas have huge flats on top that can accommodate large groups (as well as some flat spots hidden among terraced slopes). The upper camps share an outhouse at the edge of the ranch pasture. The Forest Service advises that, since these camps are the last before Mule Creek Canyon and Blossom Bar (the two toughest rapids with no flat areas for camping), campers should be prepared to share sites.

(This was not my experience after a long day's push to evacuate a possible broken leg victim—campers there claimed they had pushed early in the day to have the site to themselves. However, there is a fair site on river left among the rocks a group can squeeze into, if necessary.)

19.5: Mule Creek enters on river right. Mule Creek got its name in 1852 when an Army officer lost his mule here. There was once a bridge across the river here to accommodate mule trains. Imagine carrying glass windows for your ranch house by horse or mule, over hill and dale.

The lower camps are just below the creek and the last one, at the bend.

19.7: Mule Creek Eddy. On river right, the river slows and backs up into a large, slow, deep eddy. Depths of over 90 feet have been recorded here. Good fishing for sturgeon.

Marial is located on river right, named for Tom Billings' daughter. As many as 250 people received their mail at the Marial Post Office during the 1930s depression. Marial has a pioneer cemetery and a lodge that is popular with anglers floating the river.

Three riffles precede the entrance to Mule Creek Canyon. If your boat is not self-bailing, cheat the waves to avoid taking on extra weight before entering this tight gorge.

19.8: The narrow cleft that is **Mule Creek Canyon (Class IV)** appears ahead, the entrance guarded by a pair of ugly wrap rocks known as **The Jaws** located on river right. Plan on ferrying far left to begin the canyon, and take a deep breath. Running the canyon safely requires confidence as well as endurance and skill.

Patience is a virtue, too. Keep your group together and wait for each boat to clear narrow spots. Let faster boats go ahead of you. If you find your craft closing in too quickly, there are eddy spots beyond the entrance, against the rock walls, where you can hold up. Instruct all party members to keep arms and legs inside the boat, and watch out for paddles and oars in the tight confines (both wood oars and bones can break if smashed against cliff walls). Have rescue throw bags handy. Check to see that all life jackets are cinched down tight (powerful turbulence here can strip off inadequate or poorly fastened vests).

The first section, three rapids called The Snake, begins once you pass the Jaws safely on far left. Set up to pull away from where the current thrusts against the left cliff wall. The next current zigzags to river right and another cliff wall, requiring an oar boat to change from facing left to facing right, then pulling away. The turbulence of Mule Creek is caused by constriction. Everything seems to wash out eventually, but it's still an unpleasant swim.

The third drop has a partially-submerged boulder on river left (a big hydraulic at higher flows). Both the rock and its pour-off are dangerous, so you must change angles to face left again, and pull hard away. The rock is known as Telfer's Rock after three people who drowned here (no life jackets). Don't add your name to a rock like this!

Rock walls close in as you enter The Narrows, the second part of Mule Creek Canyon. Watch oars here, the canyon is tighter than your wing span. You must lean forward, tucking oars in, ship them, or lay back and feather them flat against the boat. A bubbling turbulent spot, sometimes called The Tea Kettle, will spin boats around. Boats 14 foot and larger should stay straight until below Coffee Pot.

The bigger boil, The Coffeepot, is just ahead. Here boats must go through one at a time, as the Coffeepot often surfs them and if too close, you can collide with the boat in front of you. There is a good eddy tucked inside a cliff wall on river left just upstream of the Coffeepot known as The Garage because you can park there. Shouts or whistles can signal when the next boat can come through.

In approaching Coffeepot, push oars forward (or dig paddles in) to gain momentum and keep the boat straight, never sideways. Ship oars promptly if you get sideways. The passage here can be as tight as 15 feet. The Coffeepot is a strange boiling eddy that can suck boaters or gear underwater, stay in the boat if possible.

Once on an April guide-training trip, I found out how tight this canyon really is. The Rogue was running lower than 1,000 cfs. We were parallel to the canyon walls, set up properly, but the perculating currents suddenly thrust the 16-foot-long raft sideways, and it got stuck between the rock walls—tight! The trainee leaned over the upstream tube to look for the rock that was holding us (no rocks, just current) and almost got sucked out of the boat (this is dangerous when a boat is stuck or just surfing, as a person could be held under water under the boat). I grabbed him and pushed him to the high side, or downstream, to hold that tube down while I fumbled for valves to let out air. The boat came through all right, but my nerves were shot.

I always get some butterflies in my stomach in Mule Creek Canyon. On my first trip, we found a kayaker sitting on the rock outcrop beside the Coffeepot. Asked if he needed help, he said he was waiting for his paddle to come back up to the surface. How long had he been waiting there? Thirty minutes! Eventually he gave up and got out his spare paddle. I always wondered where that paddle went.

On my first trip rowing solo, I saw fins like a great sea monster brush the surface ahead. With waters over 100 feet deep, I could easily imagine Nessie. Of course I had glimpsed a huge sturgeon, which look somewhat prehistoric.

21.3: A loud roar ahead is not Blossom Bar yet, just the echo of Stair Creek Falls. When the river is warm, salmon gather here to refresh in the cool waters.

Old mining gear is found on the walls along this part of the canyon. Gradually the walls open up as the river prepares for its longest drop. High over your shoulder on river left is the Devils Backbone, a ridge of jagged rock.

Changes occur with high waters. Once there was a broad gravel bar at the end of Mule Creek Canyon, where boats could be hauled up for repairs (boiling currents slamming boats into rocks has ripped rafts open. This is where I stopped and re-inflated tubes after getting stuck sideways.) Now the gravel bar has mostly gone under water, its shallows replaced by a deep pool. It comes and goes at the whim of the river.

22.6: Blossom Bar Rapid, Class IV. Scouting mandatory. Blossom Bar is a long boulder garden (rapid with large rocks scattered about, requiring lots of maneuvering). Old photographs of this rapid show that Blossom was once a virtual field of boulders, with no route whatsoever until Glen Wooldridge's dynamiting opened up a

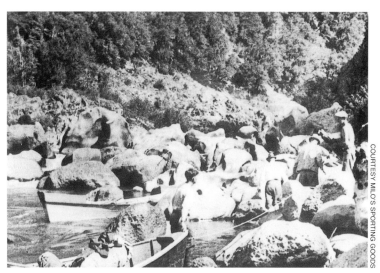

Old Blossom Bar before blasting.

route. Even today, the passage at optimum levels remains choked with rocks, and requires precise timing for a correct run. The entrance is a blind cut from river left to mid-stream, with much boulder-dodging waiting below.

Even if you know the route, someone must climb up the boulders and check to see if the route is clear of debris (wrapped boats, lines out to wrapped boats, or logs/sunken driftboats lodged in the entrance). It's quite disconcerting (as well as dangerous) to come whipping around the corner above the dreaded Picket Fence wrap rocks and find a trashed boat in your way!

What seems to be a sissy name for a major rapid simply reflects the Rogue's diversity. The first to explore and float this region noticed wild azaleas and rhododendrons in the Rogue Canyon, thus Blossom Bar. These untamed ancestors of the garden shrubs usually bloom late April into May.

Eddy out on river right. On a busy afternoon, boats will have to be shuffled in and out of these small eddies. Sometimes an entire group must tie outer boats to inner boats. (Make sure, before you leave your boat unattended, that it is securely tied.) Scout long enough to understand the route, but not so long that you lose the edge—call it adrenalin—or worse, that you lose confidence. Watch other boats go through, if you can, from both the high vantage point and at river level. You must envision a route while scouting from above, a route that begins with a blind leap of faith, rowing backwards in an oarboat.

The scout point is high on river right; be very careful scrambling over boulders in this area. Springs and mosses make footing treacherous, plus there is a lot of poison oak. From here, identify the landmarks and moves you need to make. For the traditional left run (right is an option only in high water, only for kayaks and large inflatables), the boat must ferry from the

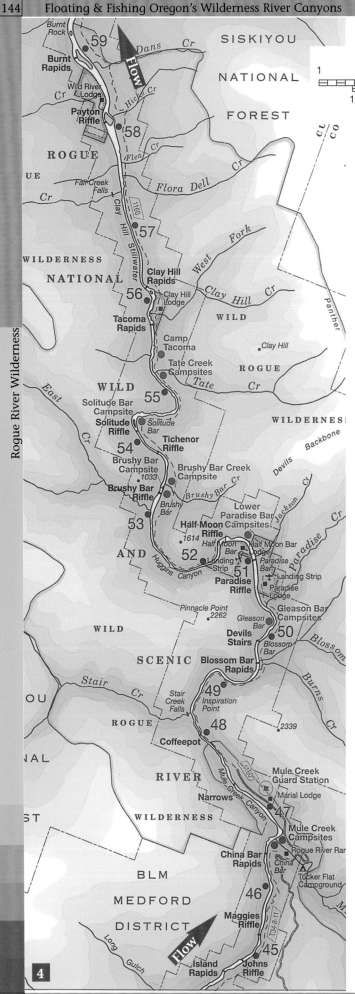

Rogue River Wilderness

stopping place on river right, to far left, before reaching the beginning of the rapid.

Next, an oarboat faces the danger, river left. At the entrance, there is an eddy at the base of the rock wall on river left where you can wait up if another boat is out of turn, or gets into trouble, but as in Coffeepot, boats should go one at a time. Identify the rocks of the Picket Fence, about 30 yards below the entrance on the left side. This is the most common place to wrap, flip or knock someone overboard, as well as the hardest place for a rescue.

With the boat angled, facing the left-side danger, float past a rock outcropping on the right of the slick (optimum to low water), not pulling until the stern has cleared. This is important, as most oar boats that strike this outcropping will be rebounded towards the Picket Fence. Once past this obstacle, begin a hard, backward pull on both oars to grab the eddy behind the entrance boulders (including the C-Rock, shaped like the letter C, which is discernable only looking back upstream). Paddle craft can reverse angle and paddle forward to make this eddy. Some boaters call this "rounding the Horn" as a sailboat would come around Cape Horn (there is a horn in Martin's Rapid on the McKenzie, a sharp entrance rock, plus The Horn Rapid on the Siuslaw).

Once in the eddy, straighten the boat to drop through a slot located between the rocks of the Picket Fence on your left and the boulders in mid-stream on your right. For a perfect run, oarboaters must immediately realign their boats to face river right again, otherwise the V-slick of this passage will carry them directly into a small rock in mid-stream, with a bigger rock behind it. (At higher water levels, the smaller rock is covered.) Inflatables usually bounce off these rocks, but driftboats won't.

Use the eddy water below the Picket Fence to help keep the oarboat to the left. Driftboats should be close to the left shore here, as much of the current now barrels into the big, rounded boulder known as Volkswagen Rock sitting in the middle of the rapid. Rafts usually survive encounters with Volkswagen's bumper, but remember if you must hit this rock, hit straight-on, never sideways, and be ready to jump to the highside. (Rafts, being heavier and clumsier than driftboats, usually don't respond as well to finesse and sometimes must be "pinballed" through a rapid.)

Once past Volkswagen, there is a small rock outcropping on river left, and a second big boulder just below this, also on river left. Don't celebrate until you are safely past this last boulder. Most water levels bring a set of rollercoaster waves to the bottom of the rapid in mid-channel; ride these out like a whitewater cowboy, with boat straight into them, not sideways. At low-medium, you may have to stay left of middle to avoid sleepers until you reach the eddy water below on river left. Now you can take a bow!

Alternate routes do exist, even at low to optimum levels. Many a raft has made the Picket Fence, only to wander to the right of Volkswagen or to get stuck on Table Rock (the big flat one) or bottomed out on a more obscure, unnamed sleeper rock.

If you get lost here, don't panic. If you can't avoid a rock, hit bow first or stern first (again, never sideways). At high levels, large inflatables and daring kayaks challenge the right side, which has more turbulence than the eddy-hopping route on the left. As the water level rises, more routes open up, such as a far-left channel right over Picket Fence (next to the left bank), or even jumping into hydraulics that were boulders at lower levels; yet the traditional run—left, cut to middle, left, cut back to middle, and dodge rocks in midchannel at end—remains the safest at nearly all levels. Bear in mind that when high water covers boulders, the resulting reversal is often not visible from upstream, except as a horizon line indicating a big drop.

At levels of 20-30,000 cfs, sometimes encountered in late winter or early spring, the huge hump of Volkswagen Rock will be totally submerged (leaving a giant reversal).

22.8: Big eddy water, river left, and slow water, river right, is where successful runners of Awesome Blossom wait for the rest of their party to make it through.

22.9: Devils Stairs, or Devil's Staircase, Class III. Strong current slams into the rock wall on river right. This rapid drops 30 feet in 300 yards, in three stages. First, set up in the V-slick and ride standing waves. (At higher water levels, a large backcurler develops here on left of center, fine for big inflatables, but should be cheated by other boats.)

Recover from the last wave promptly by angling the boat to face river right, and prepare for a hard pull. As the current hits the wall, oarboaters backferry hard to catch the slower inside current of this turn. Once past this, take the last drop in mid stream.

23.1: Gleason Bar, Gleason Creek, river left. First suitable campsites since Marial.

23.4: Paradise Creek, river right. Creek with natural stone swimming pool along trail, cascades over rock ledge into river.

23.7: Paradise Lodge. A commercial lodge, open year-round, the stopping point for jetboat trips coming upriver from Gold Beach. Motorized craft are not allowed into Blossom Bar Rapid (although I have seen a hot-dogger enter during high water levels in May. Report any violators to the Forest Service or BLM.)

Paradise has ice, drinks, fresh water, a 1550-foot airstrip, overnight lodging, plus an outdoor museum featuring photographs of the good ole days as well as retired river boats from the early 1900s. And, of course, it wouldn't be Paradise without flush toilets. Paradise is reachable by float-in and motorized craft, by aircraft,

and on foot via the Rogue River Trail. Lodge visitors often see blacktail deer and wild turkeys foraging on the lawn.

Visitors are welcome. This is a good overnight place for those who must have a hot shower, especially in off-season (reservations required). You can also get assistance in an emergency.

A long staircase leads to a flat spot atop the canyon rim and the lodge/museum. Climbers along the way are entertained by signs indicating flood water crests for various years, with the 1964 flood lapping at the lodge's deck. This short walk really puts high water into perspective. (A platform dumbwaiters supplies and handicapped patrons to the high terrace; the able-bodied climb the stairs.)

23.9: Half Moon Bar Lodge, river left. Nestled into the woods, all most boaters see as they float past is a staircase. This lodge also has an airstrip, but most guests arrive by jetboat or float-in. More visible are a set of small private cabins on river left.

Camping is available on river right, a long gravel bar with an outhouse well up the hillside. Campers are reminded they must use the available facility or set up and use their own. I have stayed at this bar in years past when thoughtless campers used prime patches of sand as their bathroom.

Half Moon Bar also makes a good lunch stop, with the main recreation using the many flat stones for skipping or building ahus (Hawaiian term for piles of rock). These strange statues are popular construction projects along the Rogue, and very biodegradable.

24.4: Half Moon Riffles. Small rapids (Class II) lead around the bar, bumping along shallows and sleeper rocks, into the mouth of Huggins Canyon.

25: Huggins Canyon. **Three Class II drops** repeat the Snake sequence from Mule Creek. This is a good place for a novice to learn how to row, sort of a Mule Creek Canyon in miniature. These can have tricky currents at higher water levels.

Now you must listen for jetboats motoring upstream. You have the right of way, but bear in mind jetboats need a deep channel and leave a big wake. Most jetboats pass slowly so as to not leave a wake, which can sweep untied boats off the shore or slam around swimmers. Both river users must show courtesy to each other (floaters should never indulge in uncouth behavior, such as mooning a jetboat; the Forest Service has been known to issue tickets for this). To be safe, pull the group's craft over to one side of the river and wait until the jetboats pass, they usually travel two or three boats together.

After the end of the entrance rapids, enjoy the canyon named for Andy Huggins (a local hunter in Glen Wooldridge's time, who lived at Half Moon Bar). This is a slow, scenic float, very warm drift in afternoon (and often with an upstream breeze). Floating in your

Rogue River Wilderness

life jacket is popular (recommended so you can be seen by jetboats from a distance). Deer and bear may be seen. The glorious flowers on the rock walls are California fuchsia. Sturgeon lurk in the deep waters here, especially in the Sturgeon Hole (25.7).

26: East Creek and cabin, river left. The cabin, once owned by World War II generals, has been removed. All that remains are a set of steps and a rock fireplace. These steps are a landmark for Brushy Bar.

26.1: Brushy Bar. A huge, high bar on river right can accommodate many campers. There are two small landing sites on river right with flat kitchen spots and trails leading up to terraced campsites and outhouses. In season, a Forest Service Guard Station about 1/4 mile into the woods is occupied by a caretaker; available in river emergencies. Brushy Bar was named after a burn in 1908 that resulted in the low and dense brush. Mining ditches from the Gold Rush days are still present.

26.3: Brushy Bar alternate camp, river left. A small sandy beach at the top of a long gravel bar on the inside of this bend has room for small groups. You must set up your own toilet facility, preferably with a portable tent as screen, since this camp is visible by campers on river right.

Bears often frequent this area. Brushy is known for both night raids on camps and daylight sightings of

bears. Once, with two groups, one on each bank of the river, we on the right saw a large black thing moving around on the left bank. A chorus of voices shouted "Bear!" to alert the others on river left, and then more shouts of, "Your side of the river, your bear!" About two minutes later, a very embarrassed woman, wearing a black sweater and pants, walked out of the bushes where we had been pointing, which was the semi-secluded site of that camp's toilet!

26.8: Tichenor Riffle, Class II, is a set of rolling waves that begins Solitude Bar (river right). The wave train ends in Decision Rock where you must decide to go right or left of the house rock in the river. Several camping areas may be found, but to find the best one, land river right just above Decision Rock. Some boats have difficulty landing here, but it's a nice site on a big spit of gravel and sand, with an outhouse up in the trees. Named after Captain William Tichenor, an Army officer traveling to Illahee to rescue settlers from an attack by Rogue Indians. Over the steep cliffs in this area, the Natives rolled rocks down onto his troops; however, this tactic only postponed their fate and soon all Rogues were put onto the Siletz Reservation. Mining equipment such as the arrastra wheel (used to break up ore to extract minerals like gold) and piles of rock tailings attest to the determination of early gold miners.

27.1: Solitude Riffle, Class II. Tichenor's Riffle continues around the spit of land, around boulders and through a chute past Decision Rock.

28.2: Long stretch of deep quiet water leads to Tate Creek, river right. Stop where Tate Creek enters the Rogue amid a jumble of boulders. From here, a bridge over the creek along the Rogue River Trail can be seen.

Hike up this hillside to the trail, then scramble up the Tate Creek streambed on a "wet-dry" hike best done in sturdy footwear. This creek drops through a series of small pools scalloped out of the streambed, framed by mosses and ferns, and ends at the Tate Creek Water slide, a thin waterfall. Scrambling, climbing and sliding are all considered hazardous by the Forest Service, so use caution.

To slide, first climb up to the top of the waterfall, via a rope tied here or through the woods to your right as you face the falls. Best to send your strongest person up first and have them secure a fresh, unfrayed rope for the others (that you then remove when you leave). People can be hoisted using a bowline knot and loop, or climb up using knots tied about a foot apart on the rope.

Sliders sit atop the waterfall (wearing a life jacket is recommended for nervous or younger sliders), block-

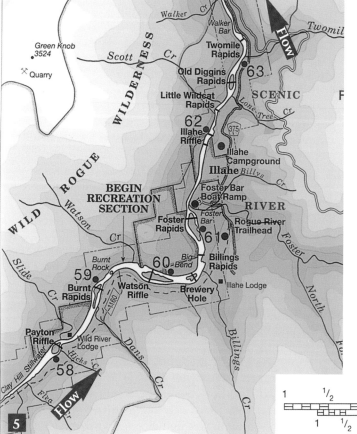

Scale 1:63,360

1"=1Mile

5

ing the water behind them into what whitewater boaters term a "butt dam". Once this water has built up enough, the slider simply wiggles their butt forward slowly, tucking in the elbows to form a narrow profile. As a certain point is reached, the butt and water both rush forward, the backed-up water propelling the slider into the cold-water pool below. Sliders should go one at a time.

28. 3: Tate Creek campsite. Much of the sand at the camp closer to Tate has washed away, so most groups prefer to camp lower and then hike back up the trail to Tate.

28.3: Tacoma Camp, right bank, followed by Tacoma Rapid (28.7, Class II+, rocky). This site is prime for large groups and has an outhouse just upriver, below the trail. Named for a mining company from Tacoma, Washington.

Bears are a concern here, so look for the electric fences to stash your food supplies. As an alternative, you can lug all your food boxes and coolers to one spot and strap them together, then have a volunteer sleep nearby, armed with pot lids to clang at marauding bears.

28.9: Clay Hill Lodge, river right. The famed Dinosaur Tree is seen on the right bank. The Lodge takes reservations for meals and sleeping quarters.

This is an area with many bears and river otter. Turtles are sometimes seen here.

29.1: Clay Hill Rapid, Class III. Enjoy this as it's one of the last big drops of your trip. The river turns sharply to the left over a rock ledge. To run, avoid the shallow far left channel around an island. Once set up on river right, stay about ten feet off the island towards the middle. Further right, the river drops over a bumpy ledge. Continue to hold your boat in the V-slick between the ledge on river right and the island on the left until you round the bend, then ride the wave train.

Lower Clay Hill (Class II, about 80 yards downstream) is a set of standing waves that end in a sleeper rock at most water levels; be ready to pull right.

29.4: Clay Hill Flats. Still waters extend for about two miles downriver, leaving time to enjoy the dramatic change of scenery from forested canyon with hard basalt rock to a more open meadow of scrub oak and grass marked by softer conglomerate rock eroded into fantastic shapes. This is almost a "moonscape" compared to the lush growth of the upper river. Potholes and undercuts were drilled out by pebbles worked around inside softer rock. Banks are studded with giant round rocks.

Boaters may curse slow current and an upstream breeze here, but the fishing is good. Both salmon and sturgeon lurk in these depths, with trout and steelhead along the shallow shores.

30.2: Fall Creek Falls, river left. A short hike brings you to this beautiful hidden falls that drops 50 feet over a ledge. Best in spring with creeks in flood.

For a good lunch spot, land where a creek sparkles above a high rock bank on river right. This is Flora Dell, a series of small but enchanting waterfalls and pools. Follow the Rogue River Trail to find the upper, larger falls. The flat rocks here are perfect for spreading out a picnic.

As you approach the end of this slow pool, watch for the Tree Rock on river left, where a persistent oak has wrapped its roots around a large boulder and appears to grow out of solid rock.

31.1: Peyton Riffle, Class II, named for the old Peyton Ranch homestead. Wild River Lodge (31.2) is on river left at the bottom of this riffle. Osprey often nest in the snags above this lodge.

Stay left here, close to the left bank, to locate the Pavement Rocks, a flat stone carved by water erosion into what seem to be individually positioned tiles. This is a cool shady spot suitable for small group lunches.

32.2: Burnt Creek Riffle, Class II. An area of big landslides. Current funnels into a V-slick on river right.

Watson Creek Stillwater. Trees here used by bald eagles and osprey. Watson Creek marks the end of the "Wild" section of the Rogue, starting the "Recreational" stretch.

32.6: Watson Riffle, Class II, leads into Big Bend, where the river turns to the right and separates around an island. Here the Rogue takes a side trip from its journey southwest to the Pacific Ocean to meander northwest, almost in a circle, with the bend finishing at Foster Bar.

Use caution in selecting channels here. Some are rocky and have strainers in them. As you drift towards a rocky island, stay left to Brewery Hole (Class I+). Jetboats usually take the blind channel on far right, at high speeds to get over the shallows. Float craft should stay left of a small boulder in the main channel. This channel is very shallow and rocky at lower levels.

Big Bend marks the site of a 30-hour battle in 1856. In the aftermath, over 1,000 Rogues were removed to the Siletz Reservation.

33.7: Billings Creek, river right, named after early-timer John Billings, who lived downriver at the mouth of the Illinois River. Illahee Lodge (chinook jargon for "land on earth"—Natives thought this land was theirs to keep and to fight for) is located on river right.

34.2: Foster Creek can be seen on river right, and the next bend is Foster Bar, also river right. You will share this take-out with other recreationists such as gold miners, campers and anglers in addition to motorized craft. Drift craft use the upper ramp sites for take-out. Cars are left in the upper parking lot, with changing rooms, bathrooms and bear-proof Dumpsters located above the parking lot.

Alternate take-out is downstream at Cougar Lane in Agness, with more facilities than the remote Foster Bar (store, gas, telephone).

Advanced Oregon Rivers

CHAPTER 9

Advanced Oregon Rivers

Snake River

THE SNAKE IN HELLS CANYON IS A 3- TO 5-DAY FLOAT trip located in the far northeastern corner of Oregon on the Oregon-Idaho border (erroneously listed as an Idaho river in many guidebooks, the launch site is on Oregon soil, as is most of the left bank).

This is a high water volume, big-water trip all season long. There are big waves and reversals. While the weather is usually scorching, the water released from the dam that feeds the last whitewater is cold enough for trout and steelhead, with bass in the few shallows and pocket water.

Hells Canyon is the deepest gorge in the nation, at over a mile deep. Summer weather is hot and dry in this desert gorge. Dam control keeps the river big; this run is the last free-flowing section with very large rapids. The flow in season is 8,000 cfs or larger. In Hells Canyon National Recreation Area, 67.5 miles are federally protected under the Wild & Scenic Rivers Act. Of these, 31.5 miles are designated "Wild." Motorized craft are grandfathered into the system, so expect to see jetboats moving up and downstream, even in the big rapids.

Fishing is excellent for trophy sturgeon (catch and release), some salmon, steelhead, trout, bass, catfish and other species. Fishing the deep waters can be harder than on smaller rivers, where fish concentrate into shallows, pocket water and underwater structures. Try for bass on the edges of the river below the dam. Poppers, hoppers and other bass lures work well. Look for steelhead at the mouths of side streams.

Wildlife includes Rocky Mountain elk, bighorn sheep, mule deer, birds of prey, and many smaller mammals. Reptiles are represented by a healthy rattlesnake population, in addition to lizards.

Begin at Hells Canyon Dam, where large, Class III to V rapids (Wild Sheep, Granite with its infamous Green Room where boaters disappear into wave troughs, Waterspout, Rush Creek) drench boats for the first day or two. Calmer conditions prevail for most of the remaining trip. Most of the gradient (9 fpm) is lost only in these rapids.

Many boaters now do 3-day trips, rather than week-long adventures, by ending at Pittsburgh Landing on river right rather than continue downstream through flat water to Heller Bar below the mouth of the Grande Ronde (river left), which takes two or more additional days.

Advance permits are required for floating during the May (Friday before Memorial Day) to September (usually ends the 10th) season. Outside the season, fall fishing can be good.

Practice your big-water skills before trying the Snake. The Rogue or North Umpqua at high levels will approximate the size of the Snake. The cfs levels are taken as released from Hells Canyon Dam.

For additional information, contacts are:

HCNRA Float Reservations (509) 758-1957
General Information (509) 758-0616
Website www.fs.fed.us/r6/w-w/hcnra.htm
Also: www.nps.gov/rivers/wsr-snake.html

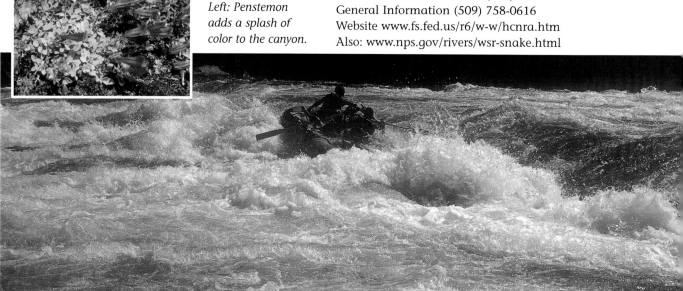

Trouble in one of the Snake's huge hydraulics.

Left: Penstemon adds a splash of color to the canyon.

Illinois River

This "rainy season" river is located in southwestern Oregon, and is a tributary of the Rogue River. It's usually done as a "technical" thrill run by whitewater experts at water levels of 1,000 to 3,000 cfs. Higher water is very dangerous, with the level of 1,500 cfs usually perfect. The main season is February to May most years.

This is a 32-mile wilderness run through a steep gorge with the Green Wall, a Class V drop against a cliff wall on river right (named for lush mosses found there).

The wild Illinois is not usually a river that is floated and fished due to the limited season, wildly fluctuating water levels, and technical rapids, but it does present a challenge to the well-prepared float-in angler. The area is one of the most isolated and rugged in Oregon outside of the desert southeastern country of the Owyhee. Rare flowers blossom in the bordering Kalmiopsis Wilderness Area.

Most limiting is that boating is usually done during the rainy season, not necessarily when fishing conditions are acceptable. However, there is a window during the levels of 600 to 1,600 cfs, achieved during a dry spell that follows a rainy spell, when fishing can be good. The water at such times has excellent clarity and is a beautiful turquoise shade.

This is a Class IV+ stream (Green Wall is considered a V, the rest of the rapids as a IV) with no exit from the deepest gorge, except by helicopter. During a late 1990s storm, boaters were trapped here by fast-rising waters and some had to be evacuated by helicopter. Two boaters perished in the extreme conditions.

The lower water levels are for the inflatable kayak, Cat-yak or small cataraft only, while the higher levels demand a bigger and more stable craft, at least 14 feet. Hydraulics at the higher levels mandate a larger craft. A very few "canyoneer" types have gone down this river at very low water levels.

The Illinois often drops to below 100 cfs in summer, which is the boating equivalent of crawling through a boulder field, while raging as high as 225,000 cfs back in 1964. Peaks of 4-8,000 occur with heavy rains and are not boatable. The flow is given at Kerby.

Most important considerations here are an advance, accurate weather forecast; excellent gear; and good boating skills. First-timers should pair up with experienced Illinois boaters. Self-issued permits are required (at Selma, the jump off place from civilization, not the launch site, Miami Bar).

Shuttles and inquiries may be made through The Galice Resort (see Rogue) and Siskyou National Forest.

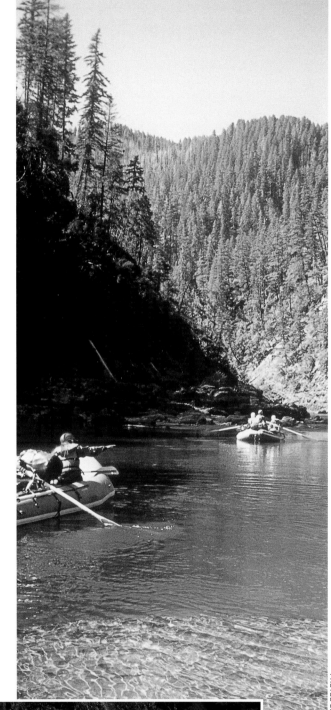

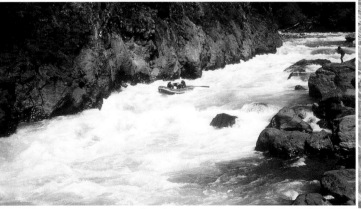

Top: A quiet moment between drops on a green and beautiful Illinois.

Lower: "The Green Wall" Class V expert run on the Illinois.

Advanced Oregon Rivers

General Information

Managing Agencies

MAPS ARE AVAILABLE FROM ALL OF THE MANAGING agencies listed here. There is a small fee charged for these maps; however, knowing where private lands, rapids, and landmarks are located is well worth this fee. I am grateful to these agencies for providing excellent maps, boating information, historical data, permit requirements, and more.

State Managing Agencies

Oregon Department of Fish & Wildlife, 2501 SW First Avenue, Portland, OR 97207 (503-872-5268). Basic information on fishing, trout-stocking dates, etc. There are seven offices but this one is the headquarters. For an agency near your river, contact the headquarters. Field officers often know where the best fishing is and what lures are working.

Oregon State Marine Board, 435 Commercial Street, NE, Salem, OR 97309 (503-378-8587). Boat license requirements, boating regulations, river safety booklets and videos. They can also confirm that the outfitter you booked to guide your family down an expert river does have a license, as required by state law. Useful pamphlet of Coast Guard-approved PFDs for use when floating whitewater.

BLM and Forest Service managing agencies are listed in the river descriptions. Contact them for current conditions (water levels, wild fires, downed logs, etc.), maps (this book is not waterproof), permit information, camping/user fees and so forth.

Grande Ronde River Managing Agency
Walla Walla Ranger District
1415 W Rose
Walla Walla, WA 99362
(509) 522-6290

Deschutes, **John Day**, **North Fork John Day** Managing Agency
BLM Prineville District
3050 NE 3rd St.
Prineville, OR 97754
(541) 416-6700
Boater passes for Deschutes River: Buy at local stores in Maupin and Madras or online at: www.boaterpass.com

General information on recreation and river conditions for the John Day and Deschutes River: www.or.blm.gov/Prineville

Owyhee River Managing Agency
BLM Vale District Office
100 Oregon St.
Vale, OR 97918
(541)473-3144
Website: www.or.blm.gov/vale

Rogue River Managing Agency
BLM Medford Resource Area
3040 Biddle Rd.
Medford, OR 97504
(541) 618 2275

Also
River Permits Office (Also Illinois River)
Rand Information Center
14335 Galice Rd.
Merlin, OR 97532
(541) 479-3735
Website: www.or.blm.gov/rogueriver. Find out which upcoming dates have spaces available during the permit system, how to apply, river conditions and bear trouble areas, etc.

Gold Beach Ranger District
Managing Agency for Illinois River

Siskiyou National Forest
1225 S. Ellensburg, Box 7
Gold Beach, OR 97444
(541) 247-6651

Snake River, Hells Canyon Managing Agency
HCNRA
PO Box 699
Clarkston, WA 99403

HCNRA Float Reservations (509) 758-1957
General Information (509) 758-0616
Website www.fs.fed.us/r6/w-w/hcnra.htm
Also: www.nps.gov/rivers/wsr-snake.html

General Boating Information:
Oregon State Marine Board
503-378-8587
435 Commercial St. NE
Salem, OR 97309
Website: www.boatoregon.com

River Forecast Center, Portland
503/261-9246 (follow the push-button-
phone directions to reach the
river levels you wish).
www.usgs.gov for all rivers
http://Oregon.usgs.gov for the state

Oregon Department of Fish & Wildlife
Main Office
2501 SW First Ave
PO Box 59
Portland, OR 97207-5268
Website: www.dfw.state.or.us

Equipment Checklists
(Including contents of first-aid and boat-repair kits for expeditions.)

Gear: what and why, tents vs. sleep out, down vs. synthetic bags, liners, gear hogs, hot shower machines.

Dry Bags are about 24" x 48" and are made for personal gear such as clothing, sleeping bag, toiletries, and so forth. I have found these large bags will not close properly if you have too much stuff in them. Since they are made of PVC, treat your dry bag kindly, don't drag or throw it around, or use it as a ground cover. Also, there is no such thing as a 100% waterproof container on any river trip. A heavy-duty garbage bag to line your dry bag, plus a separate plastic bag to seal your sleeping bag (especially a down-filled one) is a good idea. The 2-gallon zip-lock freezer bags and zippered clothing bags work well for this. I prefer a synthetic sleeping bag as they absorb less water and are warm even when wet, just wring them out!

Another good precaution is to pack every item inside Zip-lock freezer bags (socks in one, underwear in another, etc.). This lets you sort by emptying the bag onto the ground without getting everything sandy. Valuables like cameras or prescription glasses should be insured. You will want to put these into the ammo can so they don't get crushed. Keep weight and bulk in mind when selecting your gear. Inflatable pads take less room than foam pads, for example.

Items to Keep Accessible
During the Day's Float

___Waterproof sunscreen (protection factor 6 or higher strongly recommended, the sun is very intense on most river trips). Also good are special "face only" lotions to prevent stinging eyes should you get water in your face.

___Camera and film (waterproof boxes or ammo cans recommended) The disposable or "one-time use" waterproof cameras work well and are cheap (under $12, with film), Panoramic cameras take wide shots—nice for big canyons.

___Plastic bottle (1-quart to gallon milk jug) or canteen filled with clean drinking water for your personal use (mark your name on it with a felt-tip pen). Drink lots of water, especially on summer trips, so you won't dehydrate (pop doesn't do the trick). Clip the container onto your boat using a carabineer. Save beer for camp, as it also dehydrates you.

___Fishing gear: rod, reel, lures and/or flies, landing net, baits, etc. Keep these stowed in waterproof containers. I like to use a telescoping rod for trout and bass, so it can be stowed quickly when whitewater is eminent. High quality rods should be packed in rod cases to prevent breakage.

Items to Pack into Waterproof Bag

___Stuffable sleeping bag (wrap in plastic bag for additional security). Fleece sleeping bag as linen.

___Lightweight tent with ground sheet (plastic sheet or space blanket).

___Air mattress or small ensolite foam pad.

___Small pillow, or use a folded jacket.

___Small towel (cloth diaper works well).

___Extra tennis shoes or thongs for camp wear (1 pair will suffice).

___Toothbrush and toothpaste, comb, shaving gear, etc. Lip protection and skin lotion are popular, especially in the desert.

___Personal medications, feminine hygiene supplies, etc.

___Rain gear, poncho/jacket and pants (great for keeping the spray or wind off. Always bring! Oregon being famous for unexpected rain).

___Long-sleeved shirt (keeps sun off arms and shoulders).

___1 pair long pants, jeans or sweats (for camp wear).

___Warm sweater (polyester fleece is best) or jacket for eves/mornings in camp (non-bulky if possible). This, with shorts, will keep you warm 99% of the time on summer and shoulder seasons along most Oregon rivers.

___Pocket flashlight (for finding your tent in the dark), extra batteries for reading in bed.

___Hobby items (bird book, journal, binoculars, novels, magnifying glass, etc.)

To Wear on the River

___Shorts (quick-dry nylon is best) and tank top/T-shirt, or bathing suit.

General Information

___Cover-ups if you burn easily, socks for "palefoots".

___Tennis shoes or river sandals for river wear (an old pair you won't mind getting wet—shoes are mandatory for safe floating).

___Strap to secure sun/prescription glasses (Croakies or a short piece of surgical tubing from the fishing gear department).

___Hat (baseball cap or brimmed style, to shade face).

___Sunglasses (Polarized to cut glare).

___Warm gear (in cold weather): wetsuit, paddle jacket, wool sox, gloves. Fleece top and bottom for camp. Wetsuits may be rented from a dive shop.

___Rowing or paddling gloves (Fingerless gloves such as those made for bike riding or weight lifting provide good blister protection while allowing a good "feel" on the oar handles.

___Sunscreen.

___Life jacket or PFD (personal floatation device), Coast Guard Approved. The Type V vest is used by commercial outfitters for guests, offering high flotation (it also floats an unconscious person on their back). These are thick foam with a collar on the upper back to support the head. The Type III is rated for kayak/canoeists. The design is such that the user is expected to be able to swim and self-rescue, even in rapids. There is much less flotation. A guide or rescue vest has higher flotation with a slimmer profile, and often attachments for knife, rescue belt, whistle and so forth.

If in doubt, choose higher flotation. The vest will feel cumbersome at first. You can always get a second vest when you are more confident on the water.

To Be Packed with Cargo

___Beer or your favorite alcoholic beverage (Glass may break, so transfer to plastic container or use a metal flask, box wine, cans, etc. Boat sober.)

___Canned soft drinks

___Mesh bag or onion sack to keep canned drinks in (keeps your drinks together). Use these bags to pre-chill canned drinks in the river before putting them in your cooler, so they don't melt all the ice.

Always bring with you: Sense of humor. Remember you are having an adventure, and expect the unexpected!

Overnight Trip
Checklist For Group Gear

___Maps/guidebooks.

___Boats.

___Frame for oar/paddle assist.

___Oar stands and oar locks for oarboats (open oarlocks, U-shaped, are preferred by Oregon boaters; in other states, some use a pin-and-clip system that secures oars so that blades are not feathered, which can be an advantage to beginners, but prevents advanced

movements such as feathering blades and shipping oars in).

___Paddles.

___Oars & blades.

___Throwbag, bow lines, stern lines: for tying up boats, rescue, making clothes line to dry out wet stuff.

___PFDs (life jackets), at least 1 per person with one extra.

___Bail bucket (for settling murky water, as well as bailing a bucket boat).

___Scoop (optional: for water fights, washing out boat)

___Straps plus extras. Cam buckle straps over much easier to fasten and loosen than rope or "hoopie" cord.

___Camera box with tie-downs. (ammo can)

___Dry box for oar boat (packed with kitchen equipment and non-perishable food).

___Cooler for oar boat, or lunch cooler for paddle.

___Lunches packed accessible

___Charcoal and lighter fluid, matches and clicker (butane lighter).

___Tarps for rigging/de-rigging, rain protection.

___Throw-bag (mandatory safety equipment for all trips).

___First-aid kit (expedition oriented for wilderness trips, also bring a good manual).

___Repair kit(s). Patching materials, glue, solvent, sandpaper, pliers, extra oarlock and pins, wire, duct tape, screwdrivers, PVC patching for dry bags, how-to instructions.

___Foot- or hand-powered air pump for inflatables, air mattresses.

___Dry bag—at least 1 per person, with extras.

___Dunk/mesh bag for chilling pop, collecting empty cans (do not crush cans as this creates sharp edges).

___Cold trips: fire starter, matches in waterproof holder.

___Ice for coolers.

___Cook stove, gas or propane (butane doesn't work well in colder temperatures). Remember charcoal and wood fires are banned in summer on some rivers.

___Extra fuel.

___Propane tank w/tee or tree.

___Hoses (the right ones plus extra).

___Coleman lantern in ammo can (or big flashlight).

___Salvage kit: hairy trips only. This is a Z-drag kit with heavy floating rescue line, Prusik line, carabineers and pulleys. Take a "crib card" if you're not sure how to set this up.

___Extra ammo cans or rocket boxes from Army surplus, empty (to keep cameras dry, store ashes and garbage, etc.).

___Shovel/trowel (can use paddle).

___Bug candles/yellow-jacket trap, mosquito repellent.

___Everyone's personal camp gear as listed above.

___Big tarp(s).

___Roll-a-table(s).

___Big folding table(s) or fold-up camp kitchen.

___3- to 5-gallon water jugs, full if there is no launch-area water source.

___Chairs, 1 per person. You can sit on bail buckets or ammo cans.

___Solar shower: long, hot trips only.

___Cargo slings (holds cargo off floor for better boat balance).

___Cargo bags or net (helps keep small items from going overboard keeps gear dryer).

___Portable Potty, toilet paper, maybe a Peepee Teepee shelter for privacy (required on all Oregon wilderness trips).

___Portable Potty chemicals.

___Back-up stove (store generators in waterproof box, water may render them useless).

___Fire pan to contain ashes (mandatory).

___Folding grill for small group BBQ (Know fire restrictions).

___Giant fry pan for large groups.

___Big blower/generator or power inflator that uses a car battery.

___Motor/gas for reservoir tows on the Owyhee.

___Dishpans, soap, scrubbers, bleach. Sterilization of dishes is important!

___Water filter for drinking water.

___Float cushions (for chairs, IKs).

___Strainer for kitchen waste.

___Extra heavy-duty garbage bags.

___Ammonia, air horn for scaring off black bears.

___PVC pipes for building hot shower (Owyhee River only).

River Reminders
Important That Everyone In Your Party Knows This!

Drinking Water

I do not recommend drinking untreated river water. Even the cleanest of our rivers may contain a natural parasite called *Giardia* that can cause illness. For drinking and brushing teeth, use bottled water. Refill your daily container from large jugs. Most people like to bring a personal water container (even a rinsed-out plastic soda bottle). Springs are safe to drink at their source. In a pinch, a teaspoon of bleach into five gallons of river water will pretty much kill everything after an hour or so.

River water is fine for washing and bathing (do not use the bottled water for washing). Swimming or dunking yourself in the river is an excellent way to reduce the need for washing. If you want to use soap, bring only biodegradable soap and wash well away from the riverbank or any water source using a bail bucket or solar shower. Do not use soap in hot springs or side tributaries. Please help keep our rivers free from suds!

Garbage

Speaking of clean rivers, let's remember to pick up all trash we create. This includes tiny items like cigarette butts, film wrappers, nut shells, orange peels, bread twisties, etc. Boaters are required by law to remove all trash. Use zip-lock baggies on each boat to store garbage until camp is reached. Please do not throw anything into the river (except each other). Empty aluminum cans should be collected and recycled—place in bail bucket or the can bag, and do not crush cans (makes sharp edges on cans, and many recyclers won't accept them).

When fires are allowed, burn paper to reduce bulk garbage. This must be done in a firepan, and the ashes must be carried from camp to camp. Do not try to burn large trees or branches. The lowest impact fire is one made of hot, fast-burning dry driftwood. Set your pan on rocks or down on the river sand or gravel so vegetation isn't scorched. Remove any blackened rocks you find (even if this means tearing apart someone else's fire ring; it's illegal to leave them behind). Throw them into the river, where they will be Maytagged by Mother Nature.

Bathrooms

The Rogue and Deschutes have outhouses around most camps—please find them and use them whenever possible. On overnight trips elsewhere, and when no facility is available, you must bring and use your own portable potty for solid wastes only (must be agency-approved). Please use the facilities and avoid the bushes unless you are desperate (bury in 6-inch deep hole, remove toilet paper or put in hole and cover with dirt, then put a rock on top).

To cut down on weight, try not to urinate in the portable potty or put toilet paper into it (this is carried out separately in garbage bags). Install a "pee bucket" next to the "groover" (potty).

In forested areas, urinate behind bushes/trees well away from camp or waterways; in desert (Owyhee River), it's better to go at the edge of the river because it doesn't decompose otherwise.

Mother Nature

Environmental hazards along rivers vary according to terrain and climate. Brief party members on the basics of whitewater and camp safety, and point out specific hazards around camp.

Keep in mind: Poison oak is often found along river-banks, even along desert rivers. Watch out for plants with leaflets of three glossy leaves and white berries. Wash immediately after suspected contact (carry Technu poison oak remover in first-aid kit).

The deadly water hemlock is found along the Deschutes, Owyhee, and other rivers. Please do not pick or eat any plants you might find. Planning means bringing plenty of good food for everyone. If you look hard enough along any of our desert rivers (under rocks, in old shacks or outhouses, etc.) you might find nasty pests like scorpions or spiders. Rattlesnakes are found nearly everywhere in Oregon, but are timid and will not strike unless cornered or teased. Keep your eyes open, especially when you walk in grassy areas, and when picking up rocks.

You may find a tick or two in the spring or early summer—check yourself occasionally. Bring tick repellent (also good for mosquitoes) and use it if you plan on hiking off-river. In well-used camps, particularly on the Deschutes, you may encounter pests attracted to garbage. To reduce this possibility, please help keep the camp clean. Be on the lookout for yellowjackets (avoid the kitchen area, and let others know in advance if you're allergic) and, at night, skunks/black bears (they have the right-of-way!). On the whole, Oregon's river camps are clean and pleasant, free of mosquitoes and flies. A little repellent will do wonders for the few mosquitoes you may encounter. Most wild bears, cougar and bobcats are afraid of you and will run away.

Risks

Most accidents happen on shore. Please be careful getting in and out of your boats. Also, the managing agencies do not recommend climbing around on rocks, jumping into the water (no diving!), or other risky activities. Body surfing, hiking, water sliding, etc., are fun but carry risks; each person must decide if these activities are something they or their minor children should do.

River Safety "Cheat Sheet"

Always wear a Coast Guard-approved life jacket (PFD) while floating, swimming, scouting rapids. This easy step prevents 99% of all drownings. Think of the PFD as your river safety belt. Make sure the jacket is comfortably adjusted to fit your body (pull upwards to make sure it does not ride up or come off). Avoid Type II vests that may come loose in heavy hydraulics.

If thrown overboard, don't stand up. Oregon rivers have many shallows and strong currents that can knock you back down. Assume the lawn-chair position where you are sitting in the river, with feet floating on the surface (never allow feet to drag bottom, as you can have a foot caught under a rock). This is why you should wear shoes that stay on the feet, in case you have to use them to fend off rocks (use your head for this, and it will ruin your whole day!).

For rescue, a throw bag line, an outstretched paddle, or rowing towards the person for pickup is easiest. In heavy, fast or cold water, the overboard should assume more responsibility for self-rescue, and swim at an angle to the current to reach the safety of an eddy or rock, another boat, or the shoreline.

Have life lines on your boat so overboards have something to hang onto, and point them out.

To pull a swimmer back into the boat, grab them by the lapels of the PFD, never by the outstretched wrist (that can dislocate a wrist). With a heavy person, dunk them down, then haul up while you fall backwards into the boat. The push caused by their floatation device will propel them into the boat.

Limit jumping to deep water with no hidden rocks. Never dive. Boaters with asthma or heart conditions should avoid jumping into cold water, the shock can trigger an attack. The signal to be rescued immediately is waving an outstretched hand; if you're OK, pat your head.

Watch for strainers, logs, overhanging brush, bridge pillars, root wads, and other danger sites. Cheat these obstacles from a safe distance. Should you find yourself overboard and heading for a strainer, turn over and go head first, so you can chin yourself up on the strainer and not get sucked underneath. Avoid side channels around islands that are blind at the end, or small enough to have the channel blocked by a log.

Know throwbag rescue. To use, open the cord lock and hold the open mouth of the bag in your throwing hand. You can throw overhand or underhand; aim for a spot just ahead of the swimmer. Yell "Rope!" so the swimmer knows it's coming. Swimmers grab the rope, not the bag (which continues to feed out more rope).

Never wrap a rope around you or anyone else on moving water. The rope can snag on the bottom, towing you under. Cross the rescue rope over your shoulder and roll onto your back (face down, you will understand how a fishing lure works!). Many boaters carry divers' knives to cut ropes, a wise idea.

In rocky areas, if the boat is stuck, don't jump out to push until you have exhausted all other possibilities (shift weight of passengers, use a sea anchor, have a line from shore with many bodies pulling on it). If you must wade, stay upstream of the boat so you don't get crunched. Hard boats can trap boaters against rocks, so be careful.

Where strong currents hit boulders, remember your basic "highside" or "rocklike" maneuver. If broadside to a rock, all passengers and rower shift weight promptly towards the rock and/or downstream tube. The boat will often slide right off. Shrink back from the rock, and the boat may well wrap around the rock, like a wet sheet. Try to hit unavoidable rocks bow or stern first, to present less surface for the rock and currents to grab.

In reversals, keep the boat straight. Keep paddling or rowing to build momentum. Dig blades a little deeper to use the forward currents below the surface. Be prepared to highside. If overboard, get out from under the boat.

If your boat flips, locate life lines (rope around bags fastened to boat, for hanging on in such instances). Get to the outside so no one panics. Flip lines or the throwbag are attached to one side of the boat. Next, boaters use these lines to pull themselves onto the bottom of the boat. Everyone grabs the flip line and falls backward, re-righting the boat. This may be easier near shore.

Wear safety equipment on your person (or PFD) on remote rivers. Also carry signals for aircraft (flare gun, orange cloth). Three blasts on a whistle means "danger."

Dress for success. Wear wetsuits, paddle jackets, fleece and other splash gear when the water is cold. Stop to warm up your muscles often, by running up and down the shoreline.

Hard to believe, but true, that auto and airplane crashes kill more people than wild rapids. Additionally, bee stings kill more folks than bears, cougars, elk in rut, and all other wildlife. As H.D. Thoreau observed, "A man sits as many risks as he runs... Time is but the river we go fishing in..."

General Information

Bibliography & Resources

River Guidebooks

Western Whitewater, by Jim Cassidy, Bill Cross and Friar Calhoun. Covers a plethora of rivers across the West, including all the rivers mentioned here.

Soggy Sneakers: A Guide to Oregon Rivers, by the Willamette Kayak and Canoe Club. Good safety information. Oriented to small paddle boats, covers many waterways. Read between the lines to see if a suggested trip is suitable for larger, wider craft.

Paddling Oregon, by Robb Keller. Also oriented to paddle boats, covers some obscure rivers.

Oregon River Tours, by John Garren. Classic reference, but no safety or low-impact camping information.

Fishing Guide Books

Fishing in Oregon's Deschutes River, by Scott Richmond. Everything you ever wanted to know about fishing this popular trout stream.

Fishing Central Oregon, compiled by Sun Publishing. From the central Columbia south to Klamath Falls, west to the McKenzie.

Fishing Oregon, by Jim Yuskavitch. An overview of the state's fishing possibilities, including fly, lure and baits; lakes and reservoirs, as well as rivers.

Fishing in Oregon, by Madelynne Diness Sheehan. Updated frequently. An overall guide.

Flyfisher's Guide to Oregon, by John Huber. A handbook for the purist, covers lakes and reservoir fishing in addition to rivers.

Overall whitewater boating books

Whitewater Boatman, by Robert S. Wood. How a middle-aged man learned to become a river guide.

The Guide's Guide, by William McGinnis. Tips from an outfitter to his professional guide crew. Good illustrations on how to move an oar boat, recipes.

Whitewater Rafting, by William McGinnis. The classic river book, entertaining to read (the original includes no information on open oarlocks or self-bailers).

River, by Colin Fletcher. Good read of an "older" guy rowing the Colorado River solo.

The Inflatable Kayak Handbook, by Melinda Allan. A solid introduction to how IKs work.

Canoeing Basics, by Melinda Allan. All about canoes, with one chapter on whitewater.

Rafting! By Jeff Bennett. A good up-to-date beginner's manual.

Driftboats: A Complete Guide, By Dan Alsup. About the only text in this category. Classic historic photographs.

Specific River Books

Driftboater's Guide to the Upper McKenzie, by Doc Crawford. Covers the McKenzie from Leaburg Dam upstream to Olallie Campground.

John Day River: Drift and Historic Guide, by Arthur Campbell. Good reference for history of the region.

The Rogue River Guide (map format), by Vladimir Kovalik History, map, nature, geology, and so forth.

Handbook to the Rogue River Canyon, by James M. and James W. Quinn, James G. King. Good history, blow-by-blow descriptions of how to run the rapids with aerial photographs.

Handbook to the Deschutes River Canyon, same authors as above. Good history, how-to pictures.

General Reference Books

GPS Waypoints, by Michael Ferguson (Shows GPS locations of many Oregon rapids)

Oregon Geographic Names, by Lewis A. MacArthur. The last word on how places earned their names, such as Jumpoff Joe Creek.

Oregon Atlas, compilation of facts (For historic high and low water record levels)

Videos

"National Paddlesport Safety Program," Presented by the American Canoe Association. Basic safety tips.

"Let's Get Wet: The Essentials of Whitewater Rafting," by Beth Rypins and Paulo Castillo. Good for beginners, overview shots of scary big whitewater, makes fun of "rubber duckies".

Oregon Field Guide, "Owyhee River Journey" by Oregon Public Broadcasting. Occasionally shown on PBS station, trip from Rome to Leslie Gulch documented by film crew. Order for $20 from alswildwater.com.

"The Magnificent Rogue," by River Associates. Shows rapids, driftboat and raft techniques, salmon fishing.

Guide Services/Outfitters

Mah-Hah Outfitters (1-888-624-9242), guided John Day bass fishing.

Alswildwater.com (1-800-289-4534), guided bass fishing and learn to row, whitewater schools, low water trips on John Day, Owyhee, Grande Ronde; cargo raft support for kayakers and row-your-own-boats on Rogue, Deschutes, Owyhee, Grande Ronde. OPB videos of Owyhee for sale. Fall fishing on the Rogue.

River Drifters (541/395-2228 or riverdrifters.net), offers rental boats and guided trips on Deschutes River.

Helfrich Outfitters (1-800-507-9889) Fishing on Rogue, McKenzie, Idaho's Salmon.

Rogue Wilderness (1-800-336-1647 or www.wildrogue .com/) offers lodge trips on wild section of Rogue, fishing, rentals.

Morrison's Rogue River Lodge (541-476-3825) has pre-trip lodging, fishing trips.

Silver Sedge Fly Shop (541-476-2456) located near Merlin (north of Grants Pass) at 8500 Galice Road, Merlin, OR 97532.

Bi-Mart discount stores with good sporting goods and knowledgeable sales people, are in Albany, Ashland, Bend, Corvallis, Eugene, Klamath Falls, Medford, Monmouth, Oregon City, Portland, and Springfield.

The Hook Fly Shop, Sunriver Village Mall, Building 21, Sunriver OR 97707 (541-593-2358) or www.hookfish .com. Flies, fishing lessons.

Fin N Feather Fly Shop, 785 West 3rd, Prineville OR 97754 (541-447-8691). Fly patterns, especially for the Deschutes and John Day rivers.

Four Seasons Fly Shop, 10210 Wallowa Lake Highway, LaGrande OR 97850 (541-963-8420). Advice and flies for fishing the Wallowa/Grande Ronde rivers.

Numb Butt Fly Company, 380 North Highway 26, Madras, OR 97441 (541-325-5515). Fly patterns for the Deschutes River, guided trips, instruction, driftboats.

Joseph Fly Shop, 203 North Main, Joseph OR 97846 (541-432-4343) or www.eoni.com/-. Guided trips on the Grande Ronde and Wallowa, fly patterns for those rivers and Snake River.

Ashland Outdoor Store, 37 3rd Street, Ashland, OR 97520 (541-488-1202). Guided float trips, wading, instruction, flies and lures.

Fly & Field Outfitters, 143 SW Century Drive, Bend, OR 97701 (541-318-1616) or www.flyandfield.com. Fly patterns, lessons, guided trips, big fish. Courtesy photographs were provided by Steve Cook with FFO.

G. I. Joe's (sporting goods section), 63455 Highway 97 North, Bend, OR 97701 (541-388-3770). Good selection of lures, flies, rods and other fishing gear, also boating gear. Furthermore, has locations in Portland and Eugene. Sources for boats, gear

Cascade Outfitters, 800-243-1677. Mail-order rafts, catarafts, inflatable kayaks, misc. gear.

Northwest River Supplies, 800-243-1677. Mail-order rafts, inflatable kayaks, catarafts, other gear.

Koffler Boats (driftboats), 541-688-7958

Willie Boats (driftboats), 1-800-866-7775 www.willie boats.com

Jacks Plastic Welding (catarafts and paddle cats), www.jpwinc.com

Noah's River Adventures, P.O. Box 11, 53 N. Main Street, Ashland, OR 97520 (541-488-2811). Guided fishing trips on the Rogue and other rivers, whitewater including Class V Upper Klamath.

Sources for Boats, Gear

Cascade Outfitters, 800-243-1677. Mail-order rafts, catarafts, inflatable kayaks, miscellaneous gear.

Northwest River Supplies, 800-243-1677. Mail order rafts, inflatable kayaks, catarafts, other gear.

Koffler Boats (driftboats), 541-688-7958

Willie Boats (driftboats), 1-800-866-7775 www.willieboats .com

Jacks Plastic Welding (catarafts and paddle cats). www.jpwinc.com/

Luhr-Jensen, P.O. Box 297, Hood River, OR 97031. Source for special lures and fishing tips. Tech reports, patches for jackets, color catalog of fishing tackle and accessories. Cost for all this is $5.

About the Author

MELINDA ALLAN LAW HAS WORKED AS A RIVER AND fishing guide for AlsWildWater.com since the company began in 1981. Starting out as Shuttle Bunny, Shop Flunky, Head Chef and Bottle Washer, she worked her way up to rowing 16-foot-long cargo rafts piled high with gear. A Native Oregonian who grew up in Portland, Melinda loves big dogs, hot springs, pro basketball and is a card-carrying Parrothead (Jimmy Buffet fanatic). During the winter, she works as a freelance writer. Melinda has published two books on river boating (inflatable kayaks and canoes), dozens of magazine articles, and is an outdoor columnist for *The Register-Guard* newspaper in Eugene.

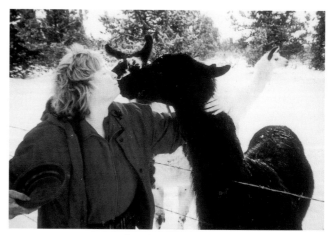

Author kissing a llama.

Oregon's Cascades; Rooster and Beacon rocks (Columbia Gorge) and Cinnamon Slab (Smith Rock State Park). She has bagged a six-point bull elk and over a dozen deer. She once backpacked solo through the rugged cliffs of the Columbia River Gorge, from Bridal Veil Falls to Mt. Defiance (highest point in the Gorge) and has scampered down sheep trails to fish the remote reaches of the Crooked River.

Melinda's greatest moment came when she yanked a 280-pound man out of the Rogue River just above Coffee Pot Rapid. Rowing an overloaded, cumbersome boat just a month after knee surgery, only sheer adrenaline landed this "fish." The man, who was a cookie salesman in real life, thanked her by saying, "I want you to have my baby!" Her response? "Ask my husband, who is doing a love scene with Meryl Streep."

Melinda can be reached at Oregonriverbum@aol.com

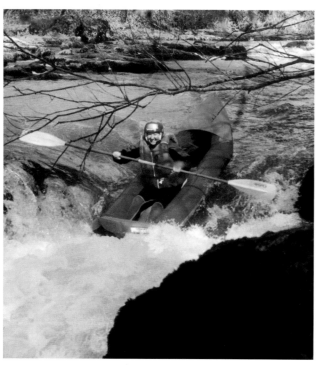

Author in IK on Row River running "Slots" section.

Melinda has taught boating classes at Lane Community College and delights in terrifying students of Al's Wild Water Adventures' spring guide school ("Pull harder, you little wimp!" has been shouted at a six-footer.)

Her river adventures include two 21-day floats on the Colorado (plus one 18-day trip); a stint working the Nenana River in Alaska (where the water temperature never exceeds 37 degrees and icebergs are common); the Idaho "Big Four" (Middle, Main and Lower Salmon, plus the Selway); and many almost-unknown creeks (Coast Fork Willamette, Row River, Mohawk River). She has logged over 10,700 river miles.

Her climbing expertise includes summits of Borah Peak (highest mountain in Idaho), South Sister in

Melinda Allan and Al Law married in Lahani, Maui, by a sailing ship's Captain!

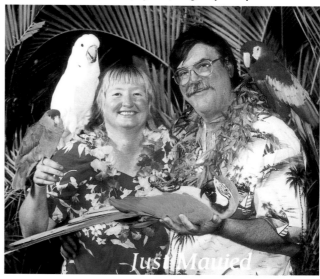

More Northwest Books

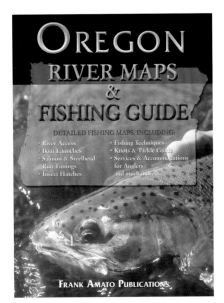

Oregon
River Maps & Fishing Guide
Frank Amato Publications

The ultimate book for Oregon anglers, *Oregon River Maps & Fishing Guide* features 37 detailed maps covering over 1000 miles of river—and that's just the beginning. Each map is packed with information, including: Roads and river access points; Drift-boat and power-boat landings; Peak fishing times for trout, salmon, steelhead, sturgeon, stripers and more; Insect hatches and hatch-timing chart; Fly-fishing and conventional tackle techniques; Fishing knots & tackle guide; Services & accommodations for anglers. Fishing guides and expert anglers from around the state have teamed up to create this essential guide to river fishing in Oregon. Learn the secrets of Oregon's best rivers, including the "inside" information you need to experience the very best fishing Oregon has to offer. 11 x 15 inches, 48 pages.

SB: $19.95   ISBN: 1-57188-317-7   UPC: 0-81127-00150-7

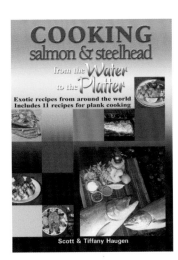

Cooking Salmon & Steelhead:
Exotic Recipes From Around the World
By Scott & Tiffany Haugen

This is not your grandmother's salmon cookbook. The long-time favorites are included and also unique yet easy-to-prepare dishes, like Cabo fish tacos and Tuscan pesto. This cookbook includes: Appetizers, soups & salads, entrees, one-dish meals, exotic tastes, marinades & rubs, outdoor cooking, pastas, stuffed fish, plank cooking, wine selection, scaling and fileting your catch, choosing market fish, cooking tips, and so much more. The Haugens have traveled to and studied cuisines in countries around the world—including the Caribbean, Asia, and Europe—your kitchen is not complete without a copy of *Cooking Salmon & Steelhead.*

Spiral SB: $24.95   ISBN: 1-57188-291-X   UPC: 0-81127-00120-0

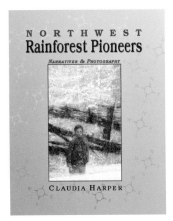

Northwest Rainforest Pioneers:
Narratives & Photography
by Claudia Harper

Have you ever wondered what everyday life was like for the early settlers in the Pacific Northwest? With interesting photo art and descriptive narratives, this unique book does a beautiful job of taking you back to these harsh times, sharing the lives and experiences of a pioneer family. Some are determined, hard-working and resourceful; others are unable to withstand the hardships and loneliness. If you are interested in the history of the Northwest, and in the reality of daily life as a Northwest pioneer, you will find yourself lost in the pages of this book. 8 1/2 x 11 inches, 72 pages.

SB: $17.95   ISBN: 1-57188-345-2   UPC: 0-81127-00179-8

More Northwest Books

NORTHWEST FLY PATTERNS & TYING GUIDE
Rainland Fly Casters

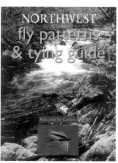

8 1/2 x 11 inches, 100 pages.
SB: $19.95
ISBN: 1-57188-283-9
UPC: 0-81127-00123-1
HB: $29.95
ISBN: 1-57188-284-7
UPC: 0-81127-00124-8
Ltd. HB: $90.00
ISBN: 1-57188-301-0

DRY FLY FISHING
Dave Hughes

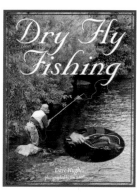

8 1/2 x 11 inches, 56 pages.
SB: $15.95
ISBN: 1-878175-68-8
UPC: 0-66066-00153-5

STEELHEAD FLOAT FISHING
Jim Butler

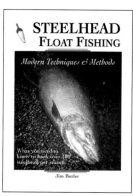

8 1/2 x 11 inches, 80 pages.
SB: $19.95
ISBN: 1-57188-322-2
UPC: 0-81127-00156-9

OREGON'S OUTBACK:
An Auto Tour Guide to Southeast Oregon
Donna Lynn Ikenberry

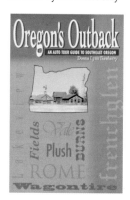

6 x 9 inches,
88 pages.
SB: $14.95
ISBN: 1-57188-043-7
UPC: 0-66066-00239-6

COLOR GUIDE TO STEELHEAD DRIFT FISHING
Bill Herzog

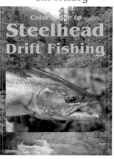

8 1/2 x 11 inches,
80 pages.
SB: $16.95
ISBN: 1-878175-59-9
UPC: 0-66066-00150-4

NYMPH FISHING
Dave Hughes

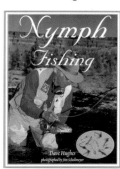

8 1/2 x 11 inches,
56 pages.
SB: $19.95
ISBN: 1-57188-002-X
UPC: 0-66066-00192-4

HATCH GUIDE FOR WESTERN STREAMS
Jim Schollmeyer

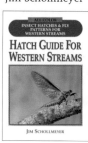

4 x 5 inches,
full-color; 196 pages;
fantastic photographs of
naturals and flies.
SB: $19.95
ISBN: 1-57188-109-3
UPC: 0-66066-00303-4

DRIFTBOATS: A COMPLETE GUIDE
Dan Alsup

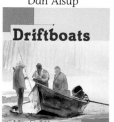

8 1/2 x 11 inches,
95 pages.
SB: $19.95
ISBN: 1-57188-189-1
UPC: 0-66066-00400-0

DRIFT BOAT FLY FISHING
A River Guide's Sage Advice
Neale Streeks

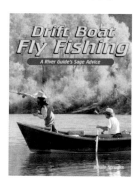

8 1/2 x 11 inches, 112 pages.
SB: $29.95
ISBN: 1-57188-016-X
UPC: 0-66066-00204-4

Lewis & Clark's Northwest Journey: "Weather Disagreeable!"
George Miller

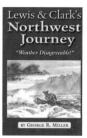

When Lewis & Clark made their epic journey to the Pacific Ocean, they found a climate that was in some ways similar to what they were used to on the East Coast, but in other respects, very different. Their clothes were rotting from the constant rain. Massive waves kept them from crossing the Columbia River. In this book, Miller examines the journals of Lewis and Clark and other members of the Corps of Discovery for key references to the weather the party experienced. It equates those weather entries to the weather patterns we know exist today. As a meteorologist, Miller has spent over 40 years wrestling with Pacific Northwest weather. He has also researched past weather events that have occurred in this part of the country over the last 200 years. With this vast knowledge, he gives great insight into the incredible difficulties the Corps of Discovery faced on their voyage west! 6 x 9 inches, 80 pages.

SB: $14.95   ISBN: 1-57188-323-1   UPC: 0-81127-00157-6